DATE DUE

MALARIA

Volume 1

MALARIA

Volume 1
Epidemology, Chemotherapy, Morphology, and Metabolism

Edited by

Julius P. Kreier

Department of Microbiology
The Ohio State University
College of Biological Sciences
Columbus, Ohio

ACADEMIC PRESS 1980
A SUBSIDIARY OF HARCOURT BRACE JOVANOVICH, PUBLISHERS
New York   London   Toronto   Sydney   San Francisco

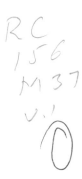

ACADEMIC PRESS, INC.
111 Fifth Avenue, New York, New York 10003

United Kingdom Edition published by
ACADEMIC PRESS, INC. (LONDON) LTD.
24/28 Oval Road, London NW1 7DX

Library of Congress Cataloging in Publication Data
Main entry under title:

Malaria.

Includes bibliographical references and index.
CONTENTS: v. 1. Epidemiology, chemotherapy,
morphology, and metabolism.
1. Malaria. I. Kreier, Julius P.
RC156.M37   616.9'362   80–21509
ISBN 0–12–426101–9 (v. 1)

PRINTED IN THE UNITED STATES OF AMERICA

80 81 82 83   9 8 7 6 5 4 3 2 1

Contents

3   Chemotherapy of Malaria
Wallace Peters

4   Morphology of Plasmodia
Masamichi Aikawa and Thomas M. Seed

5   Biochemistry of Malarial Parasites
C. A. Homewood and K. D. Neame

Index   407

List of Contributors

Numbers in parentheses indicate the pages on which the authors' contributions begin.

Masamichi Aikawa (285), Institute of Pathology, Case Western Reserve University, Cleveland, Ohio 44106

P. C. C. Garnham* (95), Imperial College Field Station, Silwood Park, Ashurst Lodge, Ascot, Berkshire SL5 7DE, England

C. A. Homewood (345), Department of Parasitology, Liverpool School of Tropical Medicine, University of Liverpool, Liverpool L69 3BX, England

K. D. Neame (345), Department of Physiology, University of Liverpool, Liverpool L69 3BX, England

Wallace Peters (145), Department of Medical Protozoology, London School of Hygiene and Tropical Medicine, London WC1E 7HT, England

Thomas M. Seed (285), Division of Biological and Medical Research, Argonne National Laboratory, Argonne, Illinois 60439

Walther H. Wernsdorfer (1), Research and Technical Intelligence, Malaria Action Programme, World Health Organization, 1211 Geneva 27, Switzerland

*Present Address: Southern Wood, Farnham Common, Slough SL2 3PA, England

Preface

The last major effort to review our knowledge of malaria was by Mark F. Boyd whose "Malariology" published by W. B. Saunders of Philadelphia in 1949 is still a valuable resource. The exquisite volume "Malaria Parasites and other Haemosporida" by P. C. C. Garnham published by Blackwell Scientific Publication of Oxford in 1966 is also a valuable review of malariology but in the author's words "is about malaria parasites and not malaria."

This three-volume treatise is appearing in a period of rising activity in malaria research. In the 1950s and 1960s and even into the 1970s funds for this research were scarce and only the hardiest of individuals remained in the field. At present malaria research is again receiving the attention it deserves. The mistaken belief common in the 1950s and 1960s that malaria would soon be eradicated by vector control and chemotherapy and that research was therefore rather pointless has been abandoned in the face of a widespread resurgence of this disease.

A variety of national and international agencies are now funding malaria research. Many individuals attracted by the possibility of funding are turning their efforts to malaria research. Biochemists, immunologists, biophysicists, and molecular biologists among others are entering the field. Many of these individuals, skilled in their specialities, know little or nothing about malaria. It is perhaps to such individuals particularly that this broad review of malariology will be of most value. Even those of us who have worked in some aspects of malaria research for some time may find the reviews of the state of the art in areas other than our own speciality of interest. Those of us actively working in a particular area may find few new facts in the reviews of the areas of our own speciality. I have, however, encouraged the authors to write critical reviews and to relate the facts reported in the literature to each other. Interpretation and speculation are discouraged by the reviewers of most scientific journals in the United States. A book such as this is thus naturally a convenient vehicle for individuals to present their thoughts as well as the facts.

The authors of the reviews of malaria research included in these volumes met in May 1979 in Mexico City with individuals doing research on the closely related disease babesiosis. Babesiosis has an effect on the development of animal husbandry somewhat similar to the effect of malaria on human societies. At this conference current research on malaria and babesiosis was reported and the similarities and differences between malaria and babesiosis were discussed. As an outgrowth of this conference a volume on babesiosis was developed, which will complement these volumes on malaria.

I extend my thanks to the co-organizers of the conference, Dr. Miodrag Ristic of the College of Veterinary Medicine of the University of Illinois with whom I edited the volume on babesiosis, and Dr. Carlos Arellano-Sota of the Instituto Nacional de Investigaciones Pecuarias in Mexico City. I particularly wish to thank the sponsors of the conference for their encouragement and help. Their support made the conference possible and made the preparation of these volumes on research in malaria and babesiosis a more pleasant task.

I particularly wish to thank John Pino, Director of Agricultural Sciences of the Rockefeller Foundation without whose early support the conference and the babesiosis volume would have been impossible. I also wish to thank Kenneth Warren, Director of Medical Sciences of the Rockefeller Foundation, Edgar A. Smith, Health Services Administrator, James Erickson, Malaria Research Officer of the United States Agency for International Development of the Department of State for their support of the conference.

In addition to the Rockefeller Foundation and the United States Agency for International Development several other organizations contributed to the support of the conference and the development of these volumes. These were The Pan American Health Organization, Parke-Davis Corporations, Merck Sharp & Dohme, Anchor Laboratories, Sandoz Ltd., Pfizer Corporation, and the Wellcome Trust.

Last but by no means least I wish to thank all the authors of the reviews that make up these volumes and Academic Press for their unfailing support.

Julius P. Kreier

Contents of Volumes 2 and 3

Contents of Babesiosis

1

The Importance of Malaria in the World

Walther H. Wernsdorfer

I. HISTORICAL REVIEW

Malaria is the accepted name denoting the disease or condition of infection in man caused by parasites belonging to the genus *Plasmodium*. Although the name malaria, which is derived from the Italian word for bad air, is not directly related to the cause of infection, it is the term commonly used, since the scientifically more appropriate term—plasmodioses—has never come into wide use.

Malaria, Vol. 1
Copyright © 1980 by Academic Press, Inc.
All rights of reproduction in any form reserved.
ISBN 0-12-426101-9

1

The term malaria was originally restricted to plasmodial infections in man, but it now includes all infections caused by organisms belonging to the family Plasmodiidae which, therefore, are commonly referred to as malaria parasites.

Human malaria is probably as old as mankind and, until very recent times, many examples of the disease influenced the course of history. The earliest indications of human disease suggestive of malaria come from ancient Egypt and are found in the Edwin Smith Surgical Papyrus, 1600 B.C. (Breasted, 1930), which describes measures to be taken against the entry of disease-laden, fever-provoking vapors into houses. The Papyrus Ebers, 1550 B.C., refers to the association of rigors, fever, and splenomegaly (Garnham, 1966). Inscriptions on the walls of the Temple of Dendera in Upper Egypt contain the word AAT, denoting an intermittent fever which recurred annually at the same season (Deaderick, 1909) and was associated with the Nile River floods (Halawani and Shawarby, 1957).

The first accurate clinical descriptions of malarial fevers were given by Hippocrates in 400 B.C. (Boyd, 1949), who mentioned the classic triad of chills, fever, and sweating and analyzed the characteristic periodicity of various forms of malaria and associated splenomegaly with the endemicity of malaria and its topographic aspects. Hippocrates recognized continued and "semitertian" fevers as the most dangerous, often fatal forms. These were probably infections caused by *Plasmodium falciparum*. He considered quartan fevers, obviously due to *P. malariae,* to be the longest lasting and least dangerous of these diseases.

Many Roman historians and writers mention fevers especially affecting populations living in the vicinity of marshes (Boyd, 1949). Celsus, in the first century A.D., gave rather precise descriptions of febrile diseases from which falciparum, vivax, and quartan malaria could be easily identified as separate entities. Galen, in the second century A.D., followed Celsus' classification. Western medicine adhered to his dicta regarding treatment of febrile diseases, including malaria, throughout the medieval era until the advent of cinchona bark.

It seems that malarial fevers were known also in ancient China and that Arab physicians, at the peak of Arab medicine during the eighth to the thirteenth century were commonly acquainted with intermittent fevers (Boyd, 1949).

Controversy still reigns regarding the occurrence of human malaria in the Americas prior to Columbus' discovery of the New World. Boyd (1949), Jarcho (1964) and Dunn (1965) came to the conclusion that human malaria was not present in the pre-Columbian era. Coatney *et al.* (1971) share this view and suggest that all forms of primate malaria now found in the New World are the outcome of post-Columbian introduction. There can be little doubt that *P. falciparum* arrived in the Americas with the Spanish and Portuguese invaders and African slaves. However, the discovery by Sulzer *et al.* (1975, 1978) of an isolated focus of hyperendemic *P. vivax* and *P. malariae,* and the conspicuous absence of *P. falciparum* in a primitive population in the Peruvian Amazon jungle, may suggest the pre-Columbian antiquity of *P. vivax* and *P. malariae* in the New World.

The earliest attempts to prevent what appears to have been malaria are contained also in the Edwin Smith Surgical Papyrus (Breasted, 1930). The Papyrus Ebers mentions the use of an oil expressed from the *Balanites* tree as a mosquito repellent (Garnham, 1966). However, these measures apparently afforded little protection and, apart from following some precautions based on experience related to the *genius epidemicus,* for a long time there were no effective means for preventing malaria and not even organized attempts to analyze the correlation between specific bioclimatic and topographic factors and the epidemic and endemic occurrence of febrile diseases. This is the more astonishing, as epidemic fevers were recognized relatively early as an obstacle to land use and as a cause of defeat of many a northern army attempting the invasion of Mediterranean countries. Garnham (1966) rightly stated that the Crusaders, faltering and turning back from the borders of the Holy Land, were defeated more by malaria than by the Saracens.

The first impetus to the treatment of malaria came in the middle of the seventeenth century with the introduction of the bark of a Peruvian tree with which the Countess of Chinchón was successfully treated for her febrile condition. Paz Soldan (1938), though, states that it was the Count and not the Countess of Chinchón who first benefited from treatment with the bark. The bark was employed in local Indian medicine as a febrifuge, although its use was apparently quite limited (Jarcho, 1964), an observation which, according to Coatney *et al.* (1971) argues against the pre-Columbian presence of human malaria in the Americas. The bark of the Peruvian tree was brought to Europe about 1640 and was soon used generally throughout western Europe for the treatment of fevers.

The botanical description of the tree yielding the Peruvian bark became known only about 100 years after introduction of the bark into Europe. Linné, in memory of the Countess of Chinchón's recovery, named (but misspelled) the new genus of the bark-yielding tree *Cinchona*. Subsequently, the bark was generally called cinchona bark or merely cinchona. The response to the latter was used as a diagnostic tool by Torti (1712), to differentiate *ex juvantibus* between malarial and nonmalarial fevers.

The large variations in the therapeutic value of different batches of cinchona stimulated chemists to isolate the active principles. In 1820, Pelletier and Caventon succeeded in extracting two alkaloids which they named quinine and cinchonine (Scott, 1939) and of which quinine was found to exert the antimalarial effect. Subsequently the use of pure quinine rapidly replaced the administration of cinchona bark, and the pure drug was also increasingly employed for the prophylaxis against malaria. While the suppressive administration of quinine has been replaced by the use of modern synthetic antimalarials, the drug has retained its value as a life-saving medicament in severe cases of falciparum malaria.

In the absence of any knowledge of the cause of transmission of malaria, the fortuitous discovery of cinchona remained for a long time the only tool which, on an individual rather than on a community scale, could be used for control of the disease which remained an enigma until the end of the nineteenth century.

Advances in pathological histology, hematology, microbiology, and parasitology, greatly aided by the development of better microscopes, brought malaria increasingly into the realm of research. The macroscopic pigmented appearance of the brain and spleen of patients who had died of malarial fever had been known in the eighteenth century, but it was Meckel (1847) who observed black granules, embedded in protoplasmic masses, in the blood of a severely ill malarious patient. Meckel's findings were subsequently confirmed by various observers.

Laveran too noticed pigment granules in the erythrocytes of malarious persons. In 1880 he observed exflagellation of a parasite which he described in 1884 and which is now known as *P. falciparum (Laverania falcipara)*. At about the same time, Gerhardt (1884) proved that malaria could be induced in healthy persons by the inoculation of blood from malarious patients. These studies and those on the morphological aspects of blood schizogony of Marchiafara and Celli (1884), and ultimately observation of the fertilization of a macrogamete by a microgamete (MacCallum, 1897), finally dispelled the myth of a miasmatic origin of malaria and other rather adventurous hypotheses of the cause of the disease. Meanwhile, the introduction by Romanowsky (1890, 1891) of a stain permitting the reproducible differential staining of blood cells, parasite cytoplasm, and chromatin greatly facilitated study of the blood parasites. The principal components of Romanowsky's stain continue to be used in the major stains of modern malariological practice, e.g., Field, Giemsa, JSB, Leishman and Wright stains.

The association between mosquitoes and malaria and the existence of a particular mechanism of transmission were long suspected even before the concept of the miasmatic origin of malaria became untenable. Roman writers frequently alluded to this association which received new attention from Lancisi (1717), Burton (1856), and King (1883), although they were all inclined to consider mosquitoes carriers of marsh miasma rather than organisms actively involved in the development of the cause of disease.

Based on his experiences with coccidia and recognizing their biological similarity to malaria parasites, Pfeiffer suggested in 1892 that the latter passed an exogenous cycle in the body of a blood-sucking insect. This view was shared by Manson (1894), who suggested that mosquitoes were the host for the malaria parasite's extrinsic development but did not, at that stage, consider the parasite's return to man through the mosquito. Stimulated by Manson's theory, Ross in India investigated the fate of malaria parasites in various mosquito species, obtaining gametocyte maturation of *P. falciparum* in *Culex* and *Aedes,* and in 1897 the production of oocysts in anopheline mosquitoes. Ross' studies on *P. falciparum* were interrupted by his transfer to Calcutta, but in 1898 he succeeded in completely elucidating the sporogony of *P. relictum* in what appears to have been *Culex pipiens fatigans.* He obtained the development of sporozoites which, through mosquito bites, proved to be infectious to healthy sparrows. By the time Ross finally had the opportunity to demonstrate the existence of the analogous sporogony of *P. falciparum* in anopheline mosquitoes in Sierra Leone in 1899 (according to Garnham, 1966), Italian workers had already succeeded in infecting a healthy volunteer with *P. falciparum* through mosquito bites (Bignami, 1899) and in elucidating the sporogony of *P. falciparum* and *P. vivax* in anopheline mosquitoes (Grassi *et al.,* 1899a; Bastianelli and Bignami, 1899). In 1899 the same group observed the development of sporogonic stages of *P. malariae* in *Anopheles claviger* (Grassi *et al.,* 1899b).

These events elucidated major parts of the life cycle of human malaria parasites as far as they were known at the turn of the century. With the identification of anopheline mosquitoes as arthropod hosts and with increasing knowledge of the habitat of the vector, the way was clear for the rapid development of malaria control methods which, for the first time, allowed direct interference with transmission. Efforts were especially directed against the aquatic stages of the anophelines, through oiling of water surfaces, the application of paris green or the use of larvivorous fish, and engineering measures such as drainage, filling of breeding places, water flow modification, and water management. Where applicable, the engineering methods, although costly, resulted in the most satisfactory and lasting results.

Mosquito abatement offered the possibility of controlling yellow fever and malaria on a large scale. In 1901 Gorgas organized a program for the control of *Aedes* and anopheline mosquitoes in Cuba, which had a dramatic impact on the incidence of yellow fever and malaria on the island. Then, 1904 saw the beginning of Gorgas' epic campaign against yellow fever and malaria in the Isthmus of Panama, where both diseases had, until then, inflicted heavy casualties on the imported labor force, seriously hampering the progress of canal construction.

By the end of 1905, mosquito abatement had led to the interruption of yellow fever transmission in Panama. Malaria was soon reduced to a negligible incidence (Gorgas, 1915) and, as a result of the efficient control of both diseases, construction work made rapid progress. After completion of the Panama Canal in 1914 the Canal Zone remained under strict mosquito control and malaria practically disappeared from the area.

At about the same time that Gorgas was working in Cuba, Watson implemented mosquito control measures in what was then British Malaya, using environmental methods, especially drainage (Watson, 1935). These measures were particularly effective in urban areas and were sufficient to free numerous towns of malaria, a state which was maintained until World War II and re-established soon after the war.

Mosquito control measures, still without residual insecticides, were also instrumental in eliminating *A. albimanus,* an invading vector, from Barbados in the late 1920s (Russell, 1952).

Besides the attack on the aquatic stages, various measures aimed at reducing human contact with adult mosquitoes were reinforced. These had formerly been merely directed against the insect nuisance and had only recently achieved new significance after the disease-carrying role of these anthropods was recognized. Such measures involved the use of mosquito nets, the screening of houses, and the wearing of apparel which gave mosquitoes only very limited access at the time of their activity. This was soon complemented by the use of pyrethrum powders—from *Chrysanthemum cinerariaefolium*—as household insecticides. These agents had a fumigant effect and the added advantage of being active against other household pests.

While these first steps toward effective malaria control were being taken, the chaos regarding the classification of malaria parasites increased and led to bitter arguments between individuals holding to distinct schools of thought. Earlier, Danilewsky (1889) had taken the view that avian and human malaria parasites belonged to one and the same species but, before the turn of the century, Italian workers established the specific identity of human and avian parasites. However, this does not detract from the importance of Danilewsky's observations on avian malaria parasites, which later became valuable experimental research models and contributed much toward elucidation of the life cycle of primate malaria parasites.

Although differential descriptions of *P. vivax* and *P. malariae* were given by Grassi and Feletti as early as as 1892, and for *P. falciparum* by Welch in 1897, it took some time before the distinct morphological, clinical, and epidemiological character of these species, and the generic name *Plasmodium* (Marchiafava and Celli, 1885), were universally recognized.

When World War I broke out, malaria control was still in its infancy; it was practically restricted to the therapeutic and prophylactic use of quinine and abatement of the aquatic mosquito stages. The application of these measures under the conditions present in the theaters of war in the eastern Mediterranean and western Asian countries posed considerable problems on both sides, one of which suffered moreover from a severe shortage of quinine. It is said that the very heavy casualties from direct war action were surpassed by losses from malaria in the campaign of the Dardanelles (Gallipoli).

The lack of quinine during World War I in Germany, caused by the blockade, stimulated a search for synthetic antimalarial drugs which, however, did not yield immediate results. The first synthetic antimalarial drug, pamaquine, was produced in 1925 (Schulemann, 1932); it was followed by mepacrine, the first synthetic blood schizontocidal drug, which was developed in 1930 (Mauss and Mietzsch, 1933).

Meanwhile, some process was also being made in developing measures for attacking adult vector mosquitoes. Pyrethrum extracts proved to be much more effective than pyrethrum powders, since they could be applied as liquid sprays. Large-scale malaria control in rural areas based on this method was successfully carried out in India, The Netherlands, and South Africa in the years preceding World War II (Russell, 1952).

Parasitological research between the world wars yielded in 1922 a description of the fourth species of human malaria parasite, *P. ovale* (Stephens, 1922).

The fate of the malaria parasite between inoculation of the sporozoite and the patency of erythrocytic forms had for a long time remained an enigma. Although Grassi's hypothesis of a specific generation of parasites between the sporozoite and the blood forms (1900) suggested the existence of parasite development outside the blood, Schaudinn's erroneous description of sporozoite penetration into erythrocytes (1903) helped to maintain the concept of an exclusively erythrocytic development of malaria parasites. The observations of Aragão de Beaupaire (1908) on *Haemoproteus columbae,* a parasite of pigeons closely related to plasmodia, proved the existence of tissue stages preceding the invasion of blood cells.

Subsequently in 1934 Raffaele discovered the exoerythrocytic schizogony of *P. elongatum* in tissue cells (1934a,b), especially the bone marrow of birds, and 2 years later he reported a similar cycle in *P. relictum* (Raffaele, 1936). James and Tate (1937) demonstrated tissue schizogony of *P. gallinaceum* in the capillary endothelium of chickens.

Schaudinn's hypothesis became increasingly untenable also with respect to human pathogenic plasmodia after Boyd and Stratman-Thomas (1934) demonstrated, through blood subinoculations from sporozoite-infected persons (*P. vivax*), that there was a period of noninfectivity starting shortly after sporozoite inoculation and ending at the moment of patency. Numerous observers repeated these studies and extended them to other *Plasmodium* species. This work was greatly aided by the availability of artificially infected patients undergoing malariotherapy for the treatment of neurospyhilis, a procedure which had been introduced on a wide scale by von Wagner-Jauregg (1922). Apart from being, at that time, the most reliable means of arresting the course of neurosyphilis, artificial infection with malaria—whether through sporozoites or through the inoculation of asexual blood forms—became an important research tool especially in the elucidation of parasitological, physiological, clinical, and epidemiological parameters. While *P. vivax* was the most widely used species, extensive experience was also obtained with *P. malariae* and the simian species *P. knowlesi*. The severe nature of *P. falciparum* infections has somewhat restricted the use of this species in malariotherapy.

World War II boosted malaria research and the development of malaria control methodology on an unprecedented scale. British and American forces applied the whole available armamentarium of control measures for the protection of their troops. Toward the end of the war, in particular, they increasingly used the chemical DDT [1,1,1-trichloro-2,2-bis(*p*-chlorophenyl)ethane], whose insecticidal properties had been discovered by Müller and Wiesmann only in 1939 (Müller, 1955), although the compound had first been synthesized by Leidler in 1874 (Russell, 1952). In Germany and in the United States drug research was promoted. This ultimately yielded the 4-aminoquinolines as blood schizontocidal drugs and improved 8-aminoquinolines as tissue schizontocidals. In addition, British scientists developed dihydrofolate reductase-inhibiting compounds of which proguanil and pyrimethamine became the most widely used.

The introduction of residual insecticides, first DDT which was soon followed by other chlorinated hydrocarbons such as dieldrin (*endo,exo*-1,2,3,4,10,10-hexachloro-6,7-epoxy-1,4,4a,5,6,8,8a-octahydro-1,4:5,8-dimethanonaphthalene) and BHC (the γ isomer of 1,2,3,4,5,6-hexachlorocyclohexane), and the availability of new potent and relatively well-tolerated, inexpensive drugs stimulated many governments to attempt eradication of the disease in their territories even before malaria eradication became a widely accepted concept. By 1948, Venezuela, Cyprus, Italy, the United States, and Mauritius had embarked on the venture of eradication, a goal which was eventually achieved by four of these countries.

In the field of basic parasitology, Garnham in 1947 demonstrated the existence of tissue forms of *Hepatocystis kochi* in the liver parenchyma cells of African monkeys. In 1948, Shortt and Garnham described the preerythrocytic development of *P. cynomolgi* and *P. vivax,* followed in 1951 by a description of the tissue stages of *P. falciparum* (Shortt *et al.,* 1951). These discoveries proved to be of considerable practical epidemiological importance and, together with the progress of malaria control methodology, the stage was set for a worldwide attack on malaria.

In 1955 and 1956 the Eighth and Ninth World Health Assemblies adopted a policy of malaria eradication (World Health Organization, 1955a, 1956), and in 1956 the Expert Committee on Malaria of the World Health Organization (WHO) prepared the appropriate technical guidelines (World Health Organization, 1957). Based on the experiences with malariotherapy which indicated the time-limited nature of infections with *P. falciparum* and *P. vivax,* the epidemiologically most important species, the committee felt that the means of mosquito control and chemotherapy available at that time would in many areas suffice to interrupt malaria transmission for such a period as was necessary to produce a complete natural disappearance of malaria in the population. Tropical Africa was not included in the concept of malaria eradication, since preliminary studies had indicated that the available methodology was inadequate under local epidemiological conditions.

Eradication programs were launched in numerous countries in the Americas, Asia, Australia, Europe, North Africa, and on islands in the Indian Ocean and the western Pacific, while efforts continued to elaborate methodologies which would permit economically feasible malaria control in tropical Africa.

It cannot be denied that confidence in the new antimalarial weapons and in the rapid initial success of malaria eradication caused a severe reduction in funds for malaria research. Malariology as a career became increasingly uncertain and unattractive and, as a result, the world was and still is, short of new methods and of qualified personnel at a time when malaria once again has taken the offensive.

The eradication effort met with various degrees of success: In more than 30 countries or territories malaria was eliminated and reintroduction effectively prevented. In many others, the mortality and morbidity caused by malaria and the prevalence of the disease were reduced to a low level. However, in a significant number of countries, initial success was followed by the maintenance of important, active foci or by a resurgence of the disease such as that having recently occurred in southern Asia. The reasons for these developments are manifold: On the one hand, political instability and financial and administrative shortcomings— sometimes expressing a lack of determination—enhanced by the inflationary price increases of equipment, insecticides, operational supplies, and fuel were responsible for inadequate operational and epidemiological coverage of the areas to be protected; on the other hand, technical problems, such as vector resistance to insecticides, vector exophily, parasite resistance to drugs, and factors related to human ecology, e.g., nomadism, labor movements, and unstable cropping, have reduced the impact of the antimalaria program.

The introduction of alternative insecticides, e.g., organophosphorus compounds and carbamates, has to some extent been outpaced by the rapid development of vector resistance. However, alternative drugs against 4-aminoquinoline-resistant *P. falciparum*, e.g., the combination of sulfonamides and pyrimethamine, and tetracyclines in association with other antimalarials, are still largely effective, and new alternative drugs are being produced.

A careful comparison of the impact of political and administrative problems with that of technical problems in areas with unstable malaria or malaria of intermediate stability shows the former to be largely responsible for the failure of a program, since there is hardly a technical problem which cannot be overcome by suitably selected and strategically applied alternative and complementary control methods. There are indications that malaria control and "decontrol" are being used as instruments to political ends; the analysis of Cleaver (1977) suggests that much of the present resurgence of malaria takes place in countries where national and foreign governments are trying to control social unrest and have resorted to the decontrol of malaria as a means of regaining political stability and growth of the economy.

Many an eradication program could have benefited from greater epidemiological and operational flexibility and the judicious use of complementary control measures; but it can be said, even about the majority of those which failed to reach the ultimate goal, that they achieved a drastic reduction in mortality and morbidity due to malaria.

In 1969 the Twenty-Second World Health Assembly adopted a revised strategy of malaria eradication and control based on a realistic assessment of the individual countries' epidemiological conditions and their potential for effective control (World Health Organization, 1969c). Consequently, the countries were grouped into those which could achieve eradication within a determined time limit and those where malaria control would need to be applied on a long-term basis. The countries of tropical Africa are part of the latter category since, in that part of the world, none of the available control tools (singly or in combination) permit the interruption of malaria transmission at a feasible cost. Here the operational priorities are set to prevent death from malaria, to curb the incidence of malaria, to reduce malaria prevalence and, ultimately, to eradicate the disease. New control tools and improved use of the classic measures—which only research can provide—will be required to achieve these objectives.

II. TAXONOMIC STATUS OF MALARIA PARASITES

There still is considerable discussion and uncertainty regarding the taxonomic status of malaria parasites, especially below the level of suborder. The classification of the phylum Protozoa introduced by the Society of Protozoologists (Honigberg *et al.*, 1964) provides a generally accepted system based on morphological and biological criteria, as well as on phylogenetic considerations. According to this classification, the malaria parasites belong to the subphylum Sporozoa, the class Telosporea (Telosporidia), and the subclass Coccidia (Coccidiomorpha).

More recently Levine (1973) included malaria parasites in the subphylum Apicomplexa, class Sporozoasida, and subclass Coccidiasina. For the sake of conformity to generally accepted terminology however, the classification and terminology proposed by the Society of Protozoologists will be adopted.

All members of the subphylum Sporozoa are parasitic. Some produce simple resistant spores, and the others have a stage in their life cycle which can be recognized as having been derived from a resistant spore; these forms contain one or more sporozoites. Sporozoa do not possess cilia or flagella, except on male gametes of certain genera, and pseudopodia are rarely formed (Baker, 1977). All

Telosporea possess sporozoites and reproduce sexually. The common characteristic of the subclass Coccidia is the intracellular nature of the trophozoites. Consensus on classification ends at the subclass level. Léger's classic division of Coccidia into the orders Coccidiida and Adeleida does not easily accommodate Haemosporidia. Garnham (1966), following the recommendation of Cheissin and Polyansky (1963), retained them as a suborder of Coccidiida in alignment with Eimeriidea. On the other hand, Baker (1977), following Levine (1961, 1973) and in accordance with the classification of the Society of Protozoologists, has divided the subclass Coccidia into the orders Protococcida and Eucoccida. The latter include three suborders, namely, Adeleina (Adeleorina), Eimeriina (Eimeriorina), and Haemosporina (Haemospororina).

The common characteristics of the order Eucoccida (Eucoccidiorida, Levine, 1961, 1973; Eucoccida, Baker, 1977) are asexual and sexual phases of reproduction, and anisogamy.

A comparison of the three suborders (Table I) shows some similarity between Adeleina and Eimeriina, on the one hand, and between Eimeriina and Haemosporina, on the other, while Adeleina and Haemosporina have very little in common apart from the general characteristics of the order.

While the status of Haemosporina (Haemosporidiidea) as a suborder does not seem to be seriously disputed—there is considerable uncertainty regarding the

TABLE I

Characteristics of the Suborders Adeleina, Eimeriina, and Haemosporina, Order Eucoccida[a]

Characteristic	Adeleina	Eimeriina	Haemosporina
Syzygy	Present	Absent	Absent
Gametocyte size in both sexes	Male, small Female, large	Equal	Equal
Number of microgametes produced by micro-gametocyte	Few	Many	Limited to eight
Zygote	Motile or not motile	Not motile	Motile
Oocyst size	Fixed	Fixed	Expanding
Spores	In some genera	In some genera	None
Sporozoites	Few, enclosed in envelope	One or few	Numerous
Tissue schizogony, dimorphism	Present	Present	Absent
Tissue schizogony, merozoites	Few	Few	Numerous
Host choice	Monoxenous and heteroxenous	Monoxenous and heteroxenous	Heteroxenous

[a] According to Garnham (1966), and Levine (1973).

division of the suborder. Garnham (1966) classifies it into three families: Plasmodiidae (Mesnil, 1899), Haemoproteidae (Doflein, 1916), and Leucocytozoidae (Fallis and Bennett, 1961). This division is justified by the numerous biological differences among the families. Only Plasmodiidae show blood schizogony and have mosquitoes as arthropod hosts. Malaria pigment is produced by Plasmodiidae and Haemoproteidae, but not by Leucocytozoidae. In the latter, gametocytes develop in leukocytes and immature red blood cells; in Plasmodiidae and Haemoproteidae gametocytes are restricted to mature erythrocytes.

However, Levine (1973) follows the unitarian approach originally proposed by Corradetti (1938) and recognizes only one family, Plasmodiidae, in the suborder Haemosporina, and aligns *Haemoproteus, Hepatocystis, Leucocytozoon,* and *Plasmodium* as genera.

Garnham's classification will be followed in this chapter in view of the rather distinct division among the families based on numerous biological criteria. In this classification, Haemoproteidae are divided into three genera—*Hepatocystis, Nycteria,* and *Polychromophilus*—and Leucocytozoidae into two genera—*Leucocytozoon* and *Akiba.* However, Plasmodiidae pose certain problems. Garnham has adopted an intermediate course between retaining all species in a single genus or grouping them into a number of separate genera. He preserves the generic name *Plasmodium* for all species and introduces subgeneric names, adopting the approach Corradetti *et al.* (1963a) had recommended earlier for avian plasmodia. Using biological criteria and host range, Garnham divides the genus *Plasmodium* into 10 subgenera, 3 comprising the mammalian, 4 the avian, and 3 the saurian plasmodia. Table II shows the major characteristics of these subgenera.

The subgenus *P. (Vinckeia)* appears to be quite heterogeneous, especially regarding host range. It is likely that biological and biochemical criteria will ultimately permit the separation of hitherto included species into several distinct subgenera.

There is considerable controversy regarding the classification of saurian plasmodia (Ayala, 1977). Telford (1974) advocated the use of selected biological and numerical parameters for the subgeneric grouping of New World saurian malaria parasites in order to fit species whose intermediate-sized schizonts would not permit their reliable inclusion in either *P. (Sauramoeba)* or *P. (Carinamoeba).* His classification, recognizing five subgenera, is summarized in Table III. The five proposed subgenera also accommodate all Old World saurian plasmodia species except *P. vastator* and *P. lygosomae.*

Ayala (1977) described the *Plasmodium* species of reptiles in five "groups," namely, *Carinamoeba, Telfordi, Tropiduri, Mexicanum,* and *Sauramoeba.* This grouping deviates in some important points from that of Telford and includes

TABLE II

Differential Characteristics of the Subgenera of _Plasmodium_[a]

Subgenus	Type species	Erythrocytic schizonts	Gametocytes	Vertebrate	Number of species known	Remarks
P. (Plasmodium)	P. (P.) malariae	Large	Round	Primates	20	
P. (Vinckeia)	P. (V.) bubalis	Small	Round	Various nonprimate mammals and lemurs	19	Very heterogeneous subgenus
P. (Laverania)	P. (L.) falciparum	Large	Elongate	Primates	2	
P. (Haemamoeba)	P. (H.) relictum	Large	Round	Birds	7	
P. (Giovannolaia)	P. (G.) circumflexum	Large	Elongate	Birds	14	
P. (Novyella)	P. (N.) vaughani	Small	Elongate or oval	Birds	7	
P. (Huffia)	P. (H.) elongatum	Large	Elongate	Birds	3	Strong attraction to immature hemopoietic system
P. (Sauramoeba)	P. (S.) agamae	Large	Round, oval, or elongate	Lizards	38	
P. (Carinamoeba)	P. (C.) minasense	Small	Round, oval, or elongate	Lizards		
P. (Ophidiella)	P. (O.) wenyoni	Small	Round or oval	Snakes	2	

[a] According to Garnham (1966).

TABLE III

Classification of Saurian Plasmodia[a]

Subgenus	Number of erythrocytic merozoites	Mean gametocyte size length × width (μm)	Sexual dimorphism	Pigment	Gametocytes	Exoerythrocytic schizogony
P. (Carinamoeba)	4–6	16–50	Absent	Always present	Erythrocytic	Thrombocytes
P. (Garnia)	10–30	45–85	Absent	Rarely visible	Erythrocytic, occasionally leukocytic	Leukocytes
P. (Sauramoeba)	7–30	35–90	Usually absent	Visibility variable	Erythrocytic, occasionally thrombocytic and lymphocytic	Thrombocytes and lymphocytes
P. (subgenus IV)	8–30	60–160	Usually present	Present	Erythrocytic	Leukocytes and/or endothelium
P. (subgenus V)	45–80	90–150	Usually present	Visibility variable	Erythrocytic	Leukocytes

[a] According to Telford (1974).

species which by definition would probably have to be placed outside the genus *Plasmodium* and consequently outside the family *Plasmodiidae*.

The classification proposed by Lainson *et al*. (1974) overcomes these difficulties. It is based on the criteria of pigment production and the location of gametocytes and schizonts. It includes most of the described malaria parasites in the genus *Plasmodium* and, by creating the family Garniidae with the subgenera *Garnia* and *Fallisia*, permits the classification of nonpigmented hemosporidia with leukocytic schizonts and gametocytes outside the genus *Plasmodium*. Nonpigmented hemosporidia with erythrocytic or leukocytic gametocytes and without circulating asexual forms are included in *Saurocytozoon* n.gen. of Leucocytozoidae.

A. Mammalian Malaria Parasites

1. Plasmodium (Plasmodium)

The 20 species of this subgenus are restricted to primates. Two species *(P. ovale* and *P. vivax)* occur naturally only in man, one is anthropozoonotic with man as the main vertebrate host *(P. malariae)*. *Plasmodium vivax* and *P. malariae* are cosmopolitan within the 16°C summer isotherm; *P. ovale* naturally occurs in tropical Africa and eastern Asia. The remaining 17 species are found either exclusively or mainly in nonhuman primates; two are restricted to tropical areas of the New World, two to Africa, and the remainder to southern and eastern Asia, with a remarkable concentration in Malaysia. Natural human infection with *P. knowlesi* was observed in Malaysia (Chin *et al*., 1965), and a doubtful infection with *P. simium* was reported from Brazil (Deane *et al*., 1966a). Several accidental laboratory infections with *P. cynomolgi* (Coatney *et al*., 1971) suggest that this infection may also be transmitted to man in nature, but morphological similarity to *P. vivax* may prevent its correct identification in the endemic areas. The distribution, natural vertebrate host, natural arthropod host, and periodicity of the species of the subgenus *P. (Plasmodium)* are summarized in Table IV.

The species of the subgenus *P. (Plasmodium)* are usually grouped according to periodicity and morphological characteristics as follows: (1) Vivax-type parasites: *P. vivax, P. cynomolgi, P. eylesi, P. gonderi, P. hylobati, P. jefferyi, P. pitheci, P. schwetzi, P. simium, P. sylvaticum, P. youngi;* (2) ovale-type parasites: *P. ovale, P. fieldi, P. simiovale;* and (3) malariae-type parasites: *P. malariae, P. brasilianum, P. inui*.

Three species stand apart: *P. knowlesi*, the only species with a 24-hour sexual cycle, and *P. coatneyi* and *P. fragile*, which are both tertian parasites. The morphological features of the last two species, except for the shape of the gametocytes, resemble those of *P. falciparum*.

TABLE IV

Species of the Subgenus *Plasmodium* (*Plasmodium*)

Species	Description	Distribution	Vertebrate host, natural	Arthropod host, natural	Periodicity of blood schizogony	Minimum duration of prepatent period	Remarks
P. (P.) brasilianum	Gonder and von Berenberg-Gossler, 1908	Brazil, Colombia, Panama, Peru, Venezuela	Various neotropic primate species	*A. (Kerteszia) cruzi*	72 hours	12 days	
P. (P.) coatneyi	Eyles et al., 1962a	Malaysia	*Macaca fascicularis*	*A. hackeri*	48 hours	10 days	
P. (P.) cynomolgi	Mayer, 1907	Tropical eastern Asia	*Macaca* and *Presbytis* spp.	Various *Anopheles* spp.	48 hours	8 days	Numerous subspecies
P. (P.) eylesi	Warren et al., 1965	Malaysia	*Hylobates lar*	Unknown	48 hours	11 days	Highly synchronous blood schizogony
P. (P.) fieldi	Eyles et al., 1962b	Malaysia	*Macaca nemestrina, M. follicularis*	*A. hackeri, A. balabacensis introlatus*	48 hours	9 days	
P. (P.) fragile	Dissanaike et al., 1965a	Southern India, Sri Lanka	*Macaca radiata, M. sinica*	*A. elegans*	48 hours	(17 days)[b]	
P. (P.) gonderi	Sinton and Mulligan, 1932	Coastal West Africa and Cameroons	*Cercocebus* and *Mandrillus* spp.	Unknown	48 hours	7 days	

Species	Authority	Distribution	Host	Vector			Remarks
P. (P.) hylobati	Rodhain, 1941	Java, Borneo	*Hylobates* spp.	Unknown	48 hours	9 days	
P. (P.) inui	Halberstaedter and von Prowazek, 1907	Tropical eastern Asia	*Macaca* spp., *Presbytis* spp.	*A. leucosphyrus, A. b. introlatus*	72 hours	11 days	*P. shortti* Bray (1963) is now considered to be a subspecies of *P. inui* (Eyles, 1963; Garnham, 1973)
P. (P.) jefferyi	Warren *et al.,* 1966	Malaysia	*Hylobates lar*	Unknown	48 hours	Unknown	
P. (P.) knowlesi	Sinton and Mulligan, 1932	Tropical eastern Asia	*Macaca* spp. and *Presbytis melalophos*	*A. hackeri*	24 hours	5½ days	Highly synchronous blood schizogony; various subspecies
P. (P.) malariae[a]	Grassi and Feletti, 1892	Cosmopolitan within 16°C summer isotherm	*Homo sapiens, Pan satyrus verus*	Numerous *Anopheles* spp.	72 hours	15 days	*P. rodhaini* Brumpt (1939) is synonymous with *P. malariae*
P. (P.) ovale[a]	Stephens, 1922	Tropical Africa, tropical eastern Asia	*Homo sapiens*	Various *Anopheles* spp.	48 hours	9 days	

(continued)

TABLE IV—*Continued*

Species	Description	Distribution	Vertebrate host, natural	Arthropod host, natural	Periodicity of blood schizogony	Minimum duration of prepatent period	Remarks
P. (P.) pitheci	Halberstaedter and von Prowazek, 1907	Borneo	*Pongo pygmaeus*	Unknown	(48 hours?)	Unknown	
P. (P.) schwetzi	Brumpt, 1939	West Africa, Cameroons, lower Congo area	*Pan satyrus, Gorilla gorilla*	Unknown	48 hours	Unknown	
P. (P.) simiovale	Dissanaike *et al.*, 1965b	Sri Lanka	*Macaca sinica*	Unknown	48 hours	(11 days)[b]	
P. (P.) simium	da Fonseca, 1951	Brazil	*Alouatta fusca, Brachyteles arachnoides*	Unknown	48 hours	(24 days)[b]	
P. (P.) sylvaticum	Garnham *et al.*, 1972	Borneo	*Pongo pygmaeus*	Unknown	48 hours	Unknown	
P. (P.) vivax[a]	Grassi and Feletti, 1890a	Cosmopolitan within 16°C summer isotherm	*Homo sapiens*	Numerous *Anopheles* spp.	48 hours	8 days	
P. (P.) youngi	Eyles *et al.*, 1964	Malaysia	*Hylobates lar*	Unknown	48 hours	Unknown	

[a] For details of geographic distribution, see Section IV.
[b] Assessed in simian species other than the natural vertebrate host.

Numerous species of nonhuman primates are receptive to infection with naturally human-pathogenic plasmodia. In most of these primate species splenectomy, sometimes complemented by other measures of immunosuppression, is required in order to induce infection. The observations of successful infection using the inoculation of infected blood or mosquito transmission are summarized in Table V. *Plasmodium knowlesi* has also been extensively used in malariotherapy. Attempts to infect humans with *P. gonderi, P. coatneyi,* and *P. fragile* by both routes of inoculation failed. Only sporozoite-induced infection was attempted with *P. eylesi, P. hylobati, P. jefferyi,* and *P. simium.* Except for a doubtful take with *P. eylesi* (Coatney *et al.,* 1971), no infection occurred in the human volunteers.

A natural infection of man with *P. simium* in Brazil was reported by Deane *et al.* (1966a) but has not been fully substantiated (Coatney *et al.,* 1971).

It is interesting to note that blacks are apparently refractory to infection with *P. cynomolgi, P. schwetzi,* and *P. inui,* analogous in fashion to their refractoriness to *P. vivax,* a phenomenon which for a long time was an enigma to epidemiologists. It is now recognized that it is probably associated with the absence of blood group substances on the host erythrocyte (Miller, 1977). A similar explanation for the difficulties experienced with infecting blacks with *P. knowlesi* (Milam and Kusch, 1938) appeared to be found in studies by Miller *et al* (1973, 1975) which also indicated that *P. knowlesi* did not invade human erythrocytes negative for Fy^a and Fy^b. However, merozoites of *P. vivax* and *P. knowlesi* appear to have other, different receptor requirements, since *P. vivax* cannot infect Old World monkeys suceptible to *P. knowlesi.* Chin *et al.* (1968), however, achieved infection of American blacks with *P. vivax* with relative ease, although this study may not contradict the work of Miller since the frequency of Duffy groups was not determined and it is known that there is a relatively high percentage of Duffy-positives among American blacks. To account for the refractoriness to *P. vivax* of Duffy-negative individuals of black African descent, for the insusceptibility to *P. knowlesi* of Duffy-negative erythrocytes from nonblack individuals, and for the ease with which infection with *P. vivax* was achieved in $Fy^a Fy^b$ negative *Aotus* (Lopez Antuñano and Palmer, 1978) it may be supposed that other unknown determinants associated with the Duffy locus have yet to be found.

The question of zoonotic or anthroponotic nature of simian malaria parasites other than *P. malariae* has been extensively discussed by Deane (1969), Juminer (1970), Coatney (1971), and Collins and Aikawa (1977). There can be no doubt that in nature man is occasionally exposed to infection with simian parasites such as *P. cynomolgi* and *P. knowlesi,* and possibly also with *P. schwetzi.* Following the assumption that *P. vivax* and *P. malariae* were introduced into South and Central America during the post-Columbian era and suspecting their synonym-

TABLE V

Experimental Infection of Nonhuman Primates by Naturally Human-Pathogenic *Plasmodium* spp.

Plasmodium spp.	Primate species successfully infected by:		Remarks
	Blood inoculation	Sporozoite inoculation[a]	
P. (P.) malariae	*Aotus trivirgatus* splenectomized and intact (Geiman and Siddiqui, 1969; Contacos and Collins, 1969)		Infections with P. (P.) malariae are naturally found in the chimpanzee (*Pan satyrus*) in which the species was described as the now obsolete P. rodhaini (Brumpt, 1939)
			Retransmission from infected Aotus to humans through A. freeborni achieved (Contacos and Collins, 1969)
P. (P.) ovale		*Pan satyrus*, splenectomized and intact [*A. gambiae*[a]], (Bray, 1957)	
P. (P.) vivax	*Aotus trivirgatus* (Porter and Young, 1966; Collins et al., 1974b)	*Aotus trivirgatus* [*A. albimanus*, A. b. balabacensis, A. freeborni, A. maculatus, A. quadrimaculatus, A. stephensi] (Ward et al., 1969; Baerg et al., 1969; Bafort and Kageruka, 1972; Collins et al., 1973a)	Cyclic retransmission of various strains of P. vivax from A. trivirgatus to *Homo sapiens* through A. albimanus has been reported by Porter and Young (1966), Young et al. (1966), Bafort and Kageruka (1972), and Collins et al. (1972)
	Ateles geoffroyi (Young and Porter, 1969)	*Ateles fusiceps* [*A. albimanus*] (Baerg et al., 1969)	
	Ateles fusiceps (Young and Porter, 1969)	*Pan satyrus* [A. b. balabacensis, A. quadrimaculatus, A. stephensi] (Ward et al., 1969)	
	Cebus capucinus (Young and Porter, 1969)		
	Hylobates lar (Cadigan et al., 1968)		
	Pan satyrus (Mesnil and Roubaud, 1917, 1920; Garnham et al., 1956)		
	Saguinus geoffroyi (Porter and Young, 1966; Porter, 1970)		

	Saimiri sciureus splenectomized (Deane et al., 1966b; Young et al., 1971)	*Saguinus geoffroyi* [*A. albimanus*] (Baerg et al., 1969) *Saimiri sciureus* [*A. albimanus*] (Young et al., 1971)	
P. falciparum	*Alouatta fusca* (Taliaferro and Taliaferro, 1934; Taliaferro and Cannon, 1934) *Ateles fusiceps* (Baerg and Young, 1970) *Alouatta villosa* (Baerg and Young, 1970; Rossan and Baerg, 1975) *Aotus trivirgatus* (Geiman and Meagher, 1967; Contacos and Collins, 1968; Geiman et al., 1969; Voller et al., 1969; Collins et al., 1974a,b; 1977) *Cebus capucinus* (Young and Baerg, 1969) *Hylobates lar* (Ward et al., 1965; Ward and Cadigan, 1966; Gould et al., 1966; Cadigan et al., 1969) *Macaca fusci*, splenectomized (Cadigan et al., 1966) *Macaca mulata siamica*, splenectomized (Cadigan et al., 1966) *Macaca nemestrina*, splenectomized (Cadigan et al., 1966) *Saguinus geoffroyi* (Porter and Young, 1967) *Saimiri sciureus* (Young and Rossan, 1969)	*Aotus trivirgatus*, splenectomized [*A. freeborni, A. stephensi, A. albimanus, A. maculatus*] (Collins and Contacos, 1972; Ward and Hayes, 1972; Collins et al., 1973c; Collins et al., 1977; Hayes and Ward, 1977) *Hylobates lar*, splenectomized [inoculation of sporozoites from *A. b. balabacensis*] (Gould et al., 1966) *Pan satyrus* [inoculation of salivary glands] (Bray, 1958)	Cyclic retransmission of various strains from *A. trivirgatus* to humans through *A. freeborni* reported by Collins et al. (1973c)

[a] Vector species used is shown in brackets.

ity with *P. simium* and *P. brasilianum*, Coatney (1971) considers the latter to be anthroponotic in origin.

With the possible exception of *P. malariae* in Africa, simian malaria is generally considered not to pose an obstacle to the control or eradication of human malaria, since the ecology of primate and invertebrate hosts form separate biological systems specific for the human and the simian hosts and parasites. This does not exclude an occasional overlap usually caused by deviation of either vertebrate or invertebrate host from the usual or representative behavioral or ecological pattern.

Simian malaria parasites, especially *P. cynomolgi* and *P. knowlesi,* are extensively used in malaria research. *Plasmodium cynomolgi,* as a vivax-type "relapsing" model, is particularly useful in basic biological and chemotherapeutic studies, while *P. knowlesi* is employed more in immunological research as well as in biological and biochemical studies where its synchronicity is of advantage.

2. Plasmodium (Laverania)

This subgenus is composed of only two species, *P. falciparum* and *P. reichenowi*. *Plasmodium falciparum* (Welch, 1897) has a wide distribution in tropical and subtropical areas within the 20°C summer isotherm and is transmitted by a large number of anopheline species and is naturally restricted to *Homo sapiens*. This species has a great number of strains and causes the clinically most serious forms of malaria.

Plasmodium reichenowi (Sluiter *et al.,* 1922) occurs in equatorial Africa within an area extending from 10°W to 30°E and 10°N to 5°S. Its natural host is *Pan satyrus,* but the invertebrate host is unknown. Blood schizogony takes 48 hours in both *P. falciparum* and *P. reichenowi*.

While there is not a single report of natural infection with *P. falciparum* in nonhuman primates, attempts to infect simians, either through blood inoculation or through mosquito bite, were successful in a wide variety of experimental hosts (see Table V) of which *Aotus trivirgatus* is now the most widely used. Cyclical retransmission of *P. falciparum* from *Aotus* to man has been achieved, confirming the value of the *Aotus* model for experimental purposes.

Attempts to infect man with *P. reichenowi* through the inoculation of infected chimpanzee blood have failed.

3. Plasmodium (Vinckeia)

This subgenus is characterized by small erythrocytic schizonts and round gametocytes; the 19 species of the group are generally stenoxenous. The subgenus occurs in widely different mammalian hosts, but individual species are usually restricted to very specific ecological niches. The various species and their distribution, natural vertebrate and arthropod hosts, and periodicity are listed in Table VI.

Although the natural arthropod hosts are not yet known in the majority of species, it appears to be quite likely that they are in all cases anopheline mosquitoes. In most species, especially those occurring in lower primates (lemurs), nonmurine rodents, and bats, the observations are largely limited to the blood forms. Future biological and biochemical investigations may lead to a new classification of the members of this heterogeneous subgenus.

It is interesting to note that none of the members of the subgenus occur in the New World. Only one species, *P. watteni,* is found on the border between the eastern palearctic and the oriental region. *Plasmodium booliati, P. bubalis, P. sandoshami,* and *P. traguli* occur in the oriental region. All other species are found in the Ethiopian zoogeographical region. Murine rodent malaria is limited to the central and western parts of tropical Africa. Malaria of bats appears to have the most marked insular distribution, with only two known microfoci in Africa, where maintenance of the species seems to depend on a delicate ecological balance.

The first species of murine rodent malaria, *P. berghei,* was described in 1948 (Vincke and Lips), and this was followed by the isolation of *P. vinckei* in 1952 (Rodhain). Both species have proved to be easily adapted to laboratory rodents, through both blood and sporozoite infection. Further investigation of rodent malarias in various parts of tropical Africa resulted in 1965 in the isolation of *P. chabaudi* (Landau) and in 1966 of *P. yoelii* (Landau and Killick-Kendrick). The latter species was initially considered a subspecies of *P. berghei* but was ultimately given species status based on the characterization of enzyme forms of the blood stages (Carter, 1973, 1978; Carter and Walliker, 1977) and of the morphological features of the sporogonic and preerythrocytic stages (Killick-Kendrick, 1974; Killick-Kendrick and Peters, 1978).

At present four type species and six subspecies are recognized: *P. berghei, P. chabaudi chabaudi, P. chabaudi adami, P. vinckei vinckei, P. vinckei petteri, P. vinckei lentum, P. vinckei brucechwatti, P. yoelii yoelii, P. yoelii killicki,* and *P. yoelii nigeriensis. Plasmodium vinckei* and *P. chabaudi* show synchronous, and *P. berghei* and *P. yoelii* asynchronous, blood schizogony.

Mice are easily infected by blood inoculation and cyclic transmission with all species and subspecies, although there are—especially with *P. berghei*—marked differences in susceptibility and course of infection in specific strains of mice. Hamsters and white rats are susceptible to blood- and sporozoite-induced infection with all subspecies of *P. berghei* and *P. yoelii* (Carter and Diggs, 1977), but generally not to blood-induced *P. vinckei* and *P. chabaudi.* The same applies to sporozoite inoculation, with the exception of *P. vinckei vinckei.*

Plasmodium berghei, P. yoelii, P. vinckei, and *P. chabaudi* were very quickly recognized as valuable laboratory models of mammalian malaria. The ease of adaptation to laboratory rodents and of establishing cyclic transmission—mainly through a rather undemanding anopheline *(A.*

TABLE VI

Species of the Subgenus *Plasmodium* (*Vinckeia*)

Species	Description	Distribution	Natural vertebrate host	Natural arthropod host	Periodicity of blood schizogony	Remarks
Plasmodia of lower primates						
P. (V.) girardi	Bück et al., 1952	Madagascar	Lemur fulvus rufus	Unknown	Probably 72 hours	P. (V.) girardi and P. (V.) lemuris may be synonymous
P. (V.) lemuris	Huff and Hoogstraal, 1963	Madagascar	Lemur collaris	Unknown	Unknown	
Plasmodia of nonmurine rodents						
P. (V.) booliati	Sandosham et al., 1965	Peninsular Malaysia	Petaurista petaurista	Unknown	Unknown	
P. (V.) watteni	Lien and Cross, 1968	Taiwan	Petaurista petaurista grandis	Unknown	Unknown	
P. (V.) anomaluri	Pringle, 1960	Tanzania	Anomalurus fraseri	Probably A. machardyi	Unknown	
P. (V.) atheruri	van den Berghe et al., 1958	Tanzania	Atherurus africanus	A. smithii vanthieli	24 hours	Primary exoerythrocytic schizogony 15 days minimum
P. (V.) landauae	Killick-Kendrick, 1973	Ivory Coast	Anomalurus peli	Unknown	Unknown	

P. (V.) pulmophilum	Killick-Kendrick, 1973	Ivory Coast	*Anomalurus peli*	Unknown	Unknown	
Plasmodia of murine rodents						
P. (V.) berghei	Vincke and Lips, 1948	Katanga	*Thamnomys surdaster, Praomys jacksoni, Leggada bella*	*A. dureni millcampsi*	22–25 hours, possibly less	All murine rodent plasmodia are extensively used for laboratory models, including cyclic transmission
P. (V.) chabaudi	Landau, 1965	Central African Republic, lower Congo (Zaire)	*Thamnomys rutilans*	Unknown	24 hours, synchronous	Recognized subspecies: *P. (V.) chabaudi chabaudi*, *P. (V.) chabaudi adami*
P. (V.) vinckei	Rodhain, 1952	Katanga, lower Congo (Zaire), Central African Republic	(*Thamnomys surdaster*),[a] *Thamnomys rutilans*	*A. dureni millcampsi* and probably *A. cinctus*	24 hours, synchronous	Recognized subspecies: *P. (V.) vinckei vinckei*, *P. (V.) vinckei petteri*, *P. (V.) vinckei lentum*, *P. (V.) vinckei brucechwatti*

(continued)

TABLE VI—*Continued*

Species	Description	Distribution	Natural vertebrate host	Natural arthropod host	Periodicity of blood schizogony	Remarks
P. (V.) yoelii	Landau and Killick-Kendrick, 1966	Central African Republic, lower Congo (Zaire), western Nigeria	*Thamnomys rutilans*	Probably *A. cinctus*	22–25 hours, possibly less	Recognized subspecies: *P. (V.) yoelii yoelii, P. (V.) yoelii killicki, P. (V.) yoelii nigeriensis*
Plasmodia of bats						
P. (V.) roussetti	van Riel *et al.*, 1951	Mont Hoyo (Zaire)	*Roussettus leachi*	Unknown	Unknown	
P. (V.) voltaicum	van der Kaay, 1964	Volta region of Ghana	*Roussettus smithi*	Probably *A. smithii*	Unknown	
Plasmodia of other mammals						
P. (V.) brucei	Garnham, 1966	Continental Tanzania, Zaire, Malawi, probably Upper Volta	*Sylvicapra grimmia*	Unknown	Unknown	
P. (V.) bubalis	Sheather, 1919	India, Pakistan	*Bubalus bubalis*	Unknown	Probably 72 hours	
P. (V.) cephalophi	Bruce *et al.*, 1913	Malawi	*Sylvicapra grimmia*	Unknown	72 hours	
P. (V.) sandoshami	Dunn *et al.*, 1963	West Malaysia	*Cynocephalus variegatus*	Unknown	Probably 72 hours	
P. (V.) traguli	Garnham and Edeson, 1962	Malaysia, Kalimantan (Indonesia)	*Tragulus javanicus*	*A. umbrosus*	Unknown	

[a] Suspected as natural host.

stephensi)—have made these parasites important and widely used tools of biological, chemotherapeutic, and immunological research.

Plasmodium berghei has also been adapted to laboratory rodents other than mice, rats, and hamsters. Hawking (1973) succeeded in infecting splenectomized monkeys of the African genera *Erythrocebus, Cercopithecus, Cercocebus,* and *Papio* with *P. berghei.* In addition, two South American monkeys, *Cebus* (two species) and *A. trivirgatus* and the Asian monkey *M. arctoides* were susceptible to *P. berghei* without splenectomy.

There have been reports that the characteristics of isolates of *P. berghei* (Jadin *et al.,* 1975) and *P. yoelii* (Yoeli and Hargreaves, 1974) may change grossly after cryopreservation. The reasons for this are unknown, but the advent of cloning in rodent plasmodia (Walliker, 1976) opens up a new field of studies which may shed light on the subject.

B. Avian Malaria Parasites

The subgenera Haemamoeba, Giovannolaia, Novyella, Huffia include 41 species which are listed in Table VII. Avian malaria parasites were among the first plasmodia to be studied (Danilewsky, 1889) and are found throughout the world.

Most species of plasmodia infecting passerine and migratory birds have a cosmopolitan distribution. The development of this wide distribution was aided by their heteroxenous character. Morphological differences in the same *Plasmodium* in different avian hosts have often caused confusion in their identification. *Plasmodium gallinaceum* and *Plasmodium juxtanucleare,* relatively stenoxenous parasites occurring in domestic fowl, have in addition a secondary cosmopolitan distribution corresponding to the cosmopolitan distribution of domestic fowl. However, domestic fowl are probably not the primary natural vertebrate hosts of the these plasmodia, but secondary to yet unidentified avians.

A limited geographic distribution of avian plasmodia is only seen in stenoxenous species affecting birds restricted to a limited habitat, e.g., *P. fallax, P. formosanum, P. garnhami, P. lophurae,* and *P. huffi.*

The morphology and biological characteristics of avian malaria parasites were extensively reviewed by Garnham (1966) and Seed and Manwell (1977).

The natural vectors of avian malaria parasites are practically all unknown, but circumstantial evidence suggests that *Culex* and *Aedes* spp. are the main arthropod hosts. According to Huff (1965) about 13 species of *Culex*, 3 of *Aedes*, 2 of *Culiseta*, and 5 of *Anopheles* have proved to be susceptible to *P. relictum.* Moreover, Corradetti *et al.* (1970) succeeded in adapting *P. gallinaceum* to *A. stephensi.* The most widely used laboratory vector for avian plasmodia is *C. pipiens.*

Avian plasmodia were the first to be extensively used as laboratory models,

TABLE VII

Species of Avian Subgenera of *Plasmodium*

Subgenus	Species	Description	Remarks
Haemamoeba	*P. (H.) cathemerium*	Hartmann, 1927	Cosmopolitan distribution; naturally occurring in passerine birds; extensively used as a laboratory model
	P. (H.) gallinaceum	Brumpt, 1935	Natural hosts are various species of jungle fowl in eastern Asia; *Gallus gallus* only secondary host; widely used as laboratory model
	P. (H.) giovannolai	Corradetti *et al.*, 1963b	Natural host *Turdus merula*
	P. (H.) griffithsi	Garnham, 1966	
	P. (H.) matutinum	Huff, 1937	Found in turkeys in Burma; natural hosts are probably other avian species
	P. (H.) relictum	Grassi and Feletti, 1891	Cosmopolitan distribution; mainly in passerine birds
			Cosmopolitan distribution; very wide (avian) host range, used as laboratory model
	P. (H.) subpraecox	Grassi and Feletti, 1892	Natural hosts are owls (Old and New World)
Giovannolaia	*P. (G.) anasum*	Manwell and Kuntz, 1965	Natural host is *Anas clypeata* (shoveller duck) from Taiwan
	P. (G.) circumflexum	Kikuth, 1931	Cosmopolitan distribution; mainly in passerine birds; used as laboratory model
	P. (G.) durae	Herman, 1941	Observed in turkeys (farm) in Kenya; natural hosts are probably wild gallinaceous birds
	P. (G.) fallax	Schwetz, 1930	Natural distribution restricted to eastern Zaire and southern Sudan (in *Syrnium nuchale* and *Numida meleagris*); adapted to turkey as a laboratory model
	P. (G.) formosanum	Manwell, 1962	Observed in *Arboriphila crudigularis* (partridge) from Taiwan
	P. (G.) gabaldoni	Garnham, 1977	Natural hosts are pigeons and ducks in Venezuela
	P. (G.) garnhami	Guindy *et al.*, 1965	Natural hosts are hoopoes in Egypt
	P. (G.) gundersi	Bray, 1962	Observed in Liberia in *Strix woodfordii nuchalis* (West African wood owl)

P. (G.) hegneri	Manwell and Kuntz, 1966	Found in European teal (*Anas c. crecca*) in Taiwan
P. (G.) lophurae	Coggeshall, 1938	Natural host is apparently the fire-backed pheasant from Borneo; adapted to ducks; extensively used as laboratory model
P. (G.) octamerium	Manwell, 1968	Found in the pintail Whydah bird (*Vidua macroura*) examined in the United States; exact origin unknown
P. (G.) pedioecetii	Schillinger, 1942	Natural hosts are gallinaceous birds in North America
P. (G.) pinottii	Muniz and Soares, 1954	Natural host is *Rhamphastos toco* (Brazilian toucan)
P. (G.) polare	Manwell, 1934	Observed in cliff swallows in North America and in falcons from Sicily
P. (N.) dissanaikei	de Jong, 1971	Observed in the rose-ringed parakeet (*Psittacula krameri manillensis*) in Sri Lanka
Novyella		
P. (N.) hexamerium	Huff, 1935	First described in the American bluebird, but naturally occurring in a variety of birds in the New World
P. (N.) justanucleare	Versiani and Gomes, 1941	Natural vertebrate host unknown; the domestic hen from which *P. justanucleare* is described is a secondary host
P. (N.) nucleophilum	Manwell, 1935 (1945)	Naturally found in catbirds and blackbirds in the New World; also recorded from *Aploxis panayensis* in Malaysia
P. (N.) paranucleophilum	Manwell and Sessler, 1971	Isolated from a South American tanager believed to have come from Brazil
P. (N.) rouxi	Sergent *et al*., 1928	Apparently cosmopolitan distribution, mainly in passerine birds
P. (N.) vaughani	Novy and MacNeal, 1904	Cosmopolitan distribution, mainly in passerine birds; *P. tenue* (Laveran and Marullaz, 1914) is considered a subspecies of *P. vaughani*; another subspecies is *P.* (Novyella) *vaughani merulae* (Corradetti and Scanga, 1973)
Huffia		
P. (H.) elongatum	Huff, 1930	Cosmopolitan distribution in a wide variety of birds, mainly passerines
P. (H.) hermani	Telford and Forrester, 1975	Found in wild turkeys (*Meleagris gallopavo*) in Florida
P. (H.) huffi	Muniz *et al*., 1951	Natural host *Rhamphastos toco* (toucan) from Brazil

e.g., *P. cathemerium, P. gallinaceum, P. relictum, P. circumflexum, P. fallax,* and *P. lophurae.* It was with avian malaria parasites that the existence of exoerythrocytic schizogony was first observed (James and Tate, 1937). The persistence of tissue schizogony after the onset of erythrocytic schizogony in avian plasmodia provided an explanation of the nature of the relapse phenomenon in malaria, as well as the failure of blood schizontocidal drugs to produce a radical cure.

The advent of rodent malaria has markedly reduced the use of avian malarias in the laboratory. However, the latter still maintain an important role of ultrastructural, biological, and immunological studies, especially in research on development of the exoerythrocytic forms and their *in vitro* culture.

C. Plasmodia and Related Parasites of Reptiles

The difficulties regarding the classification of reptilian plasmodia and related parasites were mentioned earlier in this section. In the list of species in Table VIII no attempt has been made to group the recognized reptilian plasmodia other than by zoogeographic regions. Reference is made, for subgeneric and morphological grouping, to the reviews of Garnham (1966), Ayala (1977, 1978). In Table VIII the genera *Garnia, Fallisia,* and *Saurocytozoon* are listed separately, although Telford (1973) has expressed doubts as to the validity of the former since the production of pigment is a variable character in at least some of the species included in this genus.

The classification of many saurian species is complicated by the occurrence of "blood schizogony" in blood cells other than erythrocytes, and of paraerythrocytic schizogony in blood cells instead of tissue cells. On the other hand, especially under the influence of increasing immunity, erythrocytic schizogony may be extremely short-lasting. Moreover, one and the same parasite species may, in different reptile species, considerably vary in its host cell choice.

Of the 41 reptile *Plasmodium* species and subspecies listed, only 1 is found in the palearctic region, 4 occur in Australasia, and 3 are found in the oriental region. Nine are restricted to the Ethiopian region, and about 24 species are known from the New World, mainly from the neotropic region. Only one, *P. minasense,* is found in both the oriental and neotropic regions.

The vertebrate hosts are mostly iguanids, agamids, and skinks. Only three species *P. pessoai* (Ayala *et al.,* 1978), *P. tomodoni* and *P. wenyoni,* have been found in snakes. Quite a number of species appear to be stenoxenous and, because of the limited habitat of the reptilian host, restricted in geographic distribution. Other species, such as *P. floridense, P. mexicanum, P. basilisci, A. rhadinurum,* and *A. tropiduri,* are heteroxenous and cover a wider geographic range within the neotropical region.

The vectors of reptilian malaria are unknown, but ceratopogonids,

TABLE VIII

Reptilian Malaria Parasites and Species of the Genera *Garnia, Fallisia,* and *Saurocytozoon*

Plasmodium spp.	*Plasmodium* spp. (*continued*)
Eastern palearctic species	Neotropic species (*continued*)
P. sasai	P. colombiense
Australasian species	P. diminutivum
P. egerniae	P. diploglossi
P. giganteum australis	P. floridense (also nearctic)
P. lacertiliae	P. josephinae
P. mackerrasae	P. minasense (also oriental)
Ethiopian species	P. rhadiurum (= carinii)
P. acuminatum	P. tomodoni (snakes)
P. agamae	P. torrealbai
P. fischeri	P. tropiduri
P. giganteum	P. uncinatum
P. mabuiae	P. vacuolatum
P. maculilabre	P. vautieri
P. pitmani	P. wenyoni (snakes)
P. robinsoni	*Garnia* spp. (all neotropic)
P. zonuriae	G. azurophilum
Oriental species	G. balli
P. clelandi	G. gonatodi
P. minasense (also neotropic)	G. morula
P. vastator	G. multiformis
Nearctic species	G. telfordi
P. beltrani	G. uranoscodoni
P. brumpti	G. utingensis
P. chiricahuae	*Fallisia* spp. (all neotropic)
P. floridense (also neotropic)	F. audaciosa
P. mexicanum	F. effusa
Neotropic species	F. modesta
P. achiotensis	F. simplex
P. attenuatum	*Saurocytozoon* spp. (all neotropic)
P. aurulentum	S. mabuyi
P. basilisci	S. tupinambi
P. cnemidophori	

phlebotomids, and culicine mosquitoes are suspected to play a major role. Experimentally sporogony of *P. mexicanum* has been completely followed in *Lutzomyia vexatrix occidentis,* a phlebotomid (Ayala, 1971). Oocyst formation was observed in various species of *Aedes* and *Culex,* but sporozoites were not produced.

Reptilian plasmodia never became very popular for laboratory study largely because of the more demanding care required by the experimental animals, the difficulties in establishing cyclic transmission, and the many biological characteristics that separate them from mammalian species. However, recent advances in tissue culture techniques and the ease with which reptilian cell lines can be established have led to the increasing use of reptilian parasites for *in vitro* culture studies, especially in the fields of basic biology and immunology.

III. LIFE CYCLE OF MALARIA PARASITES

Since the ultrastructure of malaria parasites will be specifically covered in Chapter 4 of this volume (Aikawa and Seed), the following description of the life cycle will generally not go into details of the fine structure. In this context, it is not intended to provide an exhaustive review—such can be found elsewhere; for example Garnham (1966) has given a comprehensive, synoptic review of the subject. The life cycles of plasmodia of nonhuman primates, rodents, birds, and reptiles were recently reviewed by Collins and Aikawa (1977), Carter and Diggs (1977), Seed and Manwell (1977), and Ayala (1977).

Malaria parasites undergo a complex life cycle alternating between vertebrate and arthropod hosts. In Fig. 1 the life cycle of *P. vivax* is shown as an example.

The sporozoite, upon inoculation by an infected mosquito, reaches the blood circulation in which it is transported to the target site or its vicinity. Possibly guided by chemotaxis and recognizing its target, it leaves the capillary lumen and enters the host cell. The latter can be a hepatocyte (as in mammalian plasmodia) or reticuloendothelial cells (as in avian plasmodia). In no case do sporozoites enter red blood cells. However, in mammalian malaria parasites there is a distinct possibility that sporozoite entry into hepatocytes is not direct, but through a reticulo-endothelial cell. Fairley's observations (1945) on *P. vivax* showed that sporozoites vanished from the circulating blood within 30 minutes after inoculation. The sporozoite's entry into the cell results in a drastic morphological change in the parasite which now appears round or oval and contains a chromatin nucleus surrounded by cytoplasm. In the course of the ensuing exoerythrocytic or tissue schizogony, the nucleus divides and the cytoplasmatic mass grows. The number of nuclear divisions and their intervals vary widely in different species. So does the ultimate size of the exoerythrocytic schizont which in some species may reach a diameter of 3 mm. After completion of the nuclear divisions, the cytoplasm segregates and merozoites are formed, consisting of a single nucleus and cytoplasm. In contrast to the erythrocytic stages, exoerythrocytic schizonts do not contain pigment. Conspicuous round vacuoles were described in the exoerythrocytic schizonts of *P. vivax,* while clefts, flocculi, or inclusions were reported in other plasmodia, which appear to be typical of the species and may permit its identification from the morphology of the exoerythrocytic schizont. *Plasmodium malariae, P. ovale,* and *P. brasilianum* are the only primate plasmodia in which the host cell nucleus is enlarged. The number of merozoites produced by one

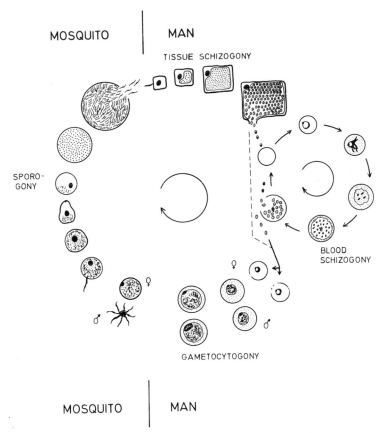

FIG. 1.   Cycle of development of *P. (Plasmodium) vivax.*

exoerythrocytic schizont is estimated to be approximately 2000 in *P. malariae,* 10,000 in *P. vivax,* 15,000 in *P. ovale,* and more than 30,000 in *P. falciparum,* roughly corresponding to 12, 14, 15, and 16 nuclear divisions. The diameter of the mature exoerythrocytic schizont is approximately 45 μm in *P. malariae,* 45 μm in *P. vivax,* 70 μm in *P. ovale,* and 60 μm in *P. falciparum.* The duration of the exoerythrocytic development of primate plasmodia roughly corresponds to the pre-patent period and is listed in Table IV. The site of primary exoerythrocytic schizogony in reptilian plasmodia is still unknown. For mammalian plasmodia, it is now generally accepted that the merozoites originating from cryptozoic schizonts, i.e., primary schizogony or exoerythrocytic schizogony arising directly from sporozoites, can only invade red cells, while those of avian plasmodia can only invade new tissue cells, giving rise to metacryptozoic schizonts, i.e., a second round of exo-erythrocytic schizogony. After having passed through at least one subsequent tissue schizogony—phanerozoic schizogony—the avian phanerozoic merozoites can ultimately invade erythrocytes.

The erythrocytic merozoites are ovoid or elongated structures and species-specific in size (the long axis in *P. falciparum* is 0.7 µm; in *P. vivax,* 1.2 µm; and in *P. ovale,* 1.8 µm). They possess an external membrane covered by a distinct surface coat which is apparently of parasitic origin (Mason *et al.*, 1977). The apical region contains the paired organelles (rhoptries) and a few micronemes which may be involved in the invasion of the erythrocyte. The nucleus and a mitochondria-like organelle are found in or near the posterior region. During invasion of the erythrocyte, the anterior end of the merozoite attaches to the erythrocyte membrane, which after thickening forms a junction with the plasma membrane of the merozoite (Aikawa *et al.*, 1978). The erythrocyte invaginates to form a parasitophorous vacuole in which the parasite eventually lies; the junction between erythrocyte membrane and plasma membrane of the merozoite assumes the form of a ring which appears to travel along the merozoite surface. During this process of invasion the surface coat of the merozoite is lost and apparently remains outside the erythrocyte.

Once within the parasitophorous vacuole, the parasite transforms rapidly into a young trophozoite which is finally surrounded by two membranes; the inner one is the original parasite membrane, and the outer one, which is contiguous with the exception of the cytostome area, is derived from the host erythrocyte. Mostly hemoglobin is ingested, probably only through the use of the cytostome, and it is digested in numerous phagosomes located in the parasite's cytoplasm to produce typical malarial pigment (hemozoin).

During this process the parasite grows; ameboid movement, initially marked in younger trophozoites, decreases when the trophozoite approaches a full-grown stage, assuming a more-or-less rounded shape. The nuclear material increases and undergoes several divisions, in mammalian species usually three to five, resulting in the appropriate number of nuclei which are situated in a cytoplasmic syncytium until it ultimately divides to form erythrocytic merozoites. The erythrocytic parasite containing many nuclei and syncytial cytoplasm is called a presegmenter or preschizont, and the parasite containing fully differentiated merozoites is called a (mature) schizont. The mature schizont bursts, liberating the individual merozoites which, in mammalian species, can only invade erythrocytes. In avian and reptile plasmodia they can also invade tissue cells and produce phanerozoic schizogony or, in the case of reptilian malaria, initiate paraerythrocytic schizogony, i.e., schizogony in blood cells other than erythrocytes.

During the process of blood schizogony the infected erythrocytes may retain their normal size, e.g., in *P. malariae* and *P. falciparum,* or become enlarged and round as in *P. vivax,* or enlarged and deformed as in *P. ovale.* Typical dots or clefts may develop in the stroma of the infected red blood cells. The choice of the human erythrocytic cell may be apparently universal, as in *P. falciparum*, or specific, e.g.. Duffy-positive young erythrocytes in *P. vivax*. The duration of blood schizogony is generally a multiple of 24 hours, usually 24, 48, or 72 hours, but there are notable exceptions, e.g., *P. gallinaceum* with a 36-hour asexual cycle. The mechanisms of synchronicity observed in some species such as *P. knowlesi* and *P. chabaudi* are largely unknown.

Growth and division synchrony of *P. berghei* in mice can be augmented by specific photoperiodic rhythms. This mechanism and vascular sequestration of parasitized erythrocytes are apparently controlled by the pineal gland. Photoperiodically augmented synchrony is lost after pinealectomy; in the pinealectomized animal it may be restored by ubiquinone and members of the vitamin K group (Arnold *et al.*, 1969a,b,c).

Upon invading a new erythrocyte the merozoite can either initiate renewed blood schizogony or develop into a female or a male gametocyte (a macrogametocyte or a microgametocyte); these gametocytes are elongated in *Laverania* and *Huffia* but round in the other mammalian and avian subgenera. The early gametocyte stages have a more solid appearance, a smaller vacuole, and less ameboid activity than the schizogonic trophozoites but exhibit a similar pattern of pigment granules. The mature macrogametocytes usually show a compact nucleus and an accumulation of pigment near the nucleus. In microgametocytes the nucleus is larger and less compact, often with a "spongy" appearance. The gametocytes are still surrounded by the host erythrocyte's membrane. Usually, the number of microgametocytes is markedly less than that of macrogametocytes. The duration of gametocytogony is not exactly known. In *P. vivax* it is assumed to be 4 days, while studies *in vitro* suggest a minimum duration of 8 days in *P. falciparum*. In a number of mammalian plasmodia, gametocytogony may be initiated directly from cryptozoic merozoites, and in avian malarias from phanerozoic merozoites. When taken up by a suitable arthropod, the gametocytes transform into gametes. Macrogametocytes shed the erythrocyte membrane and become mature macrogametes without any evident morphological change visible under the light microscope. In contrast, microgametocytes undergo a complete transformation: The nucleus divides three times, forming usually eight new nuclei which combine with cytoplasm to form microgametes having a very specific organellar structure. The exflagellated microgametes then tear free and move actively toward the macrogametes and invade them; after entry, the cytoplasmic material of the macrogamete and microgamete combine to form the zygote. Exflagellation usually takes 10–15 minutes, and microgamete entry 1 minute (Sinden and Croll, 1975; Sinden *et al.*, 1978); these processes are separated by the time required for the microgamete to reach the macrogamete and to align itself.

The zygote remains immobile for some time. After both nuclei combine, the zygote elongates to form an ookinete, the broad anterior region of which appears to be rather inflexible, containing a projecting, truncated papilla with an apical complex (Sinden, 1975). The ookinete is actively motile (Speer *et al.,* 1975). It moves toward the arthropod host's intestinal epithelium, enters it, and comes to rest beneath the basal lamina, forming an oocyst. In mammalian plasmodia, penetration of the gut epithelium by the ookinete usually takes place in the anterior part of the midgut of anopheline mosquitoes. The oocyst grows, surrounded by a smooth wall (Strome and Beaudoin, 1974). The cytoplasm maintains its syncytial structure, while there is intensive nuclear division, the speed of which is largely dependent on the environmental temperature. The pigment, carried along by the macrogamete, still remains in the oocyst. Ultimately the cytoplasm divides to form sporozoites. By this time the oocyst may have reached a diameter of 500 μm or more. The sporozoites emerge from the oocyst into the hemolymph through small individual holes or through larger openings where the oocyst wall was torn away (Sinden, 1975). In mammalian and avian plasmodia, most sporozoites—elongated, fusiform, and highly motile structures—migrate to the salivary glands of the arthropod host. They penetrate the glandular cells (Sterling *et al.* 1973) and ultimately reach the lumina of the salivary ducts from which they are able to reach the vertebrate host with the next bite of the arthropod. Sporogony, i.e., the period from gametocyte maturation until the development of infective sporozoites in the salivary glands, takes between 8 days and 8 weeks. The number of sporozoites produced by one oocyst varies according to the plasmodium species. In *P. falciparum* it is estimated to be 10,000 (Pringle, 1965), which under optimum environmental conditions indicates a 12-hour cycle of nuclear division in the oocyst. Gametocyte maturation and gamete, zygote, and ookinete formation may also take place in an a priori unsuitable host or *in vitro,* but further development is normally limited to the natural vector.

There is still controversy regarding mitotic and meiotic phases of nuclear division in plasmodia. Although some observers have described the presence of classic chromosomes, such claims have not been substantiated. This does not preclude mitotic division of nuclear material. The first division in the postzygote stage is assumed to be meiotic, accompanied by the disappearance of the nuclear membrane (Garnham, 1966). This is apparently followed by mitosis. Howells and Davies (1971) reported electron microscopic studies suggesting mitotic division in the oocyst stages of *P. berghei.* There seems to be agreement that the nucleus of sporozoites, merozoites, and gametocytes is haploid and that division during exoerythrocytic and erythrocytic schizogony is mitotic, although not typically eukaryotic, since the nuclear membrane remains intact during division.

The past decade has brought a fundamental revision of the concept of exoerythrocytic schizogony in the subgenera *Plasmodium* and *Vinckeia.* Originally it was held that the species of these subgenera underwent secondary exoerythrocytic schizogony. This would explain the relapsing nature in some of these species.

However, this hypothesis is now being questioned. The relapses in *P. cynomolgi, P. fieldi, P. ovale, P. simiovale,* and *P. vivax* are now being associated with the presence of latent cryptozoites (''hypnozoites,'' Markus, 1978), the existence of which was shown by Landau (1973) in *Grammomys surdaster* and substantiated for *P. vivax* through the clinical observations of Shute *et al.* (1976) and Ungureanu *et al.* (1976). This renders an important part of the hitherto accepted definition of the subgenus *Plasmodium* (Bray, 1963) untenable.

IV. EPIDEMIOLOGY OF HUMAN MALARIA

The epidemiology of human malaria is an example of an intricate biological system in which the parasite and its vertebrate and arthropod hosts interact in close dependence on environmental conditions.

A. The Parasite

In order to survive as a species the parasite must be present in the human host long enough and be able to offer an adequate quantum of viable gametocytes of both sexes at a time when environmental conditions are suitable for transmission. On the other hand, the parasite must be naturally adapted to a sufficiently anthropophilic mosquito species which can regularly—but not necessarily continuously—permit the completion of sporogony leading to infective sporozoites.

The natural life span of a malaria infection varies widely according to the *Plasmodium* species and the strain. *Plasmodium falciparum* averages 9–12 months, but periods of up to 3 years have been reported (Verdrager, 1964). Infections with *P. vivax* and *P. ovale* usually last not more than 4 years, but *P. malariae* infections can last for several decades—periods of over 40 years having been recorded. These periods may reflect the degree of the parasite's adaptation to man which is apparently least in *P. falciparum,* a species which often kills the host, and most accomplished in *P. malariae* which, at least in adult man, often exhibits almost commensalic features.

Natural adaptation or selection of the most suitable populations is shown by *P. vivax* at the climatogeographic limits of its distribution in the palearctic region, e.g., in *P. vivax hibernans* which apparently possesses a long incubation period allowing it to remain in the vertebrate host until the next, usually quite short, transmission period (Garnham *et al.,* 1975). Similarly, the North Korean strain of *P. vivax* often—though not regularly—shows long incubation periods which appear, however, to be also related to the quantum of the sporozoite inoculum (Shute *et al.,* 1976). The obvious explanation, that two different types of sporozoites exist, one giving rise immediately to exoerythrocytic schizogony and the other lying dormant, was originally advanced by Moshkovsky (1973) and further elaborated by Lysenko *et al.* (1977) and Rybalka *et al.* (1977). With the tropical Chesson strain of *P. vivax* the incubation period is always short, even when small inocula are used (Ungureanu *et al.*, 1976).

An epidemiologically important feature is the relatively late appearance of gametocytes in naturally acquired falciparum malaria, in no case earlier than 15 days after patency.

Moreover, studies on *P. falciparum* indicate a periodicity and strictly limited duration of the infectivity of gametocytes, which coincides with the period of highest biting activity of the vectors (Hawking *et al.*, 1971). The observations of Garnham and Powers (1974) using the *P. cynomolgi* langur strain in rhesus monkeys and *A. stephensi* or *A. atroparvus*, which showed higher infectivity at midnight as compared to midday blood meals, tend to agree with this hypothesis.

Specific adaptation of local parasite strains to particular vector species appears to be marked. Thus, *A. atroparvus* from an area near Naples, formerly a good vector of *P. falciparum* in Italy, proved to be refractory to infection with Nigerian *P. falciparum*. Similarly Kenyan *P. falciparum* failed to infect *A. labranchiae* and one strain of *A. atroparvus* from Italy, while only a low oocyst rate was found in the Volturno strain of *A. atroparvus* (Ramsdale and Coluzzi, 1975).

From studies on *P. berghei* (Vanderberg, 1975) it can be concluded that earlier crops of sporozoites are significantly less viable than older sporozoites. When considered along with the limited longevity of the vectors, this feature appears to have marked epidemiological importance. In addition skin factors may determine the number of infective sporozoites reaching the blood. Specific observations in a *P. berghei* rodent model suggest that only some 1% of the total number of inoculated sporozoites give rise to exoerythrocytic development (Vanderberg, 1977).

B. The Human Host

Genetic, physical, behavioral, and economic factors affect man's susceptibility and exposure to infection with malaria parasites.

Ethnic genetic differences in the susceptibility to particular parasite species play an important role in the distribution of *P. vivax* which is virtually absent from West and Central Africa and shows very distinct differences of incidence in Hamito-Semitic and Nilotic populations in Ethiopia (Armstrong, 1978). The distribution of *P. ovale* may suggest some relationship to ethnic factors, although at least a partial explanation should be sought in the receptivity of particular anopheline species.

Innate and physiological factors may have a marked epidemiological impact. It is known that carriers of the sickle cell gene (hemoglobin S) are less susceptible to falciparum malaria than nonsicklers (Livingston, 1971, 1976), a finding borne out by the observations of Friedman (1978) and Friedman et al. (1979). The specific advantage of the heterozygous state has apparently offset the losses caused by the lethal homozygous state and perpetuated the gene in the highly malarious areas of tropical Africa. Also, glucose-6-phosphate dehydrogenase deficiency was believed to afford an attenuation of falciparum malaria and thus a relative protection of the afflicted persons; however, the studies of Martin et al. (1979) seem to indicate that clinical evidence for protection by the homozygous or hemizygous deficient state is lacking.

In some populations it appears that different age groups have a different degree of exposure to vector bites, which expresses itself—in areas with moderate malaria transmission—in a markedly different age-specific malaria incidence. In part this may be explained by a proportionality between uncovered body surface and the probability of vector bites. The same appears to hold true for apparent sex differences in comparable groups exposed to equal risks. Although specific attraction of the vector is known to play a role, the major factors in sex differences of exposure are occupational or behavioral: in many malarious areas men stay outdoors during periods of vector activity for social or for occupational reasons.

Closely linked with and often inseparable from occupational influences are man's habits which may determine the probability of contracting malaria. Migration between malarious and nonmalarious but receptive areas may cause spread of the disease. Equally, the stay of nonmalarious persons in malarious areas exposes them to a risk—a pattern frequently found in tropical labor aggregations. The same applies to warfare, in the course of which large groups of healthy military personnel may be exposed to malaria, and the disease may be spread by massive movements of displaced civilians.

Artificially created malaria, resulting from borrow pits and inadequate water management in irrigation schemes or dam sites is on the rise. The problem confronts many tropical countries, where economic and agricultural development is not accompanied by the essential health measures, a phenomenon involving also other diseases, e.g., schistosomiasis.

Although in their strongholds malaria and its vectors do not differentiate between poor and rich or between literate and illiterate man, there are marked quantitative differences between these groups regarding vector–man and parasite–man contacts. The screening of doors and windows, the use of mosquito nets and of insecticide sprays, the prophylactic use of antimalarials, and the prompt treatment of a malarial attack are certainly in better reach of economically privileged and intellectually motivated people.

Immunity against malaria evidently influences the production of gametocytes. In areas with holo- and hyperendemic malaria, gametocyte production is highest in the young age groups with the least pronounced immunity. Frequency and intensity of gametocytemia decrease with increasing age until they reach a minimum among adults (Fig. 2). Gametocyte production in untreated, nonimmune adults is high and decreases only after long-term exposure to malaria infection. High immunity usually masks the infection. Immune malaria carriers may enter receptive areas, having escaped detection, and trigger subsequent transmission and thus be the cause of the introduction of malaria.

Artificially created malaria also includes infections induced by direct transmission, i.e., those not going through the natural vector and provoked by the transfer of asexual forms. Many of these infections, especially those with *P. malariae,* are iatrogenous, usually transmitted through blood transfusions. Such infections occur frequently in areas which have been apparently cleared of malaria but where an undetected reservoir of long-standing quartan malaria is still in existence. Usually, this type of induced malaria can be quickly and effectively controlled. In contrast, induced falciparum malaria can produce a fulminant, fatal outcome (Brooks and Barry, 1969). Such infections are relatively frequent in nonmalarious countries where people from malarious regions are accepted as blood donors and no malaria serology is carried out routinely on donor blood or no antimalarial treatment is given along with the transfusion.

Induced malaria among drug addicts is a recent though not uncommon phenomenon (Dover, 1971; Rosenblatt and Marsh, 1971; Lyman *et al.,* 1972; Friedmann *et al.,* 1973; Brown and Khoa, 1975). The majority of these cases are infections with *P. vivax.* Epidemics of induced malaria in drug addicts are not unusual. The largest on record involved 47 cases, all vivax malaria. Of the 11 described induced *P. falciparum* cases in heroin users, 8 died, usually with

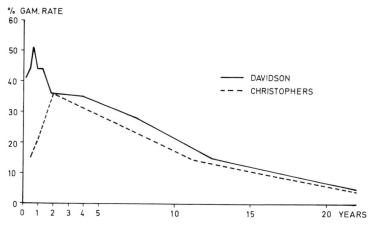

FIG. 2. Gametocytemia of *P. falciparum* as related to age in areas of high malaria endemicity. Comparison of the results of Christophers (1949) and Davidson (1955).

manifestations of cerebral malaria which can easily be confused with the state of advanced drug intoxication.

Congenital malaria is relatively rare; its occurrence seems to be associated with a state of low immunity in the mother. This may explain why most of the reports on congenital malaria come from areas where the disease is of a low endemicity.

C. The Arthropod Host

Only female anophelines are vectors of human malaria, since male anophelines do not feed on blood. Among more than 400 species of anopheline mosquitoes only 67 were found to harbor sporozoites originating from natural infection. About 28 additional species were found experimentally to be susceptible to infection with *P. falciparum, P. malariae, P. ovale,* or *P. vivax,* or to infection with several of these species (see Table IX). Only 27 species are thought to be associated with a significant degree of malaria transmission, especially in the presence of a large gametocyte reservoir.

The relative frequency of feeding on man rather than on some other animal determines the probability of a mosquito acquiring an infection and, in association with the vector's longevity, the probability of transmitting the infection to a new vertebrate host. The relative frequency of feeding on man is a composite factor reflecting the mosquito's attraction to man and the frequency of biting—in accordance with the gonotrophic cycle, since one blood meal is usually enough to support the maturation of one egg batch. The attraction to man may be rather stable in areas with little faunic fluctuation but subject to considerable variation when the availability of preferred blood hosts is changed.

The longevity of the vector, i.e., its life expectancy, determines the probability of its surviving through the time required to produce viable sporozoites. The longevity is largely dependent on environmental conditions, especially relative humidity, and on species-specific inherent factors. The duration of sporogony—which has to correlate with the vector's longevity—in turn depends on the environmental temperature. Seasonal variations in relative humidity may shorten the life expectancy of usually very potent vector species to the extent that malaria transmission ceases at temperatures which would favor rapid sporogony. This is seen, for example, with *A. gambiae* in the dry zones of the central Nile River basin (Wernsdorfer and Wernsdorfer, 1967).

Mosquito density also is a major determinant of malaria transmission, although only in a linear function. Mosquito density largely depends on the longevity of the adult mosquitoes and on the availability of suitable breeding places. The different anopheline species have very distinct ecological requirements for

TABLE IX

Arthropod Hosts of Human Malaria Parasites

Anopheles species	Sporozoite production after experimental infection with[a]				Natural infection of salivary glands
	P. m.	P. ov.	P. v.	P. f.	
A. aconitus[b]	+			+	+
A. albimanus[b]		+	+	+	+
A. albitarsis			+		+
A. algeriensis			+	+	+
A. annularis[b]	+		+		+
A. annulipes					+
A. apicimacula				+	
A. aquasalis[b]				+	+
A. argyritarsis			+		
A. atroparvus[c]		+		+	+
A. atropos	+				
A. aztecus	+		+		
A. bachmanni			+		
A. balabacensis balabacensis[c]	+	+	+		
A. bancrofti			+	+	+
A. barberi				+	
A. barbirostris			+	+	+
A. bellator			+	+	+
A. brunnipes					+
A. claviger	−		+		+
A. crucians crucians	−			+	+

Anopheles species	Sporozoite production after experimental infection with				Natural infection of salivary glands
	P. m.	P. ov.	P. v.	P. f.	
A. leucosphyrus					+
A. lindesayi	+		+	+	
A. ludlowi	+		+	+	+
A. maculatus[b]	+		+	+	+
A. maculipennis		+	+		
A. mangyanus					+
A. melas[d]	+			+	+
A. messeae[b]	+			+	+
A. minimus flavirostris[b]					+
A. minimus minimus[d]	−		+	+	+
A. moucheti	+				+
A. multicolor					
A. neomaculipalpus			+		+
A. nili				+	
A. noroestensis			+	+	+
A. nuneztovari					
A. oswaldoi guarujaensis			+	+	+
A. oswaldoi oswaldoi			+	+	+
A. pallidus			+	+	
A. pattoni			+	+	+
A. pharoensis[b]			+	+	+

Species	P. f.	P. v.	P. m.	P. ov.
A. cruzi		+	+	+
A. culicifacies[b]	+	+	+	+
A. darlingi[c]	−	+	+	+
A. d'thali		+	+	+
A. eiseni			+	+
A. farauti[c]	+	+	+	+
A. fluviatilis[d]	+	+	+	+
A. freeborni	+	+	+	+
A. fuliginosus		+		+
A. funestus[d]	+	+	+	+
A. gambiae[d] (complex)	+	+	+	+
A. hancocki		+	+	+
A. hargreavesi		+		+
A. hatori		+	+	+
A. hispaniola		+	+	+
A. hyrcanus nigerrimus	−	+	+	+
A. hyrcanus sinensis[c]	+	+	+	+
A. jamesi		+	+	−
A. jeyporiensis	+	+	+	+
A. karwari		+	+	+
A. kochi	+	+	+	+
A. koliensis		+	+	+
A. kweiyangensis		+	+	+
A. labranchiae[d]		+	+	+
A. lesteri		+	+	+
A. letifer		+	+	+
A. philippinensis[b]		+	+	+
A. plumbeus		+	+	+
A. pseudopunctipennis		+	+	+
A. pulcherrimus		+	+	+
A. punctimacula		+	+	+
A. puncipennis	+	+	+	+
A. punctulatus[b]	+	+	+	+
A. quadrimaculatus[c]	+	+		+
A. ramsayi				+
A. rhodesiensis		+	+	+
A. sacharovi[d]	+	+	+	+
A. sergenti[c]		+	+	+
A. smithi		+		+
A. splendidus	−	+	+	+
A. stephensi[b]	+	+	+	+
A. strodei		+	+	+
A. subpictus	+	+	+	+
A. sundaicus[c]		+	+	+
A. superpictus[b]	+	+	+	+
A. tesselatus		+		+
A. triannulatus		+	+	+
A. umbrosus		+	+	+
A. vagus		+	+	+
A. varuna	+	+	+	+
A. vestitipennis			+	+
A. walkeri		+	+	+
A. wilmorei			+	

[a] P. m., P. malariae; P. ov., P. ovale; P. v., P. vivax; P. f., P. falciparum.

[b] Species associated with unstable malaria.

[c] Species associated with intermediate stability of malaria.

[d] Species associated with stable malaria.

breeding, with wide variations regarding water flow, exposure to the sun, water temperature, and aquatic vegetation.

D. The Environment

Climatic and topographic features determine the ecology of both human and arthropod hosts, as well as their contact. Malaria transmission requires that infected man, i.e., the source of infection, and susceptible man be accessible to the vector which is normally confined to a flight range of up to 2 km from its breeding place. The closer the proximity of breeding places to human habitations, the higher the vector–man contact. Land vegetation, soil structure, and hydrographic features determine to a large degree the nature and the stability of potential breeding places.

The most important environmental factors influencing malaria transmission are meteorological features.

Mean temperature determines the duration of sporogony. Sporogony of *P. vivax* ceases below 16°C, that of *P. falciparum* below 20°C. At 16°C the sporogony of *P. vivax* is completed in 55 days, and at 28°C in only 7 days (Fig. 3). Sporogony does not occur at mean temperatures above 33°C. The temperature dependence of sporogony explains why *P. vivax* is not found in areas outside the 16°C summer isotherms and similarly why *P. falciparum* is restricted to areas within the 20°C summer isotherm. Certain exceptional microclimates may occa-

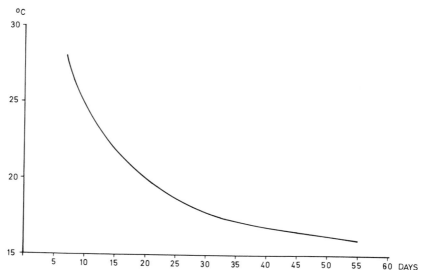

FIG. 3. Duration of sporogony of *P. (Plasmodium) vivax* at various temperatures (from W.H.O. records, Pampana, 1963).

sionally permit malaria transmission outside these limits; e.g., at high altitudes in Africa mosquitoes may shelter in warm huts, and the parasite may be able to complete sporogony under these artificial conditions.

Environmental temperature also regulates the speed of mosquito breeding. At 12°C *A. quadrimaculatus* first instar larvae take 65 days to develop to emerged adults, while only 7.3 days are required at the optimum water temperature of 31°C (Huffaker, 1944). The minimum and maximum thresholds for the development of the aquatic stages were 11° and 35°C. The threshold values are subject to wide variation in the different anopheline species and are largely in accordance with their ecological adaptation, but the temperature dependence of aquatic development is a feature common to all.

Relative humidity has a direct bearing on mosquito longevity and thus on the probability of the mosquitoe reaching an infective stage. Wernsdorfer and Wernsdorfer (1967) estimated in the central Nile River basin a daily mortality for *A. gambiae* of 5% at relative humidities of 65% and more, of 10% at 55% R.H. and of 15% at 50% R.H., at mean temperatures of 27°–30°C and night–day fluctuations of ±5°C. The longevity of *A. gambiae* at various levels of relative humidity is illustrated in Fig. 4. It is seen that significant proportions of

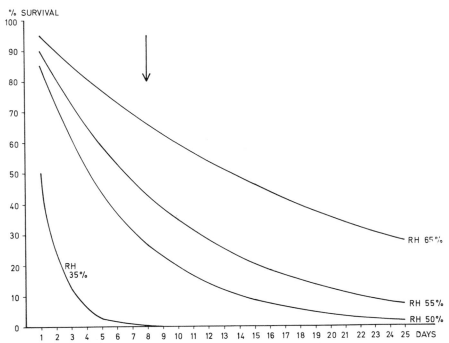

FIG. 4. Survival of *A. gambiae* in the central Nile River basin at various levels of relative humidity (Wernsdorfer and Wernsdorfer, 1967).

mosquitoes survive to potentially infective age at 50% R.H. and more. Only at daily mortalities of 50%, as observed at 35% R.H., does the proportion of mosquitoes surviving to a potentially dangerous age drop to a level well below 1%. Such conditions occur seasonally in the fringe areas of *A. gambiae* distribution in tropical Africa and on the Arabian peninsula, where such conditions may even last for the greater part of the year.

Rainfall influences malaria transmission in various ways. It may create breeding places for mosquitoes by producing surface water collections. The evaporation of large surface water sheets is apt to keep the relative humidity at high levels, thus prolonging the life span of the vector. However, the flushing of riverbeds as a result of rainfall abruptly terminates mosquito breeding in the remaining pools. Also, the biological effect of rainfall is quite different in the case of pool-breeding, stream-breeding, and well-breeding anophelines. The spacing of rainfall may often be more important than the quantity of rain. Sudden abundant rains are apt to do damage to mosquito breeding. Well-spaced lighter rains usually promote it. Therefore the "degree of wetness" (Russell *et al.*, 1963) is used as an index of rainfall distribution. This monthly index is calculated as follows:

$$\text{Degree of wetness} = \frac{\text{number of rain days in the month times total rainfall}}{\text{number of days in the month}}$$

Groundwater levels may also have a major bearing on malaria transmission, since high levels are likely to maintain mosquito breeding in seepage areas, borrow pits, and natural depressions even outside the rainy seasons.

Strong wind can be detrimental to the life of adult mosquitoes and prevent them from ovipositioning. Gentle, moist winds, however, may allow mosquitoes to lengthen their flight range much beyond the normal limits and thus to speed up a seasonal recurrence of vectors in the semiarid marginal areas of their distribution; in the Sahel zone of Africa this phenomenon aids in the building up of *A. gambiae* populations probably more than estivation.

A very specific case of a correlation between environment and malaria transmission is that between tropical dam sites and irrigation schemes and transmission. The profound changes in the ecosystems provoked by the increase in surface water, the raising of water tables, flooding, and seepage, as well as the consequent rise in relative humidity, often increase the production and the longevity of malaria vectors (Surtees, 1970). Thus semiarid and arid areas can become highly malarious, passing after some years of epidemic malaria into an apparently calmer stage of hyper- or holoendemicity. Much of the adverse effects of artificial water impoundment could be prevented by good water management, appropriate crop selection and crop cycles, and simple public health measures.

E. Parasitological and Epidemiological Parameters

In malariological practice a number of parameters are used to classify the condition of malaria in a given area, which permit a description of the epidemiological situation. For this purpose cross-sectional surveys suffice in some cases, but in the majority of areas only longitudinal observations may yield the basis for such classifications. A definition of the most essential parameters has been provided in the "Terminology of Malaria and of Malaria Eradication" (World Health Organization, 1963). The following commonly employed parameters may serve for a better understanding of the two following sections.

1. Malaria Morbidity

This is calculated on the basis of one calendar year or one complete epidemiological year and expressed as the number of malaria cases per 1000 population (unlike other diseases where morbidity is calculated on the basis of 100,000 population).

2. Malaria Mortality

This represents the number of deaths from malaria per 100,000 population during one calendar year or one epidemiological year.

3. Malaria Incidence

The malaria incidence is a dynamic measurement of the number of malaria cases occurring during a given time period in relation to the unit of population in which they occur. This allows an estimate of the monthly, quarterly, or yearly (or any other time period) incidence per any chosen unit of population, e.g., in percentage, but requires a precise mechanism for continuous, reliable parasitological examination over the chosen time period and in the selected universe.

4. Malaria Prevalence

This represents the number of malaria cases existing at any given time in relation to the unit of population in which they occur. Malaria prevalence (point prevalence) is a static measure. Depending on the seasonality and the stability of the disease, the prevalence data of the same population may differ considerably at various time points.

5. Spleen Rate

The spleen rate is the percentage of persons (usually children of 2–9 years) showing palpable enlargement of the spleen at a given time. If the spleen rate is assessed in other age groups, this should be specified, e.g., adult spleen rate if it is measured in adults.

6. Average Enlarged Spleen

This is the weighted average spleen size of those subjects with a palpably enlarged spleen in a specified age group of the population sample examined. This index is obtained by multiplying the number of individuals in each arbitrary classification of enlarged spleen by the class number, adding the products, and dividing the total by the number of individuals whose spleen is palpable. For the purpose of splenometry the classification of Hackett (1944), in which spleen size ranges between grade 0 (not enlarged) and grade 5, has become the generally accepted standard.

7. Parasite Rate

The parasite rate is the percentage of persons in a defined age group showing, on a given date, microscopically detectable malaria parasites in the peripheral blood. The parasite rate should always be defined in terms of the age group examined.

8. Parasite Count

This is the number of parasites per microliter of blood on a given slide.

9. Parasite Density

The parasite density, an epidemiological index, is the collective degree of parasitemia in a population, calculated by the use of either the geometric mean or the weighted frequencies of the individual parasite counts; e.g., by using a frequency distribution based on a geometric progression with the factor 2, as employed by Bruce-Chwatt (1958). In the former case the parasite density is expressed as a numerical value, and in the latter as a parasite density index.

10. Parasite Formula

This is a statement of the relative prevalence of each species of human malaria parasite found in a group of positive slides, e.g., the percentage of each species in the total number of infections. When slides show a mixed infection, each species is counted separately.

11. Species Infection Rate

The percentage of individuals found to be infected with any given species of *Plasmodium* is the species infection rate for that species, e.g., the vivax infection rate.

12. Gametocyte Rate

This is the percentage of individuals in a given population whose blood contains sexual forms of malaria parasites.

13. Endemicity

Malaria is endemic in a particular area when there is a constant measurable incidence of natural transmission over a succession of years. Based on the spleen rates of children and adults, endemicity is classified in the following degrees:

Hypoendemic: Spleen rate (children 2–9 years) 0–10%

Mesoendemic: Spleen rate (children 2–9 years) 11–49%

Hyperendemic: Spleen rate (children 2–9 years) constantly over 50%; adult spleen rate also high

Holoendemic: Spleen rate (children 2–9 years) constantly over 75%; adult spleen rate low.

14. Epidemicity

Malaria is epidemic when the incidence of cases in an area rises rapidly and markedly above its usual level or when the infection occurs in an area where it was not present previously.

15. Anopheline Density

The anopheline density is the number of female anophelines in relation to the number of specified shelters or hosts (e.g., per room, per trap, or per person) or to a given time period (e.g., overnight or per hour), specifying the method of collection.

16. Gonotrophic Cycle

This is one complete round of ovarian development in the mosquito, often stated in reference to the period of time required for its completion. Since one blood meal normally suffices for the maturation of one egg batch, except possibly the first, the biting cycle and gonotrophic cycle are usually parallel.

17. Host Preference

This is the preference of a mosquito for a particular type of host, e.g., human or animal, and is to be distinguished from mere readiness to feed on a particular type of host when no other is available.

18. Human Blood Index

The human blood index is the proportion of freshly fed anophelines found to contain human blood. Precipitation tests permit the specific differentiation of human and animal blood, and subgrouping of the latter.

19. Sporozoite Rate

This is the percentage of female anophelines of a given species caught in nature and found, on dissection within 24 hours of capture, to contain sporozoites in the salivary glands.

20. Infection Interval

The infection interval is the period elapsing from the time an individual is infected until this individual becomes infectious to others. In malaria, it starts at the moment of sporozoite inoculation and ends with the appearance of gameto-cytes potentially infective to mosquitoes.

21. Incubation Interval

This is the period elapsing between the occurrence of infective gametocytes in a human subject and their appearance in an infective form in a secondary case deriving from the first case. This period covers the complete life cycle of the parasite.

22. Reproduction Rate

The reproduction rate is the estimated number of malarial infections poten-tially distributed by the average nonimmune infected individual in a community where neither mosquitoes nor persons were previously infected.

F. Classification of Malaria

1. Intensity of Malaria

The frequency of splenomegaly and the degree of spleen enlargement in a community are usually good indicators of its contact with malaria unless there are other diseases which could cause splenomegaly. The higher the spleen rate and the larger the average enlarged spleen, the higher the degree of endemicity and the intensity of transmission of malaria in the area. Continuous intensive contact with the infective agent induces immunity, first marked by tolerance for the infection and later often by a conspicuous absence of malaria parasites from the peripheral blood, usually accompanied by a reduction in or the disappearannce of splenomegaly. The above-mentioned classification of endemicity into hypoen-demic, mesoendemic, hyperendemic, and holoendemic malaria reflects the in-tensity of malaria and its transmission. Attempts to arrive at a system of classification based on methods more reliable than splenometry have failed so far. Routinely available serological methods such as IFAT and passive hemagglutination tests have failed in this respect, although they have proved to be quite useful in the investigation of particular epidemiological situations such as disappearing malaria (Ambroise-Thomas *et al.*, 1976).

2. Stability of Malaria

Stable malaria is found in areas where the degree of malaria transmission is subject to very little change from season to season. It usually prevails where transmission is perennial or extends over a large period of the year and where meteorological conditions vary little over the years, thus supporting the propagation and longevity of vectors and the sporogony of the parasite in an almost regular pattern. Stable malaria is generally associated with higher degrees of endemicity, but it is occasionally found in areas with mesoendemic malaria where epidemic outbreaks show a high regularity. Epidemiologically, stability is most marked in areas with anthropophilic, long-lived vectors and temperatures permitting rapid sporogony. The density of mosquitoes is of lesser importance. *Plasmodium falciparum* is usually the predominant species.

Unstable malaria is characterized by a marked variability in incidence and is most typically found in the marginal areas of malaria distribution. Minor changes in rainfall pattern or quantity, relative humidity, temperature, and in vector deviation from the usual source of its blood meal may provoke profound changes in the epidemiological situation from month to month and from year to year. Under the conditions of unstable malaria, transmission may be absent or very low for one or more years. Unstable malaria is generally associated with *P. vivax,* but in some regions *P. falciparum* is also involved when the appropriate reservoir is available, e.g., in the Sahel zone of tropical Africa. Unstable malaria occurs mostly in areas with relatively short transmission seasons and is marked by sudden and very often intense malaria epidemics. Since the quantum of transmission varies considerably from year to year, there is no building up of immunity in the population and the epidemics maintain their devastating character. Epidemiologically, unstable malaria is most marked in areas with short-lived vectors which bite infrequently on man, and where the environmental temperature is not conducive to rapid sporogony. A high vector density is crucial to malaria transmission under these conditions.

There are innumerable epidemiological conditions between stable and unstable malaria which are termed intermediate stability. The vectors associated with the various degrees of stability and their geographic distribution are shown in Table X (see also Table IX).

G. Quantitative Epidemiology

Attempts to treat epidemiological data mathematically started shortly after discovery of the sporogonic phase in the parasite and it was Sir Ronald Ross (1911) who initiated a quantitative approach in malaria epidemiology. A comprehensive review of the history of mathematical modeling has been given by Bruce-Chwatt (1976), which is recommended to all readers interested in this subject. In the decades following Ross' earlier work, many of the factors directly or indirectly contributing to malaria were further studied and assessed. Based on a wealth of field observations, Macdonald in 1957 published ''The Epidemiology and Control of Malaria,'' which has become the classic of quantitative epidemiology of malaria. The following is a brief description of some of his

TABLE X

Distribution of Vectors Associated with Various Degrees of Stability

Type of malaria	Vector species	Geographic distribution
Stable	A. fluviatilis	Arabian peninsula and southern Asia, Kazakh SSR
	A. funestus	Tropical Africa
	A. gambiae A + B	Tropical Africa and Arabian peninsula
	A. labranchiae	Western Mediterranean
	A. melas	Littoral tropical Africa
	A. minimus minimus	Southeast Asia
	A. sacharovi	Eastern Mediterranean, Italy, Austria, USSR, Iraq, Iran
Intermediate	A. atroparvus	Littoral western Europe
	A. balabacensis balabacensis	Southeast Asia, Philippines
	A. darlingi	Mexico, Central and South America
	A. farauti	Australia, New Guinea, Southwestern Pacific islands
	A. hyrcanus sinensis	Southern Asia, Japan
	A. quadrimaculatus	North America
	A. sergenti	North Africa, western Asia, Pakistan
	A. sundaicus	Southeast Asia
Unstable	A. aconitus	India, Malaysia, Indonesia
	A. albimanus	Southern United States, Mexico, Central America, Antilles
	A. annularis	Southeast Asia, Philippines
	A. aquasalis	Central America, Antilles, Colombia
	A. culicifacies	Arabian peninsula and southern Asia
	A. maculatus	Southern Asia
	A. messeae	Europe
	A. minimus flavirostris	Indonesia, Philippines
	A. pharoensis	Africa, Asia Minor, Arabian peninsula
	A. philippinensis	Southeast Asia
	A. punctulatus	New Guinea, southwestern Pacific islands
	A. stephensi	Southern Asia, Arabian peninsula
	A. superpictus	Eastern Mediterranean, western Asia, Pakistan

concepts, with an emphasis on those factors which have a major impact on the quantum of malaria transmission.

1. Probability of Mosquito Survival

When p is the probability of surviving through 1 day, the probability of surviving through n days (i.e., the number of days required for sporogony) is p^n. The expectation of life, after surviving through n days, is $p^n/-\log_e p$.

2. Inoculation Rate

The mean daily number of bites (h) inflicted on one individual by mosquitoes infected with sporozoites which are actually infective is

$$h = mabs$$

where m denotes anopheline density in relation to man, a the average number of humans bitten by one mosquito in 1 day, b the proportion of anophelines with sporozoites in their glands which are actually infective, and s the proportion of anopheline mosquitoes with sporozoites in their salivary glands. Here a is the product of the proportion of anophelines with human blood and the average number of bites per day.

3. Reproduction Rate and Mathematical Models

While infective $(1/r;$ r, the recovery rate, is usually estimated to be 0.0125, corresponding to an estimated average of 80 days of infectivity in falciparum malaria), a case will be bitten each day by ma mosquitoes. The proportion of mosquitoes not yet infected will be

$$1 - \frac{ax}{ax - \log_e p}$$

where x denotes the proportion of people infective to mosquitoes. The proportion of mosquitoes surviving through n days is p^n, and their subsequent expectation of life is $1/-\log_e p$.

It is assumed that they will bite a human a times each day. A proportion b of these bites will be infective. Thus the reproduction rate z will be

$$z = (1 - \frac{ax}{ax - \log_e p}) \frac{ma^2 bp^n}{-r \log_e p}$$

denoting the number of secondary infections distributed by a primary case. Immunity is apt to influence the values of r and b to a considerable extent. As x approaches zero, as under conditions of very low endemicity and immunity and thus of nearly full susceptibility to infection, the basic reproduction rate z_0 becomes

$$z_0 = ma^2 bp^n / -r \log_e p$$

Thus z_0 is particularly applicable to epidemic situations in areas hitherto free of malaria or subject to a very low endemicity. In these cases it can be assumed that $r = 0.0125$ and $b = 1$. Based on this supposition, examples of basic reproduction rates are given in Table XI which illustrates the relative importance of the various basic parameters.

TABLE XI

Relative Influence of Various Epidemiological Parameters on the Basic Reproduction Rate

Situation	m	a	p	n	$-\log_e p$	z_0	Comments
1	10	0.4	0.90	8	0.105	525	Basis of comparison
2	2	0.4	0.90	8	0.105	105	m reduced to one-fifth
3	10	0.2	0.90	8	0.105	131	a reduced to one-half
4	10	0.4	0.70	8	0.357	21	Daily mortality increased threefold
5	10	0.4	0.90	16	0.105	226	Time required for sporogony doubled
6	2	0.2	0.70	16	0.357	0.0596	Lowest parameters of 2 to 5 combined
7	0.019	0.4	0.90	8	0.105	0.997	Critical m for $z_0 < 1$
8	10	0.0174	0.90	8	0.105	0.993	Critical a for $z_0 < 1$
9	10	0.4	0.51	8	0.673	0.870	Critical p for $z_0 < 1$
10	10	0.4	0.90	55	0.105	3.7	Maximum n still yields $z_0 > 1$
11	0.5	0.4	0.60	8	0.511	0.210	Situation of intervention with insecticides

Situation 1, the basis of comparison, was purposely chosen to yield a high basic reproduction rate. Conditions of this type may exist in formerly hyper- and holoendemic areas free of malaria but with "anophelism without malaria." Here the importation of a fresh malaria case—which remains untreated—will theoretically result in 525 secondary cases; in fact, somewhat fewer, since some persons will receive multiple sporozoite inoculations.

In situation 2, the mosquito density is reduced to one-fifth of its original value. The result is a linear reduction in z_0 to one-fifth of the basic rate.

A decrease in the human biting frequency to one-half of the original value—situation 3—reduces z_0 to one-quarter.

In situation 4, p is reduced from 0.90 to 0.70, i.e., the daily mosquito mortality is increased from 10 to 30% or threefold. The result is a drop in z_0 to $\frac{1}{25}$ of its original value.

Situation 5 shows the influence of prolonging n to double the original value: z_0 is only reduced to slightly less than one-half, since a considerable proportion of mosquitoes survive to day 16 (18.5% at $p = 0.90$ and $-\log_e p = 0.105$).

It is seen that a reduction in m or an increase in n exerts the least impact on the basic reproduction rate, while a reduction in the biting frequency on humans has a more marked influence. However, the increase in daily mortality, i.e., the decrease in longevity, has the most profound impact.

If the lowest parameters in situations 2 to 5 are combined (situation 6), the resulting z_0 is 0.06, which is far below the critical level ($z_0 = 1$) required for maintaining the infection in the community.

Examples 7–9 show the critical levels of m, a, and p required—in conjunction with the other standard parameters of the basic example of situation 1—in order to reduce the basic reproduction rate below 1, i.e., to a level at which the malaria will gradually, if slowly, disappear. Mosquito density would have to be reduced to less than $1/500$ and the biting frequency to less than $1/20$ of the original value, while a fivefold increase in daily mortality would achieve the same result.

Situation 10 shows that a prolongation of n, the time required for sporogony, even to its natural upper limit, does not reduce z_0 to less than 1.

Situation 11 finally shows a typical case of intervention by residual insecticides, where the daily mortality is assumed to be 40% ($p = 0.60$; $-\log_e p = 0.511$) and the mosquito density is reduced to 0.5, while the values of a and n, as in nature, are not subject to change. Here the basic reproduction rate is reduced to $z_0 = 0.210$, a level conducive to the gradual disappearance of malaria.

The basic reproduction rate has been modified to reflect also conditions of high endemicity and of equilibrium as found with stable malaria (Macdonald, 1957, 1973).

For areas with stable malaria—marked by an absence of epidemics and relatively low clinical morbidity from malaria among adolescents and adults, as well as high immunity—the reproduction rate is best expressed as the net reproduction rate (Macdonald, 1957):

$$p^n/(p^n - s)$$

The index of stability (Macdonald et al., 1973) may be calculated according to the following formula:

$$a/-\log_e p$$

The higher the frequency of biting humans, the higher the stability index. Conversely, a high $-\log_e p$, as under conditions of high daily mosquito mortality, lowers the stability index. Values of the stability index can be classified as follows: values below 0.5 indicate instability; values of 0.5–2.5 indicate intermediate stability; and values of more than 2.5 indicate stability.

The factors used for calculation of the stability index are dependent on the biting habits of the mosquito (a) and mosquito longevity $(-\log_2 p)$; this largely explains the generally marked association of particular mosquito species with specific degrees of malaria stability (see Table X).

Macdonald's approach has been applied in the field for the evaluation of epidemiological data under natural conditions and after antimalarial intervention (Wernsdorfer and Wernsdorfer, 1967; Garret-Jones and Shidrawi, 1969; Sivagnanasundaram, 1973; Pull, 1976). It has also led to the development of mathematical models able to make predictions regarding the impact of various modes of intervention. One such model was applied in a field study in northern Nigeria (Najera, 1974). The observed results were at considerable variance with the predictions of the model. These discrepancies were particularly ascribed to deficiencies of the model, to an overestimation of the effect of intervention measures in the planning of the simulation, and to imperfections in spraying coverage.

A very practical epidemiological model for evaluating the malaria inoculation rate and the risk of infections in infants has been described by Pull and Grab (1974), based on a differential equation which reflects the acquisition of the disease in time by a cohort of newborn infants:

$$dy/dt = h(1-y)$$

where y is the fraction of the infant population with proved parasitemia, h the force of infection in terms of effective contacts per unit of time and susceptible infant, and t the age. Under the initial conditions ($y = 0$ and $t = 0$) the equation becomes

$$y = 1 - \exp(-ht)$$

In applying this approach to an epidemiological study in East Africa, Pull and Grab (1974) noted satisfactory agreement between the actual and the expected curves of disease acquisition, concluding that this model could be used for simulating epidemiological processes.

A new mathematical model has been developed by Dietz et al. (1974) and applied to data collected in a field research project in the African savanna in Kano State, Nigeria. This model permits also quantitation of the influence of immunity and a description of its three major aspects, namely, loss of infectivity, loss of detectability, and increase in recovery rate. Immunity was found to increase the rate of recovery from patent parasitemia by a factor of up to 10 (Bekessy et al., 1976) and to reduce the number of episodes of patent parasitemia resulting from one inoculation. Further evaluation of the new model showed relatively good agreement of the observed data with those predicted by the model. Molineaux et al. (1978) therefore consider it epidemiologically satisfactory and fit for use in planning malaria control operations.

During the past decades malaria epidemiological models have certainly made considerable progress. However, in regard to their predictive value in decision making for intervention measures some caution is still indicated. Bruce-Chwatt (1976) rightly pointed out that the specific local conditions of host–parasite relationships and epidemiological equilibrium and thus the requirements of control are subject to a very wide variation which may not lend itself to expression in generally applicable models.

V. MALARIA IN THE WORLD

In this chapter the malaria situation is described as it presented itself from the midnineteenth century up to 1979. An account is given of the methods of malaria control and of the impact of intensified antimalarial measures in recent decades. More detail on the malaria situation prior to World War II can be found in Boyd's Malariology (1949). The material presented in Sections V, B–F is largely based on reports of the WHO Expert Committee on Malaria (1957, 1961, 1968b, 1974c; 1979b), epidemiological information on the status of malaria eradication (1962, 1966a, 1973a), information on the world malaria situation (1975a,c, 1977a, 1979a), WHO reviews on malaria eradication (1965, 1966b, 1967a, 1967b, 1968a, 1969a,b; 1970a,b; 1971a,b; 1972a,b, 1973a,b) and on the malaria situation (1974b, 1975b; 1977a,b; Noguer et al., 1976, 1978), and on personal unpublished reports.

A. Malaria Prior to the Advent of Residual Insecticides

It is believed that malaria underwent its last major expansion during the two centuries following the arrival of the conquistadores in America. After that the geographic distribution seems to have remained largely unchanged until the second half of the nineteenth century (Fig. 5). Practically all malarious areas are situated within the 16°C summer isotherms, whether these isotherms are determined by latitude or, especially in the case of the subtropics and tropics, by altitude. However, not all areas within the 16°C summer isotherms were affected, e.g., large parts of North America, Siberia, central Asia, and Australia. In most of these areas the absence or the particular bionomics of anophelines, the very short duration of the warm season, or geotopographic and meteorological conditions were and still are obviously not favorable for malaria transmission. Such conditions prevail in or near deserts in the regions close to the 16°C summer isotherm.

Apart from a few microclimatical exceptions, e.g., high-altitude conditions in the tropics, falciparum malaria was confined to areas with the 20°C summer isotherms, while in the malarious zones between the 16° and 20°C summer isotherms P. vivax was the prevailing species. Only occasionally was P. malariae found in these zones.

In the midnineteenth century malaria was endemic in large parts of the eastern United States, in the southeastern frontier region of Canada, and also on the Pacific seaboard of North America, from Vancouver to California. The malarious areas in the eastern United States were also contiguous with those in Central America. All continental territories on the Gulf of Mexico and the Caribbean Sea, and the majority of the Caribbean islands, were malarious. In South America, except for the high-altitude areas, malaria was endemic in most areas north of 32°S. In Europe malaria affected all countries on the Mediterranean Sea, Portugal, Atlantic coastal areas of France, the southeast of England, the North Sea coast of the Netherlands, Germany, and Denmark, most of the areas around the Baltic Sea, and wide areas of eastern Europe, especially in the Balkans and in

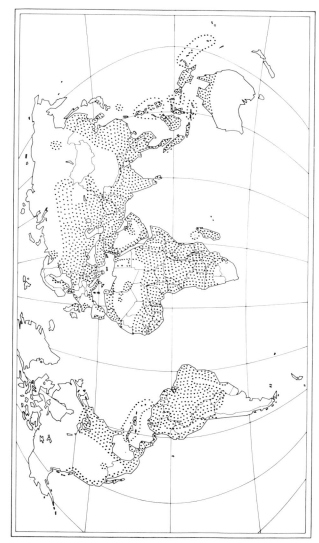

FIG. 5. Geographic distribution of malaria in the midninteenth century (malarious areas dotted).

Russia west of the Ural range. Malaria reached its northernmost distribution in the area of Archangelsk, at 64°N, near the Arctic Circle.

Practically all the countries of Asia Minor, the Arabian peninsula, and southern Asia were malarious except for areas where desert or high altitude did not permit transmission of the disease. In northern Asia extensive endemic areas existed in northern and eastern Siberia, while China, Korea, and parts of Japan were also affected. Practically all islands between the Indian and the Pacific oceans, the northern coastal areas of Australia, and the Pacific islands between the equator and 20°S, west of 170°E, were malarious.

Except for the deserts in northern and southern areas and in high-altitude regions, malaria was universally present in Africa; Madagascar was equally affected. However, the islands of Mauritius and La Réunion were free of malaria until 1867 when *A. gambiae* was introduced from Madagascar (Hackett, 1949).

It was in these areas of tropical Africa where *A. gambiae* and *A. funestus* were the main vectors and *P. falciparum* the prevalent parasite species that malaria assumed the most stable form and the highest degree of endemicity. *Plasmodium falciparum* dominated also in the tropical zones of the Americas and of southern Asia.

In spite of the seasonality of transmission, malaria was remarkably stable in some areas of southern and southeastern Asia, where *A. fluviatilis* and *A. minimus minimus* were the vectors, attaining also relatively high degrees of endemicity. In the subtropical zones of the Americas, of Asia, and around the Mediterranean, malaria was transmitted seasonally, with *P. vivax* appearing first after the start of the transmission season, followed by *P. falciparum* later in the season. This differential onset is explained by the ability of *P. vivax* to produce gametocytemia when conditions become favorable for transmission, by a relatively large gametocyte reservoir, by a lower critical temperature for sporogony, and by a relatively short incubation interval. *Plasmodium falciparum*, because of its short life span, starts usually with a low parasite reservoir, requires higher temperatures for sporogony, and has a longer incubation interval. Therefore transmission is built up more slowly. The relative predominance of *P. falciparum* in the late season may be explained by its suppression of *P. vivax* in the peripheral blood, a phenomenon similar to the relationship between *P. malariae* and *P. falciparum* in tropical Africa, where the former rises significantly during seasons of low or no transmission.

In the temperate zones malaria transmission was strictly seasonal and *P. vivax* was the prevailing or, in many areas, the only species. Conditions in these zones were usually typical of unstable malaria, and epidemics against a background of low endemicity—and therefore low immunity—determined the character of the disease.

At the end of the nineteenth century and before World War I, changing patterns of land use and animal husbandry led to a natural disappearance of malaria from areas where it was quite unstable and on the fringe of its distribution, e.g., large areas of the United States and western Europe, and the northern Baltic region.

Apart from a few areas where mainly environmental measures had brought about a reduction in malaria, the disease was able to maintain its distribution largely unchanged until after the end of World War II.

B. Social and Economic Impact of Malaria

Except in epidemics and apart from being a major cause of infant mortality in highly endemic areas of falciparum malaria, the disease is insidious rather than dramatic. Malaria causes mainly chronic suffering, results in an increased number of deaths from other causes, and lowers life expectancy (World Health Organization, 1955b). Over the centuries it has had a profound impact in curbing economic activities and social progress in the populations of vast areas throughout the world. Each year, especially in rural communities, malaria is responsible for the death of over 1 million infants and young children in tropical Africa. In the years before the introduction of intensive antimalaria operations in the second half of the twentieth century, the annual labor losses due to malaria were estimated to be 10 million workdays in Thailand and 171 million workdays in the agricultural population of India. Wide areas of arable land in Afghanistan, India, and Sri Lanka were not being cultivated, since settlers would have been exposed to a high malaria risk (World Health Organization, 1954). In the early 1950s a malaria epidemic in the Gezira irrigated area of the Sudan temporarily disabled a large part of the labor force with the result that over one-third of the cotton crop could not be harvested. This inflicted not only heavy losses on daily individual earnings, but also the government budget, which was heavily dependent on the proceeds of cotton exportation, suffered a severe reduction. At that time about $\frac{1}{100}$ of the amount of revenue lost would have been adequate to carry out effective malaria control.

Expansion of agriculture and rapid industrialization, the associated population movements, and unsuitable housing conditions expose the labor force in many tropical countries increasingly to the risk of contracting parasitic diseases (Wernsdorfer and Wernsdorfer, 1973), a trend which is aggravated by the urbanization of malaria in Africa and Asia.

Data available from India, Indonesia, the Philippines, and Colombia indicate that the cost of intensive antimalaria operations commensurate with the standards of a malaria eradication program represents approximately one-seventh to one-ninth of the cost of economic losses inflicted by the disease. In a particular agricultural area in tropical Africa it is estimated that the inhabitants spend every year, on average, the equivalent of US$8 per capita for individual antimalaria treatment, while effective prevention through appropriate malaria control measures would cost about US$2 per capita.

Nevertheless, many governments are reluctant to invest in malaria control since the immediate benefits accrue in the private sector, initially without directly visible returns to the government treasury.

Construction of the Panama Canal provides an example of the vital role of disease control, including that of malaria, in a tropical labor force, an experience which has been recently repeated at many a tropical dam or canal construction site.

Past experience shows that the success of a malaria eradication program depends on a minimum level of socioeconomic development in the country concerned. In areas with a socioeconomic status below this critical level it is necessary to take measures conducive to a general reduction in the prevalence of malaria and other endemic diseases, which in turn would lead to amelioration of the socioeconomic situation to the degree required for implementing malaria eradication.

Many governments in tropical Africa are financially not in a position to apply even a modest countrywide general disease control program (World Health Organization, 1974a). Thus it is hardly conceivable that major steps toward malaria control could be taken in this area unless a massive international drive were implemented with new control approaches, since the existing tools are clearly inadequate for such a task.

The reduction in mortality and morbidity as a result of large-scale malaria control may lead to population pressure in areas with a high reproductive potential. The number of malaria deaths prevented by control measures over the past decade is estimated to be about 50 million (Bruce-Chwatt, 1977). It will be up to health administrators and human ecologists to plan and to implement programs, with the collaboration of all strata of society, leading to a reduction in population growth to a level conducive to economic growth and social progress.

C. Methods of Malaria Control

Interruption of the chain of transmission of infected man–vector–susceptible man can theoretically be effected at any stage, whether by curing the infected human, by vector control, by protecting the susceptible man or by interrupting contact between the vector and man. The vector may be controlled by preventing breeding, by destruction of the aquatic stages, or by killing the adult forms.

1. Measures for Blocking Man–Vector Contact

These are known to be the least reliable means of malaria control since they require considerable motivation, perseverance, and financial means for their effective use. Contact can be blocked by the screening of doors, windows, and other openings of human habitations and by the use of mosquito nets, provided that man stays confined to the screened environment for the whole duration of the vector's biting activity, i.e., usually from sundown to sunrise. Outside the screened habitations some protection may be obtained from wearing apparel which leaves little skin uncovered and from using mosquito repellents, mostly containing N,N-diethyltoluamide, on uncovered body surfaces. The latter has certain disadvantages. For example, depending on climatic conditions, body surface temperature, and sweating, the protection of the repellent coat may wear off within a relatively short time, requiring a new application.

2. Vector Control

Removal of the breeding places of mosquitoes is the most effective method of malaria control where mosquito breeding is confined to water collections amenable to this type of measure, e.g., swamps, marshes, rain pools, the backwaters of rivers, seepage pools, and borrow pits. The required measures range from major engineering projects for drainage, leveling, and dredging to a simple operation such as filling. However, breeding place abatement may not be acceptable to a government or a population for environmental or economic reasons, since it changes the hydrological conditions and could modify the climatic pattern or be incompatible with the raising of customary crops.

Mosquito breeding may also be prevented by barring the access of mosquitoes to breeding places when the latter are very limited in number and suitable for screening and covering, e.g., in areas with exclusively well- or cistern-breeding anophelines.

Usually the breeding surfaces are larger. If they are not too extensive, larviciding, which has a long tradition especially in urban and periurban mosquito control, may be useful. Initially light hydrocarbons were used for this purpose. These spread easily but evaporate fast, necessitating frequent applications. The introduction of spreading agents, e.g., Triton X100, permitted the use of medium-heavy hydrocarbons which are less susceptible to evaporation. Many chemical larvicides have been used. Paris green, a selective poison for surface-feeding larvae—*Anopheles* but not *Culex* and *Aedes*—is a classic example, but its use has been discontinued. Shortly after World War II larvicidal oils were formulated with insecticides, especially dieldrin and DDT. The use of such formulations has been discouraged, since there is evidence that they exert considerable selective pressure on mosquito populations and thus accelerate the development of insecticide resistance. Abate, o,o,o',o'-tetramethyl-o,o'-thiodi-p-phenylene phosphorothioate, an organophosphorus compound (Temephos), is the only insecticide now widely used in larviciding. Operationally, it is easier to handle than larviciding oil which it has replaced in many areas. Larviciding as a malaria control measure is not effective if the breeding surfaces are too extensive, as for instance during rainy seasons in flat areas with impermeable surface soil.

Larvivorous fish, e.g., *Gambusia, Nothobranchus,* and *Tilapia* spp., may be used where breeding places are stable.

In irrigated areas larval control may be practiced through water management, usually in the form of alternating irrigation. In such schemes water is supplied at weekly or fortnightly intervals and allowed to dry up within a few days. Thus mosquitoes cannot complete the aquatic stages of development. The applicability of water management depends on the specific crop type. Cotton and many cereals do not need continuous irrigation, in contrast with some types of rice.

Imagociding became possible after the introduction of pyrethrum extracts. These are still widely used in the form of household sprays, some of which also contain a pyrethrin synergist. These sprays exert a shortlasting "knockdown" insecticidal effect.

The major breakthrough in malaria control came with the development of residual insecticides; DDT, the first residual insecticide, is still most widely used in malaria control. Its residual action extends up to 6 months. Among the other chlorinated hydrocarbons only BHC is still used in public health operations. The use of dieldrin in public health has been practically discontinued for reasons of mammalian toxicity. Chlorinated hydrocarbons are the insecticides of choice as long as vector resistance does not necessitate the use of alternatives such as organophosphorus compounds [e.g., malathion (diethyl mercaptosuccinate S-ester with O,O-dimethyl phosphorodithioate)] or carbamates [e.g., propoxur (O-isopropoxyphenyl methylcarbamate)]. The latter are more expensive than DDT, and their residual effect does not last as long, necessitating application at shorter intervals.

Residual insecticides are applied in the form of indoor sprays on walls and ceilings, using suspensions made up from water-dispersible powder formulations or water emulsions prepared from emulsion concentrates. After feeding, and while resting on sprayed surfaces, mosquitoes pick up insecticide particles and are poisoned by a neurotoxic effect. Incipient resistance is marked by a lower mortality of exposed mosquitoes, and the transience of the neurotoxic symptoms. Indoor spraying with residual insecticides is of little use in the control of exophilic mosquitoes, e.g., *Anopheles balabacensis balabacensis.* Insecticides may also induce mosquitoes to avoid sprayed surfaces, a phenomenon termed behavioristic avoidance.

3. Treatment of Malaria Cases

Malaria transmission may be reduced or even interrupted through the treatment of malaria cases, i.e., reduction or elimination of the parasite reservoir. Treatment with a 4-aminoquinoline such as chloroquine or amodiaquin, is effective against the asexual blood forms of *P. vivax, P. ovale, P. malariae,* and—where the parasites are not resistant—*P. falciparum.* 4-Aminoquinoline-resistant *P. falciparum* usually responds to a combination of sulfadoxine and pyrimethamine. Radical cure of *P. vivax* and *P. ovale* infections requires the use of primaquine, an 8-aminoquinoline, for elimination of remaining tissue forms and thus the prevention of relapses. The gametocytes of *P. falciparum* normally survive treatment with blood schizontocidal drugs, and the infectivity of the case to mosquitoes is maintained until the viability of the available gametocytes has come to a natural end. Thus, rapid sterilization of the infection and the prevention of transmission by administration of a gametocytocidal compound, e.g., primaquine, is advisable for the radical treatment of *P. falciparum* infections.

Radical treatment is indicated in all areas where the complete interruption of malaria transmission is intended and feasible, and in all malaria patients residing in nonmalarious areas (imported cases) or zones of low malaria endemicity. There is little point in giving radical treatment to patients residing in holo- or hyperendemic areas with stable malaria, since reinfection will occur within a short time. Here a single-dose treatment with a blood schizontocidal drug is usually sufficient for effectively suppressing the clinical symptoms without unduly interfering with the patient's immune response.

An up-to-date review of practical malaria chemotherapy is given by Bruce-Chwatt *et al.* (1980).

4. Drug Prophylaxis

In the absence of a causal prophylactic drug, blood schizontocidal compounds are used for the prevention of clinical malaria attacks. The most widely used are 4-aminoquinolines (chloroquine and amodiaquin) which have the largest prophylactic range. In areas with 4-aminoquinoline-resistant *P. falciparum* a combination of sulfadoxine and pyrimethamine may be used, but this will not fully suppress vivax malaria if local *P. vivax* is resistant to pyrimethamine.

Regular prophylactic administration of the available antimalarials does not exclude infection with plasmodia; it only prevents the blood forms from developing. If prophylaxis is continued for 6 weeks after leaving the malarious area, the probability is very high that infections with *P. falciparum* and *P. malariae* will be cured; however, infections with *P. vivax* and *P. ovale* may be reactivated from latent tissue forms even if prophylaxis is taken for 6 weeks after last exposure.

Mass drug prophylaxis of malaria, as a control measure, is very difficult and expensive to apply. It requires a highly organized system of regular drug distribution in order to achieve the essential coverage in space and time; the less concentrated and the more mobile the population, the less effective and the more difficult drug prophylaxis will be. However, drug prophylaxis is useful for the protection of well-organized and continuously or regularly accessible groups under special risk, e.g., armed forces, police forces, mining labor, and labor in construction camps. Information on malaria risk for international travelers and recommendations for individual malaria prophylaxis has been provided by the World Health Organization (1978a).

D. Intensive Antimalaria Operations after World War II

Recognizing the important role of malaria as a detriment to socioeconomic development, many organizations undertook intensive efforts toward control of the disease soon after the World War II. From 1948, the World Health Organization was largely involved in the international coordination of antimalaria operations. These were first oriented toward control of the disease, but in the early 1950s malaria eradication became the avowed goal in numerous countries. The Eighth World Health Assembly (1955a) decided on a policy of malaria eradication for all malarious countries with the exception of tropical continental Africa and of Madagascar, where malaria control was to remain the objective until such time as suitable and economically feasible methods would be available for complete elimination of the disease. During the following years most of the malarious countries outside tropical Africa conducted antimalaria programs which led to eradication of the disease from large areas of the world and to a considerable reduction in mortality and morbidity from it in others, accompanied by a highly significant drop in prevalence. UNICEF, UNDP, USAID, and WHO joined in the support given to antimalaria programs in many countries whose financial resources were inadequate for the task. USAID and WHO also provided technical support and promoted the building up of well-qualified personnel in the malarious countries.

Many countries have discovered that the goal of malaria eradication was not as easy to reach as anticipated. Delayed financial allocations and imperfections in technical and organizational structures resulted in epidemiological repercussions. In addition, technical obstacles such as vector resistance to insecticides and drug resistance of parasites developed, while the importance of others—which had existed before—e.g., exophilic behavior and population movements, was increasingly recognized.

The confrontation with these problems, the phasing out of UNICEF assistance, and the significant reduction in USAID and UNDP support, has discouraged many a government and slackened antimalaria operations to a point that malaria was allowed to reconquer large areas in southern Asia. Faced with these serious developments the World Health Organization (1978b) has oriented its strategy to achieve the following goals (1) reduction of malaria mortality to negligible levels, (2) alleviation of the effects of the disease on socioeconomic development, and (3) ultimate eradication of malaria whenever feasible.

This policy includes all malarious countries of the world. Some are in a position to continue the pursuit of eradication, while in most of tropical African countries the present technical and organizational means might just suffice for meeting goal 1.

It is estimated that governments, international organizations, and bilateral agencies have spent about US$2000 million on the fight against malaria between the years 1955 and 1976. A respectable sum, but quite modest if compared to the individual health-related budgets of the major industrialized nations, and minimal if compared to military expenditure, e.g., $33,448 million for health and $89,996 million for defense in the United States of America in 1976.

1. Concept of Malaria Control

Malaria control is the reduction of malaria to a level at which the disease ceases to be a major public health problem. It can be achieved through the rational use of various antimalaria measures adapted to local epidemiological conditions. Malaria control may also be applied to specific population groups or to selected areas. Thus it is quite flexible. While it is essential for planning purposes to determine realistically the feasible target level of malaria control in terms of maximum acceptable malaria mortality, morbidity, and/or prevalence, slight imperfections in application of the control measures rarely result in failure to reach the target. However, since malaria control does not eliminate the parasite reservoir, malaria transmission may be expected to build up again in the absence of suitable measures. Malaria control therefore requires a continuous effort.

2. Concept of Malaria Eradication

Malaria eradication is the "ending of the transmission of malaria and the elimination of the reservoir of infective cases in a campaign limited in time and carried to such a degree of perfection that, when it comes to an end, there is no resumption of transmission" (World Health Organization, 1957).

The strictly limited life span of *P. falciparum, P. vivax,* and *P. ovale* in humans indicates that the eradication of these species could be achieved if transmission could be interrupted during the period required for the natural disappearance of the parasites. Operationally, this theory has proved correct in many areas where essential antimalaria measures were sufficiently effective and applied with the required precision and intensity.

In order to achieve the necessary epidemiological and operational coverage in space and time malaria eradication programs are usually structured in four major phases.

a. Preparatory Phase. This requires the building up of an organizational infrastructure, including training, establishment of physical facilities for running the operations, geographic reconnaissance and census, and baseline assessment of entomological and epidemiological parameters.

b. Attack Phase.   This involves the application of attack measures on the basis of full coverage in space and time (in order to interrupt malaria transmission), the evaluation of the impact of attack measures, and the building up of epidemiological surveillance. Usually the attack measures are directed against the vector. Residual insecticides may be used for the reduction of mosquito longevity and density in areas where endophilic susceptible vectors occur. Antilarval measures may be used in areas with exophilic or insecticide-resistant vectors. The latter reduce density but not mosquito longevity. Single-round mass drug administration may be given in the beginning in order to achieve an initial drastic reduction in the parasite reservoir.

c. Consolidation Phase.   When the malaria incidence is reduced to a very low level, usually to less than 0.1 per 1000 per year, and the surveillance mechanism is functioning adequately, general attack operations may be terminated. Surveillance continues on a full-coverage basis with the following activities (1) active and passive case detection through house-to-house visits and curative health services; (2) blood sampling from all fever cases; (3) presumptive treatment, by single-dose therapy, of all fever cases; (4) radical treatment of confirmed cases; (5) epidemiological investigation of confirmed cases (to be classified as indigenous, introduced, imported, relapse, or induced) and of the communities where the infection was contracted and detected (the focus to be classified as old or new and active or inactive); (6) remedial measures, e.g., resumption of attack measures, mass radical treatment; and (7) epidemiological follow-up of cases and foci.

d. Maintenance Phase.   The consolidation phase may be terminated when no autochthonous transmission has occurred in the whole area of operations for a minimum of three continuous years and if the quality and coverage of surveillance comply with the standard criteria. Then surveillance must be replaced by vigilance, the intensity of which will depend on the degree of receptivity, i.e., the risk of resumed transmission after the importation of cases, and of vulnerability, i.e., the exposure to the importation of cases. Vigilance usually consists of measures for the detection and prompt treatment of imported infections, of monitoring and, if so indicated, of lowering the receptivity of previously malarious areas.

Unlike control, malaria eradication must essentially cover the whole population of a malarious area within the geographic boundaries of the disease. In many cases this will be a whole country or even a group of countries.

3. Development of the Antimalaria Program

At the beginning of 1950 about 143 of the 209 countries and territories on record were malarious. The population of malarious areas accounted for 64.1% of the total.

In the following years malaria eradication and control operations were undertaken in all malarious countries of the Americas and Europe and in the majority of countries and territories in Asia, Australia, the Pacific islands, North Africa, Mauritius, and La Réunion. The global development of these operations is illustrated in Fig. 6. Between 1957 and 1972 the population of malarious areas was increasingly brought under protection from malaria risk. By 1972 about 40.5% of the population originally under risk lived in areas which were freed from the disease. The percentage dropped to 22.2% in 1978, since large areas of India were reinvaded by malaria. This development is also reflected in a worldwide relative increase in autochthonous malaria cases between 1972 and 1976. All regions except the eastern Mediterranean recorded increasing malaria incidence, which was most marked in Southeast Asia where the 1976 incidence was almost $3\frac{1}{2}$ times as high as that observed in 1972 (Fig. 7).

The proportion of population living in areas without specific antimalaria measures, mostly in tropical Africa, has remained largely unchanged since 1972.

In spite of the gloomy picture projected by the above data it must be recognized that in the countries which have attempted, but not yet achieved eradication, mortality and morbidity from malaria, as well as its prevalence, have been generally reduced to a small fraction of what they were prior to the start of operations. In Central America the annual number of deaths from malaria dropped from over 40,000 in the late 1940s to less than 400 in 1978. Similar reduc-

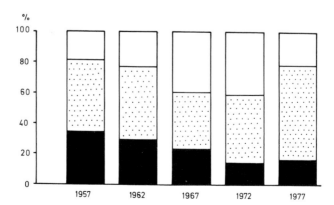

FIG. 6. Status of the antimalaria program, 1957–1977, based on the total world population under malaria risk in 1960 (excluding China). Open area, population in areas freed from malaria; dotted area, population under malaria risk, protected; shaded area, population under malaria risk, not protected.

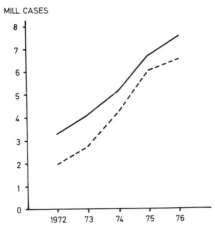

FIG. 7. Number of autochthonous malaria cases in areas under surveillance outside tropical Africa (solid line) and in Southeast Asia (broken line), 1972–1976.

tions were reported from large parts of South America and Asia. Even in India, where malaria reached a new peak incidence of nearly 7 million cases in 1976, i.e., roughly $\frac{1}{20}$ of what it was preoperationally, the number of deaths from malaria recorded in 1976 was only 37.

From Table XII it can be seen that 37 (26%) of the 142 originally malarious countries have achieved and maintained malaria eradication. Most of these are in Europe and in the Americas. Australia has become malaria-free, Europe as well, apart from a few small foci in Greece and European continental Turkey. A

TABLE XII

Status of Malaria Eradication in the World (1978)[a]

Status	Africa	America	Asia	Europe	Australia and Oceania	Total
No. of countries and territories	54	49	45	38	23	209
No. of nonmalarious countries (1950)	5	16	4	21	20	66
No. of malarious countries (1950)	49	33	41	17	3	143
No. of countries freed from malaria	2	12	6	15	1	37
No. of countries still malarious (1978)	47	21	35	2	2	106

[a] Countries that eradicated malaria between 1950 and 1978: Africa: Mauritius and La Réunion; America: Chile, Cuba, Dominica, Grenada and Carriacou, Guadeloupe, Jamaica, Martinique, Puerto Rico, St. Lucia, Trinidad and Tobago, United States of America, U.S. Virgin Islands; Asia: Brunei, Lebanon, Taiwan, Hong Kong, Japan, Israel, Macao; Europe: Albania, Bulgaria, Byelorussian SSR, Czechoslovakia, Cyprus, France, Hungary, Italy, Netherlands, Poland, Portugal, Romania, Spain, Ukrainian SSR, Yugoslavia; Australia and Oceania: Australia.

comparison of Figs. 5 and 9 (see later) shows that malaria has receded mainly from the temperate zones and some subtropical areas where it was relatively unstable, while it has maintained its presence in the tropics—in the Americas and in Asia generally at greatly reduced levels.

4. Constraints of Antimalaria Operations

Malaria has been eliminated from numerous countries in the temperate zones and in the subtropics where the disease was relatively unstable and not very deeply entrenched. Vector control measures, case treatment, and surveillance were very well within the means of the countries concerned and were applied with a high degree of precision.

In some countries, financial, administrative, political, and operational difficulties have impeded the proper running of antimalaria programs, although the available technical methodology would have permitted the complete interruption of malaria transmission. In others again, e.g., in tropical Africa, none of the available, financially and logistically feasible technologies is adequate to produce a complete interruption of malaria transmission or even a major reduction in malaria prevalence, since environment, vector, and parasite show a high degree of harmony not seen elsewhere.

In addition to these basic obstacles, a number of technical problems developed, which were either preexisting but appreciated only after a significant reduction in malaria or associated with the unduly prolonged application of antimalaria measures.

First, the resistance of anophelines, especially to chlorinated hydrocarbons, is already widespread in the majority of main vector species. There may be several explanations for this, but there is evidence that the agricultural use of insecticides has contributed significantly to the occurrence of this resistance. Multiresistance of malaria vectors also occurs but is still quite rare, although of great epidemiological importance where it is present. Nevertheless, vector resistance is not a universal phenomenon, and residual indoor spraying is still effective in many parts of the world.

Second, exophilic behavior of malaria vectors is also an obstacle to intensive malaria control, especially in areas where mosquito breeding is widespread. Under these circumstances house spraying with residual insecticides is quite useless, and other vector control methods may hardly be feasible.

Third, parasite resistance to antimalaria drugs is seriously impeding malaria control operations in parts of southeastern Asia and South America where *P. falciparum* is resistant to 4-aminoquinolines (see Fig. 8). There are strong indications that chloroquine-resistant *P. falciparum* infections occur also in Kenya and Tanzania. Again, in several areas affected by resistance, the latter is still comparatively infrequent and of a rather low degree, so that 4-aminoquinolines may still be clinically useful but of rather limited use as malaria control tools.

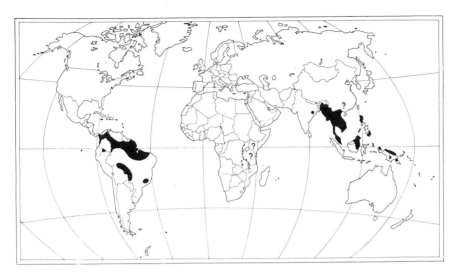

FIG. 8. Geographic distribution of 4-aminoquinoline-resistant *P. (Laverania) falciparum.* Areas with resistant *P. falciparum* are shaded.

Factors related to human ecology, especially population movements and outdoor sleeping, may jeopardize the success of antimalaria operations. Other obstacles to malaria control include the temporary, often seasonal inaccessibility of population groups, the inadequate development of the health service infrastructure, and the rising cost of insecticides, larvicides, drugs, motor vehicle operation, and materials required for the running of the operations, which has outrun the financial capabilities of some governments.

E. Present Malaria Situation in the World

At the beginning of 1979 about 2128 million persons were living in originally malarious areas of the world, representing 65% of the total world population of 3287 million not including China. Table XIII shows that over 80% of the population of Africa and Asia and a significant proportion of Americans and Europeans were orginally exposed to malaria risk, while Australia and Oceania were largely free of the disease. Eradication operations have eliminated malaria from large parts of the Americas and from Australia, and almost completely from Europe and the Asian part of the USSR. In contrast, only a very small fraction of African and Asian countries has become malaria-free. In the areas still under malaria risk all populations are protected in Europe and the Asian parts of the USSR, and well over 90% in America, Asia, and Oceania, but only 10% in tropical Africa south of the Sahara which remains the world's epicenter of malaria. The distribution of malaria in the world is shown in Fig. 9.

TABLE XIII

Status of Antimalaria Operations (Mid-1978)[a]

Population	Africa	America	Asia[b]	Australia and Oceania	Europe[c]	Total
Total	437.00	586.21	1458.13	19.18	786.22	3286.74
Areas where malaria was never indigenous	62.05	366.13	252.50	18.40	459.94	1159.02
Percentage of total	14.2	62.5	17.3	95.9	58.5	35.26
Originally malarious areas	374.95	220.08	1205.63	0.78	326.28	2127.72
Percentage of total	85.8	37.5	82.7	4.1	41.5	64.74
Areas freed from malaria	9.37	106.82	71.38	0.48	283.71	471.76
Percentage of population originally at risk	2.5	48.54	5.9	61.6	87.0	22.17
Areas still at risk	365.58	113.26	1134.25	0.30	42.57	1655.96
Percentage of population originally at risk	97.5	51.46	94.1	38.4	13.0	77.83
Protected areas	95.14	98.06	1048.84	0.30	42.57	1284.91
Percentage of population still at risk	26.6	86.6	92.5	100.0	100.0	77.6
Non-protected areas	270.44	15.20	85.41	—	—	371.05
Percentage of population still at risk	73.4	13.4	7.5	0	0	22.4

[a] Population figures in millions.

[b] Including European continental Turkey, but excluding China and Taiwan (no recent data available).

[c] Including the Asian part of the U.S.S.R.

1. Africa

Parts of northern and southern Africa were naturally nonmalarious, whereas some—e.g., parts of Libya and the Republic of South Africa—have become malaria-free as a result of eradication operations. Malaria has been reduced to a very low incidence in most of the North African countries. Morocco, Algeria, Tunisia, and Libya are in far advanced stages of malaria eradication; local transmission of *P. falicparum* has been practically interrupted, and as a result *P. vivax* remains the prevailing species. In Egypt the average parasite prevalence recently fluctuated around 0.1%, almost exclusively *P. vivax*.

In the Republic of South Africa only 5.0% of the population are still under malaria risk. In these areas the parasite rate was 1.7% in 1977, with *P. falciparum* as the prevailing species.

All countries of tropical continental Africa, as well as Madagascar, are malarious. The parasite rate in children exceeds 50% in most areas, with *P. falciparum* representing between 80 and 99% of the parasite formula, followed by *P. malariae* (1–36%) and, especially in West Africa, *P. ovale* (0–11%). The geo-

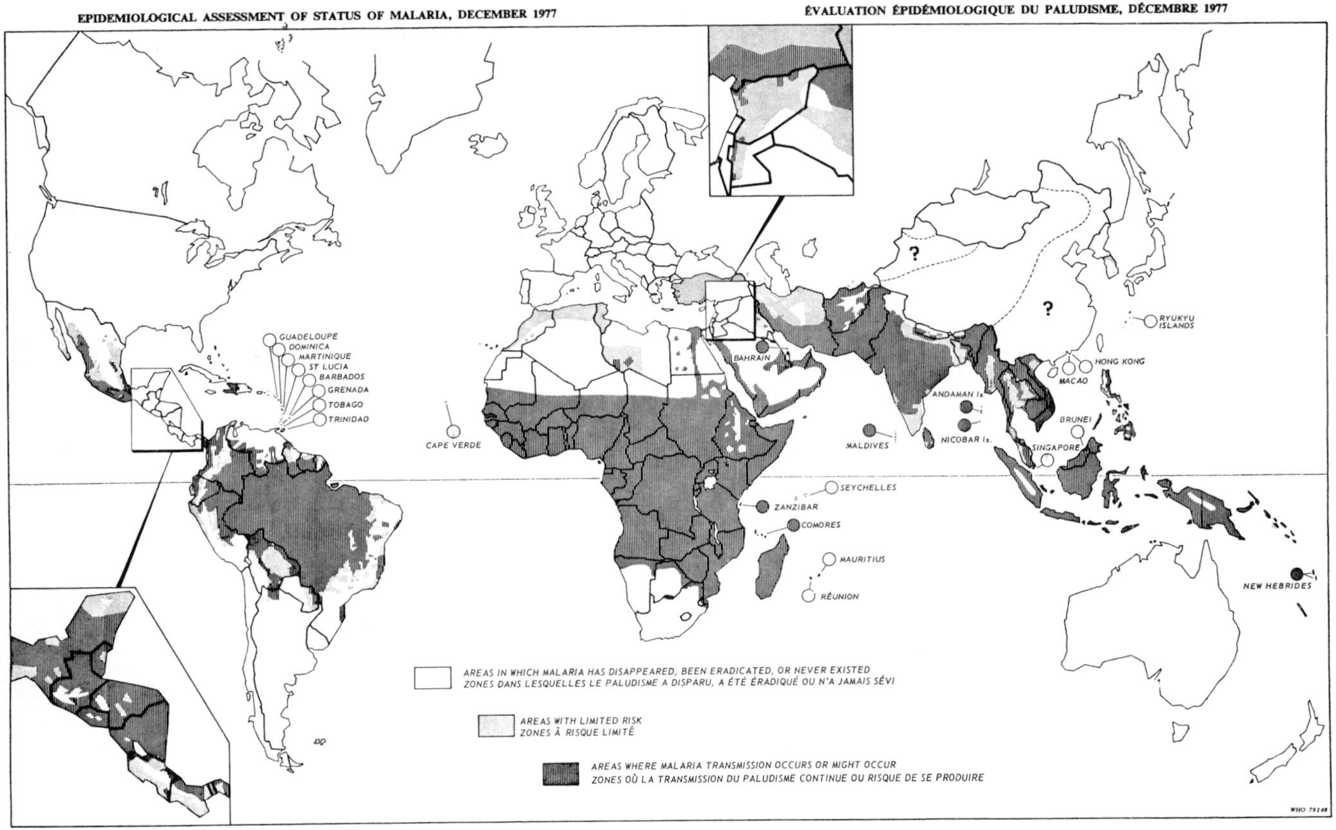
EPIDEMIOLOGICAL ASSESSMENT OF STATUS OF MALARIA, DECEMBER 1977
ÉVALUATION ÉPIDÉMIOLOGIQUE DU PALUDISME, DÉCEMBRE 1977
GUADELOUPE
DOMINICA
MARTINIQUE
ST LUCIA
BARBADOS
GRENADA
TOBAGO
TRINIDAD
CAPE VERDE
BAHRAIN
MALDIVES
ANDAMAN Is
NICOBAR Is.
SEYCHELLES
ZANZIBAR
COMORES
MAURITIUS
RÉUNION
HONG KONG
MACAO
BRUNEI
SINGAPORE
RYUKYU ISLANDS
NEW HEBRIDES
?
?
AREAS IN WHICH MALARIA HAS DISAPPEARED, BEEN ERADICATED, OR NEVER EXISTED
ZONES DANS LESQUELLES LE PALUDISME A DISPARU, A ÉTÉ ÉRADIQUÉ OU N'A JAMAIS SÉVI
AREAS WITH LIMITED RISK
ZONES À RISQUE LIMITÉ
AREAS WHERE MALARIA TRANSMISSION OCCURS OR MIGHT OCCUR
ZONES OÙ LA TRANSMISSION DU PALUDISME CONTINUE OU RISQUE DE SE PRODUIRE
WHO 79148

Map published in WHO *Weekly Epidemiological Record* No. 22, 1979 — Carte publiée dans le *Relevé épidémiologique hebdomadaire* de l'OMS N° 22, 1979.

FIG. 9. Epidemiological status of malaria in December 1977 (courtesy W.H.O.).

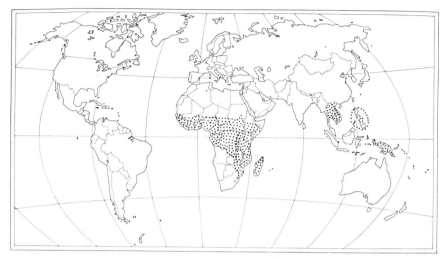

FIG. 10. Geographic distribution of *P. (Plasmodium) ovale* (dotted areas).

graphic distribution of *P. ovale* is shown in Fig. 10. *Plasmodium vivax* is practically absent in West and Central Africa; in tropical Africa its distribution is limited to eastern and southern regions with Hamito-Semitic and Caucasian population groups. Malaria remains deeply entrenched in tropical Africa where it is predominantly hyper-and holoendemic and where *A. gambiae* and *A. funestus* are the main vectors, the former being largely resistant to chlorinated hydrocarbons. These potent vectors are responsible for maintaining a high degree of stability of malaria. Chloroquine-resistant *P. falciparum* of the R-I type has occured in Kenya and Tanzania (CDC Atlanta, 1978; Fogh *et al.*, 1979; Kean, 1979; Stille, 1979). Malaria has been eradicated in the islands of Mauritius and La Réunion. Following a devastating cyclone, however, a small epidemic occurred in the mid-1970s in Mauritius, originating from cases imported from Madagascar; since then malaria has been eliminated again, but new foci occurred following a cyclone in 1979.

2. America

In continental America only Canada and Uruguay were naturally free of malaria (the status of the early twentieth century). Malaria has been eradicated from the United States of America, Cuba, Jamaica, Puerto Rico, the Antilles, Chile, and parts of Argentina, Brazil, the Dominican Republic, and Venezuela. In Grenada, where malaria was eradicated by 1962, a survey in February 1978 showed 47 cases of quartan malaria but no other *Plasmodium* species (World Health Organization, 1978c). Remedial measures have since then been implemented. Malaria risk still exists in Mexico, all Central American countries, Haiti, parts of the Dominican Republic, and parts of all South American countries except Chile and Uruguay. All countries pursue malaria eradication, but some population groups in Colombia, Ecuador, El Salvador, Guatemala, Haiti, Honduras, Nicaragua, and Peru are still unprotected. The total number of confirmed malaria cases in the Americas in 1977 was 394,000, with a relatively high incidence in Colombia, Guatemala, Haiti, and Honduras. About 369,000 cases occurred in areas in the attack phase, 20,000 cases were detected in areas under consolidation, and nearly 5000 imported cases were recorded in areas which were originally nonmalarious or freed from malaria.

The United States has maintained a malaria-free status but has been exposed to a heavy importation of cases from abroad: 610 of the 616 cases reported in 1978 were imported, while 3 were induced through blood transfusions, 2 transmitted congenitally and 1 induced by kidney transplantation. The largest sections affected were tourists, students and teachers, business persons, and missionaries, the majority of which contracted infections in Asia (52%) and Africa (29%). About 64% of the cases showed infections with *P. vivax,* 19% with *P. falciparum,* 7% with *P. malariae,* and 2% with *P. ovale* (CDC, 1979). In Mexico malaria has continued to affect mainly the Yucatan Peninsula and the southern and the western coastal parts of the country, but there has been a further reduction in malaria incidence, with a virtual absence of *P. falciparum.* Except for Belize, the Canal Zone, Costa Rica, the Dominican Republic, and Panama, where malaria incidence is relatively low, the disease has maintained rather high levels in the rest of Central America and Haiti. The situation has markedly deteriorated in Haiti, Honduras, and Nicaragua, whereas an important reduction in malaria incidence, especially of *P. falciparum* infections, was recently observed in El Salvador. In 1977, most cases in continental Central America were caused by *P. vivax* (on average 94%), but 99.97% of the Haitian cases were falciparum infections. The Dominican Republic is exposed to a heavy importation of falciparum cases from Haiti. The major problem of malaria control in Central America is the insecticide resistance of malaria vectors, which is especially serious in El Salvador where *A. albimanus* has become resistant to all operational insecticides. In South America, French Guiana and Venezuela have been able to keep malaria well under control, and Argentina, Brazil and Paraguay have made further progress toward malaria eradication. The malaria situation has slightly deteriorated in Bolivia, Colombia, Ecuador, and Peru; an epidemic increase was observed in Guyana and in Surinam. In all malarious countries except Argentina, Peru, and Paraguay, *P. falciparum* still represents a significant proportion of the infections—between 13% in Bolivia and 96% in Surinam. The situation is aggravated by the chloroquine resistance of *P. falciparum* in the majority of South American countries (see Fig. 8).

3. Asia

Kuwait and Mongolia are the only naturally malaria-free countries in Asia. Brunei, Hong Kong, Israel, Japan, Lebanon, Macao, Taiwan, and apparently also North Korea have achieved and maintained malaria eradication and, following intensive malaria control or eradication measures, considerable reduction in malaria has been obtained in Asia Minor, Iran, Pakistan, India, Nepal, Bangladesh, Thailand, and the Philippines. However, the slackening of control measures, political and martial events, and their sequelae have recently led to a deterioration of the malaria situation in many parts of Asia.

In Turkey, malaria was eradicated from the European continental part and the incidence in the Asian part reduced to 1293 cases by 1970. In the absence of adequate control measures the malaria incidence rose subsequently to 115,385 cases, mainly *P. vivax*, in 1977.

Jordan has managed to maintain effective control of malaria in spite of the Israeli-Arab conflict, but Syria has recently experienced a sharp rise in malaria to more than 2000 cases in 1977. This is in part associated with the developments in Turkey. Iraq has continued to pursue malaria eradication; the annual parasite incidence in 1976 was high at 0.7 per thousand, but it dropped to 0.4 per thousand in 1977; more than 99% of the infections were caused by *P. vivax*. The malaria situation in the countries of the Arabian peninsula is largely unchanged. Malaria prevalence is usually below 10%, except for Democratic Yemen where it reaches up to 60% in some localities. *Plasmodium falciparum* accounts for approximately one-half of the parasite formula in these areas. In Iran and Afghanistan the situation has remained largely static, with an annual parasite incidence of $1.9^0/oo$ in the former and an average parasite rate of 0.44% in the latter (1977). *Plasmodium vivax* prevails in Afghanistan (99%), and *P. falciparum* is responsible for 21% of the infections in Iran.

After a significant initial success of eradication operations in the 1960s in Pakistan, antimalaria measures were interrupted following the Indo-Pakistan conflict and the ending of vital bilateral assistance to the program. After malaria had been nearly eradicated in the early 1960s the malaria situation in India was similar in many ways to that of Sri Lanka, where a premature phasing out of antimalaria measures and an inappropriate reduction of surveillance resulted in a countrywide malaria epidemic with a peak incidence of more than 1 million cases, mostly *P. vivax*. In India the incidence dropped to an all-time low of 60,000 cases in 1966 but reached a new peak of over $6\frac{1}{2}$ million in 1976. Although more than 90% of these infections were caused by *P. vivax*, the absolute number of *P. falciparum* infections was nevertheless a reason for concern, and consequently the Indian government took measures toward strengthening control as a consequence of which the number of cases dropped to 4.7 million in 1977 and 4.1 million in 1978. Following the epidemics of the late 1960s malaria became endemic again in large parts of Sri Lanka, where the average parasite rate was 28% in 1977; 4.1% of the infections were caused by *P. falciparum,* and almost all of the remainder by *P. vivax.*

Nepal also recorded in 1977 a rise in malaria cases, 14% of which were infections with *P. falciparum;* the average parasite rate was 0.8%. Initially, Bangladesh managed to preserve the gains of the antimalaria campaign rather well in spite of the political and military struggles of the early 1970s. However, in the eastern region exophilic *A. b. balabacensis* and chloroquine-resistant *P. falciparum* pose a problem, and in 1977 the average parasite rate rose to 2.1%, with some 43% of all infections caused by *P. falciparum.*

In eastern Asia, antimalaria operations have been countrywide in Thailand, Malaysia, the Philippines, and Singapore, whereas in Indonesia, Burma, and Papua New Guinea, they have been limited to only parts of the countries; little information is available on the situation in Kampuchea and Laos, but in Viet Nam a vigorous antimalaria campaign was resumed soon after the end of the military conflict. While further progress was made in Malaysia, Java (Indonesia), and parts of the Philippines and Papua New Guinea, the operations in Burma and Thailand succeeded only in preventing further deterioration.

In 1977 the most important reservoir level was found in Papua New Guinea, with parasite rates varying between 14% and 76%, according to altitude. Relatively high parasite rates also prevailed in Sabah and in the unprotected areas of Indonesia. Burma recorded an average parasite rate of 5.1% while rates in Java (Indonesia) and Sarawak were considerably lower. The annual parasite incidence in 1977 was lowest in peninsular Malaysia with 1.3%oo and highest in the Philippines with 10.3%oo; Thailand occupied an intermediate position. *Plasmodium falciparum* is usually the prevailing species with a range between 40% of all infections in Indonesia and 77.4% in peninsular Malaysia. In the Republic of Korea, malaria is on the verge of elimination. Data from China became only recently available, showing an incidence of 6.2 million cases for 1977 and 3.1 million for 1978. *P. vivax* is the prevalent species, but also *P. falciparum* occurs at a significant level in the south.

Besides tropical Africa, eastern Asia appears to be the only area of natural distribution of *P. ovale.* Locally contracted infections have been described from China, the Philippines, Papua New Guinea, Thailand, and Viet Nam.

Many of the countries in eastern Asia are afflicted with chloroquine-resistant *P. falciparum* (see Fig. 8), and the frequency and degree of resistance are higher than in South America. The epicenter of drug resistance is in Burma, Thailand, Laos, Kampuchea, and Viet Nam, but the Philippines, Malaysia, and southern China are also already widely affected. The present eastern limit of resistance is in Solomon Islands, whereas the western limit in Asia is situated in the State of Orissa, India (Rooney, 1979).

4. Europe

Seventeen European countries were malarious in the late 1940s, 15 of which have now achieved malaria eradication (see Table XII). In Europe all countries except Greece and European continental Turkey are now free of malaria. In Greece a small focus in the area of Haematia has remained, but it appears that this focus is at last on the verge of elimination. The USSR has eradicated malaria, except for a small area in the Asian region, adjacent to Afghanistan, where strict antimalaria measures and surveillance are maintained in order to prevent a massive reintroduction of malaria into other areas. Europe is, however, exposed to the extensive, ever-increasing importation of malaria from abroad. This is best illustrated by the example of the United Kingdom, where the number of imported cases has risen continuously from 134 cases in 1970 to 1528 cases in 1977. This phenomenon can in part be ascribed to increased business, tourist, and student travel, but it mainly reflects the rising malaria incidence in India and Pakistan. In 1977 nearly 3000 malaria cases were imported into Europe (excluding the USSR). Even the smaller countries are exposed, e.g., 48 cases were recorded in Switzerland. The true figure for imported cases is estimated to be considerably higher than the reports suggest, since many a case may be missed by practitioners who have little acquaintance with the symptomatology of malaria. The situation is somewhat precarious in southern Europe, where the receptivity is highest. The possibility of epidemics starting from imported cases is ever present as evidenced by the small, but rapidly controlled, outbreak of 1973–1974 in Corsica.

5. Australia and Pacific Islands

Australia has achieved and maintained malaria eradication, although the country is exposed to importation of many cases (2269 between 1969 and 1978), especially from Papua New Guinea. A few foci with indigenous transmission were detected in 1973 and 1977 in the Torres Strait Islands and North Queensland, but these were soon brought under control.

Malaria control is pursued in the New Hebrides where the parasite rate in the various islands was 0–14%, with an average of 10% *P. falciparum* among the positive slides. In the Solomon Islands *P. falciparum* represents 30% of all infections; the annual parasite incidence rose from 17.3‰ in 1975 to 52.4‰ in 1977.

In summary it can be stated that the present world malaria situation does not give cause for complacency. The lessons of Southeast Asia clearly show that the slackening of antimalaria measures has serious consequences not easily overcome. They may be taken as an example of the need for administrative and political stability and last, but not least, for the lasting determination required for the pursuit of malaria eradication.

F. Major Research Needs for the Improvement of Malaria Control

The present malaria situation clearly calls for improved and wider use of available control tools and for the development of new tools and methods which would allow the reduction and ultimately the elimination of malaria. These methods should be available at a cost within the reach of countries hitherto fully exposed to the onslaught of malaria.

Such development can only be expected from research in the laboratory and in the field, be it related to chemotherapy, immunology, epidemiology, disease control, or supportive studies on parasite and host biology.

It would be wrong to give absolute priority to one research discipline to the neglect of others, since past experience has shown that reliance on one or two selected control methods is usually not enough to bring about a lasting reduction in or the elimination of parasite reservoirs in areas with stable malaria. It is these areas on which attention will have to be focused in the future. It is these areas which will also have to be increasingly involved in malaria research. Traditional approaches to the problem in some areas of chemotherapy and vector control are still valid, as are innovative lines of research, such as the improved use of existing drugs through lysosomotropic or sustained-release systems, the development of malaria vaccines, and the search for new vector control methods, e.g., the use of insect pathogens or genetic control.

The recent renaissance of malaria research under the auspices of governmental agencies and services, especially in the United States and Great Britain, and of international organizations such as the UNDP–World Bank–WHO Special Programme for Research and Training in Tropical Diseases, provides an opportunity for expanding and accelerating the research effort with the aim of developing the tools and methods required for ultimately mastering malaria in the world.

ACKNOWLEDGMENTS

The author would like to thank Drs. P. I. Trigg and D. Muir, World Health Organization, Geneva, for their critical review of the manuscript, and the World Health Organization for permission to reproduce Graph WHO 79148, Fig. 9 in this chapter, and to quote from the "Terminology of Malaria and of Malaria Eradication."

REFERENCES

Aikawa, M., Miller, L. H., Johnson, J., and Rabbege, J. (1978). Erythrocyte entry by malarial parasites: A moving junction between erythrocyte and parasite. *J. Cell Biol.* **77,** 72–82.

Ambroise-Thomas, P., Wernsdorfer, W. H., Grab, B., Cullen, J., and Bertagna, P. (1976). Etude séro-épidémiologique longitudinale sur le paludisme en Tunisie. *Bull. W. H. O.* **54,** 355–367.

Aragão de Beauparie, H. (1908). Über den Entwicklungsgang und die Übertragung von *Haemoproteus columbae*. *Arch. Protistenkd.* **12**, 154–167.

Armstrong, J. C. (1978). Susceptibility to *vivax malaria* in Ethiopia. *Trans. R. Soc. Trop. Med. Hyg.* **72**, 342–344.

Armstrong, J. C., Asfaha, W., and Palmer, T. T. (1976). Chloroquine sensitivity of *Plasmodium falciparum* in Ethiopia, I. Results of an *in vivo* test. *Am. J. Trop. Med. Hyg.* **25**, 2–9.

Arnold, J. D., Lalli, F., and Martin, D. C. (1969a). Augmentation of growth and division synchrony and of vascular sequestration of *Plasmodium berghei* by the photoperiodic rhythm. *J. Parasitol.* **55**, 597–608.

Arnold, J. D., Berger, A., and Martin, D. C. (1969b). The role of the pineal in mediating photoperiodic control of growth and division synchrony and capillary sequestration of *Plasmodium berghei* in mice. *J. Parasitol.* **55**, 609–616.

Arnold, J. D., Berger, A., and Martin, D. C. (1969c). Chemical agents effective in mediating control of growth and division synchrony of *Plasmodium berghei* in pinealectomized mice. *J. Parasitol.* **55**, 617–625.

Ayala, S. C. (1971). Sporogony and experimental transmission of *Plasmodium mexicanum*. *J. Parasitol.* **57**, 598–602.

Ayala, S. C. (1977). *In* "Parasitic Protozoa" (J. P. Kreier, ed.) Vol. 3, pp. 267–309. Academic Press, New York.

Ayala, S. C. (1978). Checklist, host index, and annotated bibliography of *Plasmodium* from reptiles. *J. Protozool.* **25**, No. 1, 87–100.

Ayala, S. C., Moreno, E., and Bolanos, R. (1978). *Plasmodium pessoai* sp. n. from two Costa Rican snakes. *J. Parasit.* **64**, No. 2, 330–335.

Baerg, D. C., and Young, M. D. (1970). *Plasmodium falciparum* infection induced in the black spider monkey, *Ateles fusiceps,* and black howler monkey, *Alouatta villosa*. *Trans. R. Soc. Trop. Med. Hyg.* **64**, 193–194.

Baerg, D. C., Porter, J. A., Jr., and Young, M. D. (1969). Sporozoite transmission of *Plasmodium vivax* to Panamanian primates. *Am. J. Trop. Med. Hyg.* **18**, 346–350.

Bafort, J. M., and Kageruka, P. (1972). Mosquito transmission of *Plasmodium vivax* from night monkey to night monkey. *Ann. Soc. Belg. Med. Trop.* **52**, 235–236.

Baker, J. R. (1977). Systematics of parasitic protozoa. *In* "Parasitic Protozoa" (J. P. Kreier, ed.), Vol. 1, pp. 35–57. Academic Press, New York.

Bastianelli, G., and Bignami, A. (1899). Sullo sviluppo dei parassiti della terzana nell'*Anopheles claviger*. *Atti Soc. Studi Malar.* **1**, 28–49.

Bekessy, A., Molineaux, L., and Storey, J. (1976). Estimation of incidence and recovery rates of *Plasmodium falciparum* parasitaemia from longitudinal data. *Bull. W. H. O.* **54**, 685–693.

Bignami, A. (1899). Come si prendono le febbri malariche. *Boll. R. Accad. Med., Roma* **25**, 17–46.

Boyd, M. F., ed. (1949). "Malariology." Saunders, Philadelphia, Pennsylvania.

Boyd, M. F., and Stratman-Thomas, W. K. (1934). Studies on benign tertian malaria. 1. Some observations on inoculation and onset. *Am. J. Hyg.* **20**, 488–493.

Bray, R. S. (1957). Studies on malaria in chimpanzees. IV. *Plasmodium ovale*. *Am. J. Trop. Med. Hyg.* **6**, 638–645.

Bray, R. S. (1958). Studies on malaria in chimpanzees. VI. *Laverania falciparum*. *Am. J. Trop. Med. Hyg.* **7**, 20–24.

Bray, R. S. (1962). On the parasitic protozoa of Liberia. VII. Haemosporidia of owls. *Arch. Inst. Pasteur Alger.* **40**, 201–207.

Bray, R. S. (1963). The malaria parasites of anthropoid apes. *J. Parasitol.* **49**, 888–891.

Breasted, J. H. (1930). "The Edwin Smith Surgical Papyrus." Univ. of Chicago Press, Chicago, Illinois.

Brooks, M. H., and Barry, K. G. (1969). Fatal transfusion malaria. *Blood* **34**, 806–810.

Brown, J. D., and Khoa, N. Q. (1975). Fatal falciparum malaria among narcotic injectors. *Am. J. Trop. Med. Hyg.* **24**, 729–733.

Bruce, D., Harvey, D., Hamerton, A. E., and Bruce, Lady M. E. (1913). *Plasmodium cephalophi* sp. nov. *Proc. R. Soc. London, Ser. B* **87**, 45–47.

Bruce-Chwatt, L. J. (1958). Parasite density index in malaria. *Trans. R. Soc. Trop. Med. Hyg.* **52**, 389–391.

Bruce-Chwatt, L. J. (1976). Mathematical models in the epidemiology and control of malaria. *Trop. Geogr. Med.* **28**, 1–8.

Bruce-Chwatt, L. J. (1977). Der geomedizinische Hintergrund der Malariaausrottung. *Ther. Ggw.* **116**, 2166–2181.

Bruce-Chwatt, L. J., Black, R., Canfield, C. J., Clyde, D. F., Peters, W., and Wernsdorfer, W. H. (1980). ''Chemotherapy of Malaria.'' WHO, Geneva.

Brumpt, E. (1935). Paludisme aviaire: *Plasmodium gallinaceum* n.sp. de la poule domestique. *C.R. Hebd. Seances Acad. Sci.* **200**, 783–786.

Brumpt, E. (1939). Les parasites du paludisme des chimpanzés. *C. R. Seances Soc. Biol. Ses Fil.* **130**, 837–840.

Bück, G., Coudurier, J., and Quesnel, J. J. (1952). Sur deux nouveaux plasmodiums observés chez un lémurien de Madagascar splénectomisé. *Arch. Inst. Pasteur Alger.* **30**, 240–243.

Burton, R. F. (1856). ''First Footsteps in East Africa.'' Longmans, Green, New York.

Cadigan, F. C., Jr., Spertzel, R. O., Chaicumpa, V., and Puhomchareon, S. (1966). *Plasmodium falciparum* in non-human primates (macaque monkeys). *Mil. Med.* **131**, 959–960.

Cadigan, F. C., Jr., Ward, R. A., and Puhomchareon, S. (1968). Transient infection of the gibbon with *Plasmodium vivax* malaria. *Trans. R. Soc. Trop. Med. Hyg.* **62**, 295–296.

Cadigan, F. C., Jr., Ward, R. A., and Chaicumpa, V. (1969). Further studies on the biology of human malarial parasites in gibbons from Thailand. *Mil. Med.* **134**, 757–766.

Carter, R. (1973). Enzyme variation in *Plasmodium berghei* and *Plasmodium vinckei*. *Parasitology* **66**, 297–307.

Carter, R. (1978). Studies on enzyme variation in the murine malaria parasites *Plasmodium berghei, P. yoelii, P. vinckei* and *P. chabaudi* by starch gel electrophoresis. *Parasitology* **76**, 241–267.

Carter, R., and Diggs, C. L. (1977). Plasmodia of rodents. *In* ''Parasitic Protozoa'' (J. P. Kreier, ed.), Vol. 3., 359–465. Academic Press, New York.

Carter, R., and Walliker, D. (1977). Biochemical markers for strain differentiation in malarial parasites. *Bull. W. H. O.* **55**, 339–345.

CDC, Atlanta (1978). Chloroquine-resistant malaria acquired in Kenya and Tanzania - Denmark, Georgia, New York. *Morbid. Mortal. Wkly Rep.* **27**, 463–464.

CDC, Atlanta (1979). Malaria Surveillance. Annual Survey 1978. US Department of Health, Education, and Welfare, USPHS, CDC, Atlanta.

Cheissin, E. M., and Polyansky, G. I. (1963). On the taxonomic system of protozoa. *Acta Protozool.* **1**, 327–352.

Chin, W., Contacos, P. G., Coatney, G. R., and Kimball, H. R. (1965). A naturally acquired quotidian-type malaria in man transferable to monkeys. *Science* **149**, 865.

Chin, W., Contacos, P. G., Collins, W. E., Jeter, M. H., and Alpert, E. (1968). Experimental mosquito transmission of *Plasmodium knowlesi* to man and monkey. *Am. J. Trop. Med. Hyg.* **17**, 355–358.

Christophers, Sir R. (1949). ''Endemic and epidemic prevalence'' *In* ''Malariology'' (M. F. Boyd, ed.), pp. 698–721. Saunders, Philadelphia, Pennsylvania.

Cleaver, H. (1977). Malaria and the political economy of public health. *Int. J. Health Serv.* **7**, 557–579.

Coatney, G. R. (1971). The simian malarias: Zoonoses, anthroponoses, or both? *Am. J. Trop. Med. Hyg.* **20**, 795–803.

Coatney, G. R., Collins, W. E., Warren, McW., and Contacos, P. G. (1971). "The Primate Malarias." US Dept. of Health, Education and Welfare, NIH, NIAID, Bethesda, Maryland.

Coggeshall, L. T. (1938). *Plasmodium lophurae,* a new species of malaria parasite pathogenic for the domestic fowl. *Am. J. Hyg.* **27**, 615–618.

Collins, W. E., and Aikawa, M. (1977). Plasmodia of non human primates. *In* "Parasitic Protozoa" (J. P. Kreier, ed.), Vol 3. 467–492 Academic Press, New York.

Collins, W. E., and Contacos, P. G. (1972). Transmission of *Plasmodium falciparum* from monkey to monkey by the bite of infected *Anopheles freeborni* mosquitoes. *Trans. R. Soc. Trop. Med. Hyg.* **66**, 371–372.

Collins, W. E., Contacos, P. G., Krotoski, W. A., and Howard, W. A. (1972). Transmission of four Central American strains of *Plasmodium vivax* from monkey to man. *J. Parasitol.* **58**, 332–335.

Collins, W. E., Contacos, P. G., Stanfill, P. S., and Richardson, B. B. (1973a). Studies on human malaria in *Aotus* monkeys. I. Sporozoite transmission of *Plasmodium vivax* from El Salvador. *J. Parasitol.* **59**, 606–608.

Collins, W. E., Neva, F. A., Chaves-Carpallo, E., Stanfill, P. S., and Richardson, B. B. (1973b). Studies on human malaria in *Aotus* monkeys. II. Establishment of a strain of *Plasmodium falciparum* from Panama. *J. Parasitol.* **59**, 609–612.

Collins, W. E., Miller, L. H., Glew, R. H., Contacos, P. G., Howard, W. A., and Wyler, D. J. (1973c). Transmission of three strains of *Plasmodium falciparum* from monkey to man. *J. Parasitol.* **59**, 855–858.

Collins, W. E., Stanfill, P. S., Skinner, J. C., Harrison, A. J., and Smith, C. S. (1974a). Studies on human malaria in *Aotus* monkeys. IV. Development of *Plasmodium falciparum* in two subspecies of *Aotus trivirgatus. J. Parasitol.* **60**, 335–338.

Collins, W. E., Skinner, J. C., Richardson, B. B., Stanfill, P. S., and Contacos, P. G. (1974b). Studies on human malaria in *Aotus* monkeys. V. Blood-induced infections of *Plasmodium vivax. J. Parasitol.* **60**, 393–398.

Collins, W. E., Warren, McW., Skinner, J. C., Chin, W., and Richardson, B. B. (1977). Studies on the Santa Lucia (El Salvador) strain of *Plasmodium falciparum* in *Aotus trivirgatus* monkeys. *J. Parasitol.* **63**, 52–56.

Contacos, P. G., and Collins, W. E. (1968). Falciparum malaria transmissible from monkey to man by mosquito bite. *Science* **161**, 56.

Contacos, P. G., and Collins, W. E. (1969). *Plasmodium malariae:* Transmission from monkey to man by mosquito bite. *Science* **165**, 918–919.

Corradetti, A. (1938). Osservazioni sul ciclo schizogonico dei plasmodi nelle cellule dei tessuti e proposta di una unova classificazione degli Haemosporidiidea. *Riv. Parassitol.* **2**, 23–36.

Corradetti, A., and Scanga, M. (1973). The *Plasmodium vaughani*-complex. *Exp. Parasitol.* **34**, 344–349.

Corradetti, A., Garnham, P. C. C., and Laird, M. (1963a). New classification of the avian malaria parasites. *Parassitologia* **5**, 1–4.

Corradetti, A., Verolini, F., and Neri, G. (1963b). *Plasmodium (Haemomoeba) giovannolai* n.sp. parassita di *Turdus merula. Parassitologia* **5**, 11–18.

Corradetti, A., Dojmi di Delupis, G. L., Palmieri, C., and Piccione, G. (1970). Modello sperimentale, realizzato con *Plasmodium gallinaceum* e *Anopheles stephensi,* per selezionare popolazioni di plasmodio adatte a vivere in un vettore apparentemente refrattario, e per selezionare popolazioni di vettore suscettibili a un plasmodio apparentemente inadatto a vivere in esso. *Parassitologia* **12**, 81–99.

da Fonseca, F. (1951). Plasmodio de primata do Brasil. *Mem. Inst. Oswaldo Cruz* **49**, 543–551.

Danilewsky, B. (1889). "La parasitologie comparée du sang," Vols 1–2. Karl Richer, St. Petersburg.

Davidson, G. (1955). Further studies of the basic factors concerned in the transmission of malaria. *Trans. R. Soc. Trop. Med. Hyg.* **49**, 339–350.

Deaderick, W. H. (1909). "A Practical Study of Malaria." Saunders, Philadelphia, Pennsylvania.

Deane, L. M. (1969). Plasmodia of monkeys and malaria eradication in Brazil. *Rev. Latinoam. Microbiol.* **11**, 69–73.

Deane, L. M., Deane, M. P., and Ferreira Neto, J. (1966a). A naturally acquired human infection by *Plasmodium simium* of howler monkeys. *Trans. R. Soc. Trop. Med. Hyg.* **60**, 563–564.

Deane, L. M., Ferreira Neto, F., and Silveira, I. P. S. (1966b). Experimental infection of a splenectomized squirrel-monkey, *Saimiri sciureus,* with *Plasmodium vivax. Trans. R. Soc. Trop. Med. Hyg.* **60**, 811–812.

de Jong, A. C. (1971). *Plasmodium dissanaikei* n.sp. a new avian malaria parasite from the rose-ringed parakeet of Ceylon, *Psittacula krameri manillensis. Ceylon J. Med. Sci.* **20**, 41–45.

Dietz, K., Molineaux, L., and Thomas, A. (1974). A malaria model tested in the African savannah. *Bull. W. H. O.* **50**, 347–357.

Dissanaike, A. S., Nelson, P., and Garnham, P. C. C. (1965a). Two new malaria parasites, *Plasmodium cynomolgi ceylonensis* subsp. nov. and *Plasmodium fragile* sp. nov., from monkeys in Ceylon. *Ceylon J. Med. Sci.* **14**, 1–9.

Dissanaike, A. S., Nelson, P., and Garnham, P. C. C. (1965b). *Plasmodium simiovale* sp. nov., a new simian malaria parasite from Ceylon. *Ceylon J. Med. Sci.* **14**, 27–32.

Doflein, F. (1916). "Lehrbuch der Protozoenkunde," 5th ed. Fischer, Jena.

Dover, A. S. (1971). Malaria in a heroin user. *J. Am. Med. Assoc.* **215**, 1987.

Dunn, F. L. (1965). On the antiquity of malaria in the Western Hemisphere. *Hum. Biol.* **37**, 385–393.

Dunn, F. L., Eyles, D. E., and Yap, L. F. (1963). *Plasmodium sandoshami,* a new species of malaria parasite from the Malayan flying lemur. *Ann. Trop. Med. Parasitol.* **57**, 75–81.

Eyles, D. E. (1963). The species of simian malaria: Taxonomy, morphology, life cycle, and geographical distribution of the monkey species. *J. Parasitol.* **49**, 866–887.

Eyles, D. E., Fong, Y. L., Warren, M., Guinn, E., Sandosham, A. A., and Wharton, R. H. (1962a). *Plasmodium coatneyi,* a new species of primate malaria from Malaya. *Am. J. Trop. Med. Hyg.* **11**, 597–604.

Eyles, D. E., Laing, A. B. G., and Fong, Y. L. (1962b). *Plasmodium fieldi* sp. nov., a new species of malaria parasite from the pig-tailed macaque in Malaya. *Am. Trop. Med. Parasitol.* **56**, 242–247.

Eyles, D. E. Fong, Y. L., Dunn, F. L., Guinn, E., Warren, M., and Sandosham, A. A. (1964). *Plasmodium youngi* n.sp., a malaria parasite of the Malayan gibbon, *Hylobates lar lar. Am. J. Trop. Med. Hyg.* **13**, 248–255.

Fairley, N. H. (1945). Chemotherapeutic suppression and prophylaxis in malaria. *Trans. R. Soc. Trop. Med. Hyg.* **38**, 311–355.

Fallis, A. M., and Bennett, G. F. (1961). Sporogony of *Leucocytozoon* and *Haemoproteus* in simuliids and certapogonids and a revised classification of the Haemosporidiida. *Can. J. Zool.* **39**, 215–228.

Fogh, S., Jepsen, S., and Effersøe, P. (1979). Chloroquine resistant *P. falciparum* malaria in Kenya. *Trans. R. Soc. Trop. Med. Hyg.* **73**, 228–229.

Friedman, M. J. (1978). Erythrocytic mechanism of sickle cell resistance to malaria. *Proc. Natl. Acad. Sci. U.S.A.* **75**, 1994–1997.

Friedmann, C. T. H., Dover, A. S., Roberto, R. R., and Kearns, O. A. (1973). A malaria epidemic among heroin users. *Am. J. Trop. Med. Hyg.* **22**, 302–307.

Friedman, M. J., Roth, E. F., Nagel, R. L., and Trager, W. (1979). *Plasmodium falciparum:* physiological interactions with the human sickle cell. *Exp. Parasitol.* **47**, 73–80.

Garnham, P. C. C. (1947). Exo-erythrocytic schizogony in *Plasmodium kochi* Laveran: A preliminary note. *Trans. R. Soc. Trop. Med. Hyg.* **40,** 719–722.

Garnham, P. C. C. (1966). "Malaria Parasites and Other Haemosporidia." Blackwell, Oxford.

Garnham, P. C. C. (1973). Second roundtable discussion on taxonomic problems relating to malaria parasites. *J. Protozool.* **20,** 37–42.

Garnham, P. C. C. (1977). A new malaria parasite of pigeons and ducks from Venezuela. *Protistologica* **13,** 113–125.

Garnham, P. C. C., and Edeson, J. F. B. (1962). Two new malaria parasites of the Malayan mouse deer. *Riv. Malarial.* **41,** 3–10.

Garnham, P. C. C., and Powers, K. G. (1974). Periodicity of infectivity of plasmodial gametocytes: The "Hawking phenomenon." *Int. J. Parasitol.* **4,** 103–106.

Garnham, P. C. C., Lainson, R., and Gunders, A. E. (1956). Some observations on malaria parasites in a chimpanzee, with particular reference to the persistence of *Plasmodium reichenowi* and *Plasmodium vivax*. *Ann. Soc. Belge Med. Trop.* **36,** 811–821.

Garnham, P. C. C., Rajapaksa, N., Peters, W., and Killick-Kendrick, R. (1972). Malaria parasites of the orang-utan *(Pongo pygmaeus)*. *Ann. Trop. Med. Parasitol.* **66,** 287–294.

Garnham, P. C. C., Bray, R. S., Bruce-Chwatt, L. J., Draper, C. C., Killick-Kendrick, R., Sergiev, P. G., and Maryon, M. (1975). A strain of *Plasmodium vivax* characterized by prolonged incubation: Morphological and biological characteristics. *Bull. W. H. O.* **52,** 21–32.

Garrett-Jones,   and Shidrawi, G. R. (1969). Malaria vectorial capacity of a population of *Anopheles gambiae:* An exercise in epidemiological entomology. *Bull. W. H. O.* **40,** 531–545.

Geiman, Q. M., and Meagher, M. J. (1967). Susceptibility of a New World monkey to *Plasmodium falciparum* from man. *Nature (London)* **215,** 437–439.

Geiman, Q. M., and Siddiqui, W. A. (1969). Susceptibility of a New World monkey to *Plasmodium malariae* from man. *Am. J. Trop. Med. Hyg.* **18,** 351–354.

Geiman, Q. M., Siddiqui, W. A., and Schnell, J. V. (1969). Biological basis for susceptibility of *Aotus trivirgatus* to species of plasmodia from man. *Mil. Med.* **134,** 780–786.

Gerhardt, G. (1884). Über Intermittensimpfungen. *Z. Klin. Med.* **7,** 372–377.

Gonder, R., and von Berenberg-Gossler, H. (1908). Untersuchungen über die Malariaplasmodien der Affen. *Malar. Int. Arch. Leipzig* **1,** 47–56.

Gorgas, W. C. (1915). "Sanitation in Panama." Appleton, New York.

Gould, D. J., Cadigan, F. C., Jr., and Ward, R. A. (1966). Falciparum malaria: Transmission to the
· gibbon by *Anopheles balabacensis*. *Science* **153,** 1384.

Grassi, B. (1900). Studi di uno zoologo sulla malaria. *Mem. R. Accad. Lincei* **3,** 299–502.

Grassi, B., and Feletti, R. (1890a). Parassiti malarici negli uccelli: Nota preliminaria. *Boll. Mens. Accad. Gioenia Sci. Nat. Catania* **13,** 3–6.

Grassi, B., and Feletti, R. (1890b). Parasites malariques chez les oiseaux. *Boll. Mens. Accad. Gioenia Sci. Nat. Catania* **13,** 297–300.

Grassi, B., and Feletti, R. (1891). Nuova contribuzione allo studio della malaria. *Boll. Mens. Accad. Gioenia Sci. Nat. Catania* **16,** 16–20.

Grassi, B., and Feletti, R. (1892). Contribuzione allo studio dei parassiti malarici. *Atti Accad. Gioenia Sci. Nat. Catania* **5,** 1–81.

Grassi, B., Bignami, A., and Bastianelli, G. (1899a). Ciclo evolutivo delle semilune nell' *Anopheles claviger*. *Atti Soc. Studi Malar.* **1,** 14.

Grassi, B., Bignami, A., and Bastianelli, G. (1899b). Resoconto degli studi fatti sulla malaria durante il mese di Gennaio. *Atti Accad. Naz. Lincei, Cl. Sci. Fis., Mat. Nat., Rend.* [5] **8,** 100–104.

Guindy, E., Hoogstraal, H., and Mohamed, A. H. H. (1965). *Plasmodium garnhami* sp. nov.

from the Egyptian hoopoe (*Upupa epops major* Brehm). *Trans. R. Soc. Trop. Med. Hyg.* **59**, 280-284.

Hackett, L. W. (1944). Spleen measurements in malaria. *J. Natl. Malar. Soc.* **3**, 121-134.

Hackett, L. W. (1949). Distribution of malaria. *In* "Malariology" (M. F. Boyd, ed.), pp. 722-735. Saunders, Philadelphia, Pennsylvania.

Halawani, A., and Shawarby, A. A. (1957). Malaria in Egypt. *J. Egypt. Med. Assoc.* **40**, 753-792.

Halberstaedter, L., and von Prowazek, S. (1907). Untersuchungen über die Malariaparasiten der Affen. *Arb. Kais. Gesundheitsamte* **26**, 37-43.

Hartmann, E. (1927). Three species of bird malaria, *Plasmodium praecox, P. cathemerium* n.sp. and *P. inconstons* n.sp. *Arch. Protistenkd.* **60**, 1-18.

Hawking, F. (1973). Infectivity of *Plasmodium berghei* and of *Babesia rodhaini* to various primates. *Am. J. Trop. Med. Hyg.* **22**, 163-167.

Hawking, F., Wilson, M. E., and Gammage, K. (1972). Evidence for cyclic development and short-lived maturity in the gametocytes of *Plasmodium falciparum*. *Trans. R. Soc. Trop. Med. Hyg.* **65**, 549-559.

Hayes, D. E., and Ward, R. A. (1977). Sporozoite transmission of falciparum malaria (Burma-Thau strain) from man to *Aotus* monkey. *Am. J. Trop. Med. Hyg.* **26**, 1841-1845.

Herman, C. M. (1941). *Plasmodium durae,* a new species of malaria parasite from the common turkey. *Am. J. Hyg.* **34** (c), 22-27.

Honigberg, B. M., Balamuth, W., Bovee, E. C., Corliss, J. O., Gojdics, M., Hall, R. P., Kudo, R. R., Levine, N. D., Loeblich, A. R., Jr., Weiser, J., and Wenrich, D. H. (1964). A revised classification of the phylum protozoa. *J. Protozool.* **11**, 7-20.

Howells, R. E., and Davies, E. E. (1971). Nuclear division in the oocyst of *Plasmodium berghei*. *Ann. Trop. Med. Parasitol.* **65**, 451-459.

Huff, C. G. (1930). *Plasmodium elongatum* n.sp., an avian malarial organism with an elongate gametocyte. *Am. J. Hyg.* **11**, 385-391.

Huff, C. G. (1935). *Plasmodium hexamerium* n.sp. from the bluebird inoculable to canaries. *Am. J. Hyg.* **22**, 274-277.

Huff, C. G. (1937). A new variety of *Plasmodium relictum* from the robin. *J. Parasitol.* **23**, 400-404.

Huff, C. G. (1965). Susceptibility of mosquitoes to avian malaria. *Exp. Parasitol.* **16**, 107-132.

Huff, C. G., and Hoogstraal, H. (1963). *Plasmodium lemuris* n.sp. from *Lemur collaris* E. Geoffroy. *J. Infect. Dis.* **112**, 233-236.

Huffaker, C. B. (1944). The temperature relations of the immature stages of the malarial mosquito *Anopheles quadrimaculatus* Say, with a comparison of the developmental power of constant and variable temperature in insect metabolism. *Ann. Entomol. Soc. Am.* **37**, 1-27.

Jadin, J., Timperman, G., and de Ruysser, F. (1975). Comportement d'une lignée de *P. berghei* aprés préservation à basse température pendant plus de dix ans. *Ann. Soc. Belge Med. Trop.* **55**, 603-608.

James, S. P., and Tate, P. (1937). New knowledge of the life-cycle of malaria parasites. *Nature (London)* **139**, 545-546.

Jarcho, S. (1964). Some observations on disease in pre-historic North America. *Bull. Hist. Med.* **38**, 1-18.

Juminer, B. (1970). Le paludisme est-il une anthropozoonose? *Arch. Inst. Pasteur Tunis* **47**, 229-241.

Kean, B. H. (1979). Chloroquine-resistant falciparum malaria from Africa. *J. Am. Med. Ass.* **241**, 395.

Kikuth, W. (1931). Immunobiologische und chemotherapeutische Studien an verschiedenen Stämmen von Vogelmalaria. *Zentralbl. Bakteriol., Parasitenkd., Infektionskr. Hyg., Abt. 1:Orig.* **121**, 401-409.

Killick-Kendrick, R. (1973). Parasitic protozoa of the blood of rodents. III. Two new malaria parasites of anomaliurine flying squirrels of the Ivory Coast. *Ann. Parasitol. Hum. Comp.* **48**, 639–651.

Killick-Kendrick, R. (1974). Parasitic protozoa of the blood of rodents: A revision of *Plasmodium berghei. Parasitology* **69** (2), 225–237.

Killick-Kendrick, R., and Peters, W. (1978). "Rodent Malaria." Academic Press, New York.

King, A. F. A. (1883). Insects and disease—Mosquitoes and malaria. *Pop. Sci. Mon.* **23**, 644.

Kouznetsov, R. L., Rooney, W., Wernsdorfer, W. H., Gaddal, A. A., Payne, D., and Abdalla, R. E. (1979). Assessment of the sensitivity of *Plasmodium falciparum* to antimalarial drugs at Sennar Sudan: use of the *in vitro* microtechnique and the *in vivo* method. WHO/MAL/79.910, WHO, Geneva.

Lainson, R., Landau, I., and Shaw, J. J. (1974). Further parasites of the family Garniidae (Coccidia: Haemosporidiidae) in Brazilian lizards: *Fallisia effusa* gen. nov., sp. nov. and *Fallisia modesta* gen. nov., sp. nov. *Parasitology* **68**, 117–125.

Lancisi, G. M. (1717). "De noxiis paludum effluviis corumque remediis." Salvioni, Roma.

Landau, I. (1965). Description de *Plasmodium chabaudi* n.sp., parasite de rongeurs africains. *C. R. Hebd. Seances Acad. Sci.* **260**, 3758–3761.

Landau, I. (1973). Diversité des mécanismes assurant la pérennitéde l'infection chez les sporozoaires coccidiomorphes. *Mem. Mus. Natl. Hist. Nat., Paris, Ser. A* **77**, 1–62.

Landau, I., and Killick-Kendrick, R. (1966). Note préliminaire sur le cycle évolutif des deux *Plasmodium* de rongeur *Thamnomys rutilans* en République Centre Africaine. *C. R. Hebd. Seances Acad. Sci., Groupe 12* **262**, 1113–1116.

Laveran, A. (1884). "Traité des fièvres palustres." Doin, Paris.

Laveran, A., and Marullaz, M. (1914). Sur deux hémamibes et un toxoplasma *Liothrix luteus. Bull. Soc. Pathol. Exot.* **7**, 21–25.

Levine, N. D. (1961). "Protozoan Parasites of Domestic Animals and Man," 1st ed. Burgess, Minneapolis, Minnesota.

Levine, N. D. (1973). "Protozoan Parasites of Domestic Animals and Man," 2nd ed. Burgess, Minneapolis, Minnesota.

Lien, J. C., and Cross, J. H. (1968). *Plasmodium (Vinckeia) watteni* sp.n. from the Formosan flying squirrel, *Petaurista petaurista grandis. J. Parasitol.* **54**, 1171–1174.

Livingstone, F. B. (1971). Malaria and human polymorphisms. *Annu. Rev. Genet.* **5**, 33–64.

Livingstone, F. B. (1976). Haemoglobin history in West Africa. *Hum. Biol.* **48**, 487–500.

Lopez-Antunano, F. J., and Palmer, T. T. (1978). Sensitivity of Duffy negative erythrocytes in *Aotus* monkeys to *Plasmodium vivax. Trans. R. Soc. Trop. Med. Hyg.* **72**, 319.

Lyman, D. O., Boese, R. J., and Shearer, L. A. (1972). Malaria among heroin users. *Health Serv. Rep.* **87**, 545–549.

Lysenko, A. Ya., Beljaev, A. E., and Rybalka, V. M. (1977). Population studies of *Plasmodium vivax.* 1. The theory of polymorphism of sporozoites and epidemiological phenomena of tertian malaria. *Bull. W.H.O.* **55**, 451–549.

MacCallum, W. G. (1897). On the flagellated form of the malarial parasite. *Lancet* **2**, 1240–1241.

Macdonald, G. (1957). "The Epidemiology and Control of Malaria." Oxford Univ. Press, London and New York.

Macdonald, G. (1973). *In* "Dynamics of Tropical Disease" (L. J. Bruce-Chwatt and V. J. Glanville, eds.), p. 159 Oxford Univ. Press, London and New York.

Manson, P. (1894). On the nature and significance of the crecetic and flagellated bodies in malarial blood. *Br. Med. J.* **2**, 1306–1308.

Manwell, R. D. (1934). Avian malarial infections in classroom material. *Science* **79**, 544–545.

Manwell, R. D. (1935). *Plasmodium vaughani* (Novy & MacNeal). *Am. J. Hyg.* **21**, 180–187.

Manwell, R. D. (1945). How many speices of avian malaria parasites are there? *Am. J. Trop. Med.* **15**, 365–380.

Manwell, R. D. (1962). A new species of avian *Plasmodium*. *J. Protozool.* **9**, 401–403.

Manwell, R. D. (1968). *Plasmodium octamerium* n.sp., an avian malaria parasite from the pintail Whydah bird *Vidua macroura*. *J. Protozool.* **15**, 680–685.

Manwell, R. D., and Kuntz, R. E. (1965). A new species of *Plasmodium* from the Formosan shoveller duck (*Anas clypeata* L.). *J. Protozool.* **12**, 101–104.

Manwell, R. D., and Kuntz, R. E. (1966). *Plasmodium hegneri* n.sp. from the European teal *Anas c. crecca* in Taiwan. *J. Protozool.* **13**, 437–440.

Manwell, R. D., and Sessler, G. J. (1971). *Plasmodium paranucleophilum* n.sp. from a South American tanager. *J. Protozool.* **18**, 629–632.

Marchiafava, E., and Celli, A. (1884). Sulle alterazioni dei globuli rossi nella infezione da malaria e sulla genesi della melanemia. *Arch. Clin. Ital.* **14**, 265–268.

Marchiafava, E., and Celli, A. (1885). Nuove ricerche sulla infezione malarica. *Arch. Sci. Med.* **9**, 311–340.

Markus, M. B. (1978). Terminology of invasive stages of protozoa of the subphylum apicomplexa (sporozoa). *South Afr. J. Sci.* **74**, 105–106.

Martin, S. K., Miller, L. H., Alling, D., Okoye, V. C., Esan, G. J. F., Osunkoya, B. O., and Deane, M. (1979). Severe malaria and glucose-6-phosphate dehydrogenase deficiency: A re-appraisal of the malaria G-6-PD hypothesis. *Lancet* 1(8115), 524–526.

Mason, S. J., Aikawa, M., Shiroishi, T., and Miller, L. H. (1977). Further evidence for the parasitic origin of the surface coat on malaria merozoites. *Am. J. Trop. Med. Hyg.* **26**, 195–197.

Mauss, H., and Mietzsch, L. (1933). Atebrin, ein neues Heilmittel gegen Malaria. *Klin. Wochenschr.* **12**, 1276–1278.

Mayer, M. (1907). Über Malaria beim Affen. *Med. Klin.* **3**, 579–580.

Meckel, H. (1847). Über Schwarzer Pigment in der Milz und im Blute einer Geisteskranken. *Z. Psychiatr.* **4**, 198–226.

Mesnil, F. (1899). Essai sur la classification et l'origine des sporozoaires. *Cinquante Soc. Biol.* pp. 258NS–274NS.

Mesnil, F., and Roubaud, E. (1917). Sur la sensibilité du chimpanzé au paludisme humain. *C. R. Hebd. Seances Acad. Sci.* **165**, 39–41.

Mesnil, F., and Roubaud, E. (1920). Essais d'inoculation de paludisme au chimpanzé. *Ann. Inst. Pasteur, Paris* **34**, 466–480.

Milam, D. F., and Kusch, E. (1938). Observations on *Plasmodium knowlesi* malaria in general paresis. *South. Med. J.* **31**, 947–949.

Miller, L. H. (1977). Hypothesis on the mechanism of erythrocyte invasion by malaria merozoites. *Bull. W. H. O.* **55**, 157–162.

Miller, L. H., Dvorak, J. A., Shiroishi, T. and Durocher, J. R. (1973). Influence of erythrocyte membrane components on malaria merozoite invasion. *J. Exp. Med.* **138**, 1597–1601.

Miller, L. H., Mason, S. J., and Dvorak, J. A. (1975). Erythrocyte receptors for (*Plasmodium knowlesi*) malaria: Duffy blood group determinants. *Science* **189**, 561–563.

Molineaux, L., Dietz, K., and Thomas, A. (1978). Further epidemiological evaluation of a malaria model. *Bull. W. H. O.* **56**, 565–571.

Moshkovsky, Sh. D. (1973). (Explanation for the difference of incubation type and features of alternation of acute periods of tertian malaria associated with different strains of *Plasmodium vivax*). *Med. Parazitol. Parazit. Bolezni* **42**, 393–400.

Müller, P. (1955). "DDT. Das Insektizid Dichlordiphenyltrichloräthan und seine Bedeutung," pp. 14–23, Birkhäuser, Basel.

Muniz, J., and Soares, R. (1954). Nota sôbre un parasita do gênero *Plasmodium* encontrado no

Ramphastos toco Müller, 1776, "Tucano-açu", e differente do *Plasmodium huffi: Plasmodium pinottii* n.sp. *Rev. Bras. Malariol. Doencas Trop.* **6,** 611–617.

Muniz, J., Soares, R., and Batista, S. (1951). Sôbre una espécie de *Plasmodium* parasita do *Ramphastos toco* Müller, 1776, *Plasmodium huffi* n.sp. *Rev. Bras. Malariol. Doencas Trop.* **3,** 339–356.

Najera, J. A. (1974). A critical review of the field application of a mathematical model of malaria eradication. *Bull. W. H. O.* **50,** 449–457.

Noguer, A., Wernsdorfer, W., and Kouznetsov, R. (1976). The malaria situation in 1975. *WHO Chron.* **30,** 486–493.

Noguer, A., Wernsdorfer, W., Kouznetsov, R., and Hempel, J. (1978). The malaria situation in 1976. *WHO Chron.* **32,** 9–17.

Novy, F. G., and MacNeal, W. J. (1904). Trypanosomes and bird malaria. *Am. Med.* **8,** 932–934.

Omer, A. H. S. (1978). Response of *Plasmodium falciparum* in Sudan to oral chloroquine. *Am. J. Trop. Med. Hyg.* **27,** 853–857.

Palmer, T. T., Twonby, L. B., Yigzaw, M., and Armstrong, J. C. (1976). Chloroquine sensitivity of *Plasmodium falciparum* in Ethiopia. II. Results of an *in vitro* test. *Am. J. Trop. Med. Hyg.* **25,** 10–13.

Pampana, E. (1963). "A Textbook of Malaria Eradication," 1st ed. Oxford Univ. Press, London and New York.

Paz Soldan, C. E. (1938). "Las tertianas del Condo de Chinchón." Ediciones de la Reform Medica, Lima.

Pfeiffer, R. (1892). "Beiträge zue Protozoen-Forschung. I. Die Coccidien-Krankheit bei Kauinchen." Hirschwald, Berlin.

Porter, J. A., Jr. (1970). Infections of *Plasmodium vivax* in *Saguinus geoffroyi. J. Protozool.* **17,** 361–363.

Porter, J. A., Jr., and Young, M. D. (1966). Susceptibility of Panamanian primates to *Plasmodium vivax. Mil. Med.* **131,** 952–958.

Porter, J. A., Jr., and Young, M. D. (1967). The transfer of *Plasmodium falciparum* from man to the marmoset *Saguinus geoffroyi. J. Parasitol.* **53,** 845–846.

Pringle, G. (1960). Two new malaria parasites from East African vertebrates. *Trans. R. Soc. Trop. Med. Hyg.* **54,** 411–414.

Pringle, G. (1965). A count of the sporozoites in an oocyst of *Plasmodium falciparum. Trans. R. Soc. Trop. Med. Hyg.* **59,** 285–288.

Pull, J. H. (1976). La notion de risque dans les maladies parasitaires avec référence particulière au paludisme. *Rev. Epidemiol., Med. Soc. Sante Publique* **24,** 221–229.

Pull, J. H., and Grab, B. (1974). A simple epidemiological model for evaluating the malaria inoculation rate and the risk of infection in infants. *Bull. W. H. O.* **51,** 507–516.

Raffaele, G. (1934a). Un ceppo italiano di *Plasmodium elongatum. Riv. Malariol.* **13,** 3–8.

Raffaele, G. (1934b). Sul comportamento degli sporozoiti nel sangue dell'ospite. *Riv. Malariol.* **13,** 395 and 705.

Raffaele, G. (1936). Presumibili forme iniziali di evoluzione di *Plasmodium relictum. Riv. Malariol.* **15,** 318–324.

Ramsdale, C. D., and Coluzzi, M. (1975). Studies on the infectivity of tropical African strains of *Plasmodium falciparum* to some southern European vectors of malaria. *Parassitologia* **17,** 39–48.

Rodhain, J. (1941). Sur un *Plasmodium* du gibbon *Hylobates lensciscus* Geoff. *Acta Biol. Belg.* **1,** 118–123.

Rodhain, J. (1952). *Plasmodium vinckei* n.sp. un deuxième *Plasmodium* parasite de rongeurs sauvages au Katanga. *Ann. Soc. Belge Med. Trop.* **32,** 275–280.

Romanowsky, D. L. (1890). K voprosu o stroyenii chuzheyadnikh malyarii; Zur Frage über den Bau der Malariaparasiten; The structure of malaria parasites. *Vrach, St. Petersburg* **11**, 1171–1173.

Romanowsky, D. L. (1891). Zur Frage der Parasitologie und Therapie der Malaria. *St. Petersb. Med. Wochenschr.* **16**, 297–307.

Rooney, W. (1979). Chloroquine-resistant falciparum malaria in the Sate of Orissa, India. WHO/ MAL/79.914, WHO, Geneva.

Rosenblatt, J. E., and Marsh, V. H. (1971). Induced malaria in narcotic addicts. *Lancet* 2 189–190.

Ross, R. (1897). On some peculiar pigmented cells found in two mosquitoes fed on malarial blood. *Br. Med. J.* **2**, 1786–1788.

Ross, R. (1898). "Report on the Cultivation of Proteosoma, *Labbé,* in Grey Mosquitoes." Govt. Press, Calcutta.

Ross, R. (1911). "The Prevention of Malaria," 2nd ed. Murray, London.

Rossan, R. N., and Baerg, D. C. (1975). Development of falciparum malaria in a Panamanian subspecies of howler monkey. *Am. J. Trop. Med. Hyg.* **24**, 1035–1036.

Russell, P. F. (1952). "Malaria: Basic Principles Briefly Stated." Blackwell, Oxford.

Russell, P. F., West, L. S., Manwell, R. D., and Macdonald, G. (1963). "Practical Malariology." Oxford Univ. Press, London and New York.

Rybalka, V. M., Beljaev, A. E., and Lysenko, A. Ya. (1977). Population studies of *Plasmodium vivax.* 2. Distribution of manifestations in foci of tertian malaria. *Bull. W.H.O.* **55**, 551–556.

Sandosham, A. A., Yap, L. F., and Omar, I. (1965). A malaria parasite, *Plasmodium (Vinckeia) booliati* sp. nov., from a Malayan giant flying squirrel. *Med. J. Malaya* **20**, 3–7.

Schaudinn, F. (1903). Studien über krankheitserregende Protozoen. II. *Plasmodium vivax,* der Erreger des Tertianfiebers beim Menschen. *Arb. Kais. Gesundheitsamte* **19**, 169–250.

Schillinger, J. E. (1942). Diseases of wildlife and their relationship to domestic livestock. *In* "Yearbook of Agriculture, USDA," pp. 1217–1225. US Govt. Printing Office, Washington, D.C.

Schulemann, W. (1932). Synthetic antimalarial preparations. *Proc. R. Soc. Med.* **25**, 897–905.

Schwetz, J. (1930). Sur un plasmodium aviaire à formes de division allongées—*Plasmodium fallax* n.sp. *Arch. Inst. Pasteur Alger.* **8**, 289–296.

Scott, H. H. (1939). "A History of Tropical Medicine." Arnold, London.

Seed, T. M., and Manwell, R. D. (1977). Plasmodia of birds. *In* "Parasitic Protozoa" (J. P. Kreier, ed.), Vol. 3., 311–357 Academic Press, New York.

Sergent, E., Sergent, E., and Catanei, A. (1928). Sur un parasite nouveau du paludisme des oiseaux. *C. R. Hebd. Seances Acad. Sci.* **186**, 809–810.

Sheather, A. L. (1919). A malaria parasite in the blood of a buffalo. *J. Comp. Pathol. Ther.* **32**, 223–226.

Shortt, H. E., and Garnham, P. C. C. (1948). The pre-erythrocytic development of *Plasmodium cynomolgi* and *Plasmodium vivax. Trans. R. Soc. Trop. Med. Hyg.* **41**, 785–795.

Shortt, H. E., Fairley, N. H., Covell, G., Shute, P. G., and Garnham, P. C. C. (1951). The pre-erythrocytic stages of *Plasmodium falciparum. Trans R. Soc. Trop. Med. Hyg.* **44**, 405–419.

Shute, P. G., Lupascu, Gh., Branzei, P., Maryon, M., Constantinescu, P., Bruce-Chwatt, L. J., Draper, C. C., Killick-Kendrick, R., and Garnham, P. C. C. (1976). A strain of *Plasmodium vivax* characterized by prolonged incubation: The effect of numbers of sporozoites on the length of the prepatent period. *Trans. R. Soc. Trop. Med. Hyg.* **70**, 474–481.

Sinden, R. E. (1975). The sporogonic cycle of *Plasmodium yoelii nigeriensis:* A scanning electron microscope study. *Protistologica* **11**, 31–39.

Sinden, R. E., and Croll, N. A. (1975). Cytology and kinetics of microgametogenesis and fertilization in *Plasmodium yoelii nigeriensis. Parasitology* **70**, 53–65.

Sinden, R. E., Canning, E. U., Bray, R. S., and Smalley, M. E. (1978). Gametocyte and gamete development in *Plasmodium falciparum*. *Proc. R. Soc., Ser. B* **201**, 375–399.

Sinton, J. A., and Mulligan, H. W. (1932). A critical review of the literature relating to the identification of the malarial parasites recorded from monkeys of the families Cercopithecidae and Colobidae. *Rec. Malar. Surv. India* **3**, 357–380.

Sivagnanasundaram, C. (1973). Reproduction rates of infection during the 1967–1968 *P. vivax* epidemic in Sri Lanka (Ceylon). *J. Trop. Med. Hyg.* **76**, 83–86.

Sluiter, C. P., Swellengrebel, N. H., and Ihle, J. E. (1922). "De dierlijke Parasieten van den Mensch en van onze Huisdieren," 3rd ed. Scheltema & Holkema, Amsterdam.

Speer, C. A., Rosales-Ronquillo, M. C., and Silverman, P. H. (1975). Motility of *Plasmodium berghei* ookinetes *in vitro*. *J. Invertrbr. Pathol.* **25**, 73–78.

Stephens, J. W. W. (1922). A new malaria parasite of man. *Ann. Trop. Med. Parasitol.* **16**, 383–388.

Sterling, C. R., Aikawa, M., and Vanderberg, J. P. (1973). The passage of *Plasmodium berghei* sporozoites through the salivary glands of *Anopheles stephensi:* An electron microscope study. *J. Parasitol.* **59**, 593–605.

Stille, W. (1979). Chloroquine-resistente Malaria tropica nach Kenia-Reise. *Deutsche Medizinische Wochenschrift* **104**, 954–955.

Strome, C. P. A., and Beaudoin, R. L. (1974). The surface of the malaria parasite. I. Scanning electron microscopy of the oocyst. *Exp. Parasitol.* **36**, 131–142.

Sulzer, A. J., Cantella, R., Colichon, A., Gleason, N. N., and Walls, K. W. (1975). A focus of hyperendemic *Plasmodium malariae—P. vivax* with no *P. falciparum* in a primitive population in the Peruvian Amazonian jungle: Studies by means of immunofluorescence and blood smear. *Bull. W. H. O.* **52**, 273–278.

Sulzer, A. J., Sulzer, K. R., Cantella, R. A., Colichon, H., Latorre, C. R., and Welch, M. (1978). Study of coinciding foci of malaria and leptospirosis in the Peruvian Amazon area. *Trans. R. Soc. Trop. Med. Hyg.* **72**, 76–83.

Surtees, G. (1970). Effects of irrigation on mosquito populations and mosquito-borne diseases in man, with particular reference to ricefield extension. *Int. J. Environ. Stud.* **1**, 35–42.

Taliaferro, W. H., and Cannon, P. R. (1934). Transmission of *Plasmodium falciparum* to the howler monkey, *Alouatta* sp. II. Cellular reactions. *Am. J. Hyg.* **19**, 335–342.

Taliaferro, W. H., and Taliaferro, L. G. (1934). The transmission of *Plasmodium falciparum* to the howler monkey, *Alouatta* sp. I. General nature of infections and morphology of the parasites. *Am. J. Hyg.* **19**, 318–334.

Telford, S. R., Jr. (1973). Saurian malarial parasites from Guyana: Their effect upon the validity of the family Garniidae and the genus *Garnia*, with descriptions of two new species. *Int. J. Parasitol.* **3**, 829–842.

Telford, S. R., Jr. (1974). The subgeneric groups of New World saurian malarias. *Proc. Int. Congr. Parasitol. 3rd, 1974* Sect. A 1 (11).

Telford, S. R., Jr., and Forrester, D. J. (1975). *Plasmodium (Huffia) hermani* sp.n. from wild turkeys *(Meleagris gallopavo)* in Florida. *J. Protozool.* **22**, 324–328.

Torti, F. (1712). "Therapeutice specialis ad febres quasdam perniciosas." Soliani, Mutinae.

Ungureanu, E., Killick-Kendrick, R., Garnham, P. C. C., Branzei, P., Romanescu, C., and Shute, P. G. (1976). Prepatent periods of a tropical strain of *Plasmodium vivax* after inoculations of tenfold dilutions of sporozoites. *Trans. R. Soc. Trop. Med. Hyg.* **70**, 482–483.

van den Berghe, L., Peel, E., Chardôme, M., and Lambrecht, F. L. (1958). Le cycle asexué de *Plasmodium atheruri* n.sp. du porc-épic *Atherurus africanus centralis* au Congo belge. *Ann. Soc. Belge Med. Trop.* **38**, 971–976.

Vanderberg, J. P. (1975). Development of infectivity by the *Plasmodium berghei* sporozoite. *J. Parasitol.* **61**, 43–50.

Vanderberg, J. P. (1977). *Plasmodium berghei:* quantitation of sporozoites injected by mosquitoes feeding on a rodent host. *Exp. Parasitol.* **42**, 169–181.

van der Kaay, H. J. (1964). Description of a new plasmodium *Plasmodium voltaicum* sp. nov. found in a fruit bat, *Roussettus smithi,* in Ghana. *Ann. Trop. Med. Parasitol.* **58**, 261–264.

van Riel, J., Hiernaux-l'Hoest, D., and Hiernaux-l'Hoest, J. (1951). Description of a *Plasmodium* found in a bat, *Roussettus leachi. Parasitology* **41**, 270–273.

Verdrager, J. (1964). Observations on the longevity of *Plasmodium falciparum,* with special reference to findings on Mauritius. *Bull. W. H. O.* **31**, 747–751.

Versiani, V., and Gomes, B. F. (1941). *Plasmodium juxtanucleare,* parasita da galinha doméstica (Notas adicionais). *Rev. Bras. Biol.* **3**, (1), 231–233.

Vincke, I. H., and Lips, M. (1948). Un nouveau *Plasmodium* d'un rongeur sauvage du Congo, *Plasmodium berghei* n.sp. *Ann. Soc. Belge Med. Trop.* **28**, 97–104.

Voller, A., Richards, W. H. G., Hawkey, C. M., and Ridley, D. S. (1969). Human malaria *(Plasmodium falciparum)* in owl monkeys *(Aotus trivirgatus). J. Trop. Med. Hyg.* **72**, 153–160.

von Wagner-Jauregg, J. (1922). Treatment of general paralysis of inoculation of malaria. *J. Neurol. & Ment. Dis.* **55**, 369–375.

Walliker, D. (1976). *In* "Genetic Aspects of Host-parasite Relationships" (A. E. R. Taylor and R. Muller, eds.), Symp. Br. Soc. Parasitol., Vol. 14, 25–44 Blackwell, Oxford.

Ward, R. A. and Cadigan, F. C., Jr. (1966). The development of erythrocytic stages of *Plasmodium falciparum* in the gibbon *Hylobates lar. Mil. Med.* **131**, 944–951.

Ward, R. A., and Hayes, D. E. (1972). Sporozoite transmission of falciparum malaria (Vietnam, Smith strain) from monkey to monkey. *Trans. R. Soc. Trop. Med. Hyg.* **66**, 670–671.

Ward, R. A., Morris, J. H., Gould, D. J., Bourke, A. T. C., and Cadigan, F. C., Jr. (1965). Susceptibility of the gibbon *Hylobates lar* to *Plasmodium falciparum. Science* **150**, 1604–1605.

Ward, R. A., Rutledge, L. C., and Hickman, R. L. (1969). Cyclical transmission of Chesson vivax malaria in subhuman primates. *Nature (London)* **224**, 1126–1127.

Warren, M., Bennett, G. F., Sandosham, A. A., and Coatney, G. R. (1965). *Plasmodium eylesi* n.sp., a tertian malaria parasite from the white-handed gibbon, *Hylobates lar. Ann. Trop. Med. Parasitol.* **59**, 500–508.

Warren, M., Coatney, G. R., and Skinner, J. C. (1966). *Plasmodium jefferyi* n.sp. from *Hylobates lar* in Malaysia. *J. Parasitol.* **52**, 9–13.

Watson, M. (1935). "Some Pages from the History of the Prevention of Malaria (Finlayson Lecture)." Alex. MacDougal, Glasgow.

Welch, W. H. (1897). Malaria: Definitions, synonyms, history and parasitology. In: Loomis & Thompson's *Syst. Pract. Med.* **1**, 17.

Wernsdorfer, G., and Wernsdorfer, W. H. (1967). Malaria im mittleren Nilbecken und dessen Randgebieten. *Z. Tropenmed. Parasitol.* **18**, 17–44.

Wernsdorfer, G., and Wernsdorfer, W. H. (1973). Arbeitsmedizinische Aspekte in den Entwicklungsländern. *Müench. Med. Wochenschr.* **115**, 1321–1328.

World Health Organization (1954). First Asian Malaria Conference. *WHO Chron.* **8**, 117–128.

World Health Organization (1955a). Resolution WHA 8:30. *Off. Rec. W. H. O.* **63**, 31.

World Health Organization (1955b). Malaria: A world problem. *WHO Chron.* **9**, 31–100.

World Health Organization (1956). Resolution WHA 9.61. *Off. Rec. W. H. O.* **71**, 43.

World Health Organization (1957). Sixth Report of the Expert Committee on Malaria. *W.H.O., Tech. Rep. Ser.* **123**.

World Health Organization (1961). Eighth Report of the Expert Committee on Malaria. *W.H.O., Tech. Rep. Ser.* **205**.

World Health Organization (1962). Epidemiological information on the status of malaria eradication. *Wkly. Epidemiol. Rec.* **37**, 498–502.

World Health Organization. (1963). ''Terminology of Malaria and of Malaria Eradication.'' WHO, Geneva.

World Health Organization (1965). Malaria eradication in 1964. *WHO Chron.* **19**, 339–353.

World Health Organization (1966a). Status of malaria eradication during the year 1965. *Wkly. Epidemiol. Rec.* **41**, 541–547.

World Health Organization (1966b). Malaria eradication in 1965. *WHO Chron.* **20**, 286–300.

World Health Organization (1967a). Status of malaria eradication during the year 1966. *Wkly. Epidemiol. Rec.* **42**, 345–354.

World Health Organization (1967b). Malaria eradication in 1966. *WHO Chron.* **21**, 373–388.

World Health Organization (1968a). Status of malaria eradication during the year 1967. *Wkly. Epidemiol. Rec.* **43**, 423–436.

World Health Organization (1968b). Fourteenth Report of the Expert Committee on Malaria. *W.H.O., Tech. Rep. Ser.* **382.**

World Health Organization (1969a). Status of malaria eradication during the year 1968. *Wkly. Epidemiol. Rec.* **44**, 535–546.

World Health Organization (1969b). Malaria eradication in 1968. *WHO Chron.* **23**, 513–523.

World Health Organization (1969c). Resolution WHA 22.39. *Off. Rec. W. H. O.* **176**, 18 and Annex 13.

World Health Organization (1970a). Status of malaria eradication during the year 1969. *Wkly. Epidemiol. Rec.* **45**, 429–445.

World Health Organization (1970b). Malaria eradication in 1969. *WHO Chron.* **24**, 395–403.

World Health Organization (1971a). Status of malaria eradication during the year 1976. *Wkly. Epidemiol. Rec.* **46**, 293–305.

World Health Organization (1971b). Malaria eradication in 1970. *WHO Chron.* **25**, 498–504.

World Health Organization (1972a). Status of malaria eradication during the year 1971. *Wkly. Epidemiol. Rec.* **47**, 353–368.

World Health Organization (1972b). Malaria eradication in 1971. *WHO Chron.* **26**, 485–496.

World Health Organization (1973a). Status of malaria eradication during the year 1972. *Wkly. Epidemiol. Rec.* **48**, 329–340.

World Health Organization (1973b). Malaria eradication and other antimalaria activities in 1972. *WHO Chron.* **27**, 516–524.

World Health Organization (1974a). Malaria control in countries where time-limited eradication is impracticable at present. *W.H.O., Tech. Rep. Ser.* **537.**

World Health Organization (1974b). The malaria situation in 1973. *WHO Chron.* **28**, 479–487.

World Health Organization (1974c). Sixteenth Report of the Expert Committee on Malaria. *W.H.O., Tech. Rep. Ser.* **549.**

World Health Organization (1975a). Six-monthly information on the world malaria situation January–December 1973. *Wkly. Epidemiol. Rec.* **50**, 53–69 and 76–86.

World Health Organization (1975b). The malaria situation in 1974. *WHO Chron.* **29**, 474–481.

World Health Organization (1975c). Information on the world malaria situation January–December 1974. *Wkly. Epidemiol. Rec.* **50**, 377–390, 402–406, and 410–419.

World Health Organization (1977a). Information on the world malaria situation January–December 1975. *Wkly. Epidemiol. Rec.* **52**, 21–34, 45–51, and 66–73.

World Health Organization (1977b). Information on the world malaria situation January–December 1976. *Wkly. Epidemiol. Rec.* **52**, 325–327, 333–339, 341–347, 349–353, 359–362, and 366–370.

World Health Organization (1978a). Information on malaria risk for international travellers. *Wkly. Epidemiol. Rec.* **53**, 181–186 and 189–196.

World Health Organization (1978b). Malaria control—A reoriented strategy. *WHO Chron.* **32**, 226–236.

World Health Organization (1978c). Malaria surveillance. A *Plasmodium malariae* outbreak. *Wkly Epidem. Rec.* 53, 240.

World Health Organization (1979a). Information on the World Malaria Situation January-December 1977. *Wkly Epidem. Rec.* 54, 105–107, 114–119, 133–135, 146–149, 162–166, 170–175.

World Health Organization (1979b). Seventeenth Report of the Expert Committee on Malaria. *Techn. Rep. Ser.* **646.**

Yoeli, M., and Hargreaves, B. J. (1974). Brain capillary blockage produced by a virulent strain of rodent malaria. *Science* **184,** 572–573.

Young M. D., and Baerg, D. C. (1969). Experimental infections of *Plasmodium falciparum* in *Cebus capucinus* (white faced capuchin) monkeys. *Mil. Med.* **134,** 767–771.

Young, M. D., and Porter, J. A., Jr. (1969). Susceptibility of *Ateles fusiceps, Ateles geoffroyi* and *Cebus capucinus* monkeys to *Plasmodium vivax. Trans. R. Soc. Trop. Med. Hyg.* **63,** 203–205.

Young, M. D., and Rossan, R. N. (1969). *Plasmodium falciparum* induced in the squirrel monkey, *Saimiri sciureus. Trans. R. Soc. Trop. Med. Hyg.* **63,** 686–687.

Young, M. D., Porter, J. A., Jr., and Johnson, C. M. (1966). *Plasmodium vivax* transmitted from man to monkey to man. *Science* **153,** 1006–1007.

Young, M. D., Baerg, D. C., and Rossan, R. N. (1971). Sporozoite transmission and serial blood passage of *Plasmodium vivax* in squirrel monkeys *Saimiri sciureus). Trans. R. Soc. Trop. Med. Hyg.* **65,** 835–836.

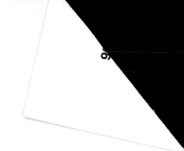

2

Malaria in Its Various Vertebrate Hosts

P. C. C. Garnham

Malaria, Vol. 1
Copyright © 1980 by Academic Press, Inc.
All rights of reproduction in any form reserved.
ISBN 0-12-426101-9

I. COMMON FEATURES

A. General Characteristics of Malaria as a Disease

The clinical picture of malaria is well known in man, and some of its features are also seen in lower primates; they are less discernible in other mammals, a few characters may be found in birds, but practically none are visible in reptiles. This progressive diminution of common characters in members of the animal kingdom indicates the potential value of the different forms of animal malaria as models for the human disease; the higher apes are likely to be the most useful, and the reptiles the least. But the clinical picture of the human disease comprises the classic division into (physical) signs and (subjective) symptoms; the latter are ascertained by questioning the patient and can no more be obtained in animals than in children before they can talk.

The clinical aspects of the disease as a rule are easily recognized, but there are many exceptions, and a well-known aphorism is that "malaria may assume protean forms." The primary result of malaria is the rupture of infected erythrocytes and the escape of a "toxic" substance into the bloodstream. The toxin gives rise to a sequence of events, which in man is as follows: a feeling of chilliness, shivering, headache, and a rise in temperature up to 39°–41°C; after about 6 hours the paroxysm ends with profuse sweating, the headache disappears, and the sufferer waits for the next bout after the characteristic quotidian, tertian, or quartan interval that is inevitable in the absence of treatment. The symptoms are, of course, inapparent in animals, and even the measurements of pyrexia are inadequate because of the wide fluctuations of temperature in normal animals. Nevertheless, certain effects of a malaria infection are found in all animals, e.g., anemia from the direct or indirect destruction of red blood corpuscles, enlargement of the spleen, and the deposition of malaria pigment in various organs and tissues of the body. Details of the biochemical and pathological changes are given in this volume, Chapters 1 and 5 and Volume 2, Chapter 2.

Immunity has a profound effect on the clinical course of an infection. It may be natural or acquired, and neither treatment of an individual case nor prophylaxis in the community can be satisfactorily conducted unless the details of the immune status are fully appreciated. The subject of clinical malaria must be viewed against this all-important background. Racial features are highly significant; e.g., the avian parasite *Plasmodium gallinaceum* produces only a mild disease in the "country fowls" of Sri Lanka but causes devastating epizootics in exotic breeds imported into the island; *P. falciparum* is relatively mild in the indigenous inhabitants of holoendemic areas in Africa but is severe or fatal in Caucasian immigrants or in Africans from malaria-free localities; *P. knowlesi* gives rise to chronic infections in its natural host, *Macaca fascicularis (irus)*, but is uniformly fatal to *M. mulatta* (the rhesus monkey). Special genetic conditions, such as the presence of Hemoglobin S, the absence of the Duffy factor, and a deficiency of certain enzymes (e.g. glucose-6-phosphate dehydrogenase) greatly affect the severity of certain species of *Plasmodium* infections in man and some of these are considered briefly in Section II,A,1 and 2). The age of the host is of general importance in practically all forms of malaria; this has been studied particularly in human and avian malaria, and examples are discussed in Section II,F.

B. Periodicity

The time factor in malaria, as in most examples of infective diseases, is of prime clinical interest. For malaria there is the characteristic incubation period. In some diseases, however, there is no "biological" incubation period, i.e., no interval during which the infective agent has to undergo a course of development before reaching maturity. For this reason, it is necessary, to use terminology which describes these events, and in addition to the rather vague expression "incubation period," the more explicit term "prepatent period" has been introduced. The incubation period is defined (World Health Organization, 1963) as the "time elapsing between the initial malaria infection in man and the first clinical manifestation"; the prepatent period is defined (Garnham, 1966) as "the minimal time elapsing between the initial sporozoite infection and the first appearance of parasites in the erythrocytes." In experimental malaria, and for a true understanding of the disease, it is essential to consider the prepatent period, which is fixed and characteristic in each species of parasite. In practice, the prepatent period is determined by observing parasites in thick blood films, but their actual appearance can only be demonstrated with certainty by the inoculation of large quantities of blood (the "isodiagnosis" of Sergent, 1963). The incubation period is the first appearance of symptoms after infection and may be of considerable length, though it is usually at least 2 days longer than the prepatent period, during which interval parasites have multiplied sufficiently in the blood to reach a certain "pyrogenic threshold level."

In mosquito-transmitted infections, the prepatent period of human malaria is never less than 5 days (in *P. falciparum*), though a few doubtful records 3–4 days have been published (de Sanctis Monaldi, 1953). Precise dates may be valuable in taking the history of a patient in relation to exposure to bites. On the other hand, in unnatural methods of transmission when the blood forms of the parasite have been inoculated, as among drug addicts by syringe passage (Most, 1940), in blood transfusions, or in malaria therapy (see Section II,B), there is no true prepatent period because (theoretically) the parasites could immediately become detectable by the subinoculation of blood into a susceptible host. The incubation period in these cases varies according to the number of parasites introduced. Congenital malaria, in which parasites pass from an infected mother transplacentally to the fetus or from blood during parturition, is a rare event in man; the clinical features are discussed in Section II,A,3.

The natural prepatent period corresponds exactly to the duration of growth of the sporozoite into the mature exoerythrocytic schizont, its rupture, and the simultaneous invasion of the blood by its merozoites. The minimum duration should be measured, because within a few hours the great majority of the schizonts of primate species reach maturity and only a few stragglers may persist for several more days. The more quickly developing rodent species have an equally characteristic periodicity, as probably do also avian species; the latter present more difficulties because two generations (cryptozoic and metacryptozoic) have to undergo development during the prepatent period.

The periodicity of "fever" has been described since the time of Hippocrates, and its significance was determined in human malaria by Golgi (in the so-called Golgi cycles corresponding to the maturation of erythrocytic schizonts of the three common human species). Apart from the existence of two or more broods of parasites, giving rise to double tertian or triple quartan infections with quotidian fever, some species exhibit little periodicity, the schizonts apparently having failed to follow a specific timetable. Such aperiodic infections are particularly seen in rodent malaria and in some avian species. Periodicity is apt to be lost in fulminating infections.

No satisfactory explanation has been found for the ability of all the schizonts to mature at about the same time. The commonest cycle in primate malaria is one of 48 hours; there is a special and smaller group of quartan malarias in which the blood cycle occupies 72 hours, and a single primate species—*P. knowlesi*—which has a cycle of 24 hours. These periodicities bear some relationship to the duration of other stages of the life cycles—the length of sporogony in the mosquito and the exoerythrocytic stage in the liver. Table I compares the figures for a few typical species.

Some investigators (e.g., Hawking *et al.*, 1968) have tried to link the periodicity of gametocytes with the time of day when mosquitoes are most active and

TABLE I

Duration of Developmental Stages in Human Malaria Parasites

Species	Exoerythrocytic schizogony (days)	Erythrocytic schizogony (days)	Sporogony minimum (days)
P. vivax	8	2	8
P. ovale	9	2	12
P. falciparum	5½	2	9
P. malariae	15	3	16

capable of providing a site for the next stage of development of the parasite. Other workers (e.g., Taliaferro and Taliaferro, 1934; Demina, 1959) associated periodicity with light and darkness and were able to prolong the cycles of primate and avian malaria parasites, respectively. Garnham (1966) has suggested that shortly before maturation of the blood schizonts there is a profound alteration in the metabolic requirements of the parasite; it requires DNA in large quantities, and it can be postulated that the precursor of DNA is produced periodically by the host, e.g., via hormones or through the night–day stimulus. It could also be assumed that this explains the *synchronicity* of development, for the growing parasites would have to wait until the DNA became available before they could begin their final schizogony, and then they would all partake of this substance together.

The phenomenon of periodicity provides good criteria for the diagnosis of species of *Plasmodium;* it allows a preliminary classification into three main categories (quotidian, tertian, and quartan) and provides specific features of interest in regard to sporogonic and tissue stages of the parasites; small but constant modifications in the duration of these various stages are also useful for the separation of some subspecies.

Although periodicity of a well-defined nature is emphasized, like all biological phenomenon it is not absolutely constant, and the 48-hour duration of erythrocytic schizogony may be 49 hours in some strains of *P. ovale.* Some early authors even used the expression "subtertian malaria" for a special type of *P. falciparum* infection in which schizogony in the blood was thought to take 36 instead of 48 hours.

C. Relapses

Of the four prominent clinical characters of malaria (namely, the paroxysm, periodicity, splenomegaly, and relapse), the last-mentioned is the most mysterious, its nature remaining incompletely explained until very recently. Coatney (1976) and Garnham (1977a) discussed this question in some detail and emphasized two points. First, relapses in primate malaria are due to the survival in the liver of dormant sporozoites which become reactivated by an unknown trigger after a certain interval. Second, a true relapse is confined to a few species of malaria parasites.

Late or delayed forms of primate malaria parasites had been seen in the liver since 1948 when Shortt and Garnham described exoerythrocytic schizonts of *Plasmodium cynomolgi cynomologi* 102 days after inoculation of sporozoites; they were about 35 μm in diameter, often with a slightly crinkled, convoluted border, and the nuclei were in a state of division. Similar forms were found in chimpanzees inoculated with *P. vivax,* the most delayed being found by Rodhain 275 days after sporozoites had been inoculated. During the 30 years since their first demonstration, such late or relapse forms were seen from time to time, but little more light was thrown on the phenomonon; however the theory of successive cycles of development in the liver was replaced by the theory that the sporozoite or its immediate successor remained dormant in a parenchyma cell.

Searches for resting forms were always unsuccessful until Krotoski *et al.* (1980), working with *P. cynomologi bastianellii,* at last revealed by immunofluorescent technique (and later by Giemsa staining) the present of uninucleate bodies, 7 days and 50 days after the inoculation of sporozoites, in biopsies of the liver. The "hypnozoites" lay inside parenchyma cells, were oval in shape and measured a mean of 4.5 μm in the earlier and 6.6 in the latter; the nuclei were invariably single and stained deeply with Giemsa. These hypnozoites are assumed to be the long- sought latent forms which ultimately become reactivated and cause relapses. The large multinucleate parasites, present both in this material (at 102 days) and occasionally in the past, represent the hypnozoites after reactivation.

A relapse is defined as a renewed manifestation of malarial infection separated from previous manifestations of the same infection by an interval greater than the 48 or 72 hours between the paroxysms. This is a general term for all types of recrudescences; a true or biological relapse unfortunately may not be a clinical phenomenon. However, it is essential to understand it in order to differentiate between relapses and recrudescences for which a different form of therapy is required. A recrudescence is defined (by World Health Organization, 1963) as a renewed manifestation of infection believed due to the survival of erythrocytic forms. Recrudescences may recur in infections of any species of malaria parasite.

The special characters of relapses (and recrudescences) are discussed separately under the individual species, but the following characters are common to the phenomena in general. (1) Relapses can only occur after sporozoite induction of the infection and are absent in blood-induced disease; and (2) relapses cannot be prevented by treatment of the primary attack or by prophylaxis with quinine or other blood schizonticides (e.g., chloroquine). There are several interesting parasitological features of relapses which are only briefly mentioned here; e.g., relapses only occur in infections in which the parasitized corpuscles are stippled with Schuffner's dots; there are no parasites in the blood between relapses; gametocytes may be found in the blood on the first day of the relapse; the "relapse exoerythrocytic schizont" sometimes has a crinkled envelope in primate malaria or even a cyst wall in avian malaria (*Leucocytozoon simondi,* Desser *et al.*, 1968).

The clinical picture in a relapse is much the same as that of the primary infection except that the fever is tertian from the start (instead of quotidian which frequently characterizes *P. vivax* infections). Later relapses tend to be less severe than earlier ones.

D. Cause of Death

Some forms of malaria are peculiarly lethal to their vertebrate hosts, of which the following are examples: *P. falciparum* in man, *P. knowlesi* in rhesus monkeys, *P. berghei* in mice, *P. elongatum* in canaries, and *P. floridense* in some lizards.

There is a profound difference in the cause of death in human and avian malaria. Obstruction of the cerebral vessels occurs in both, but in *P. falciparum* infections death is due to blockage by an accumulation of erythrocytic schizonts in the lumen, while in *P. gallinaceum* the exoerythrocytic schizonts grow in the capillary endothelial cells and obstruct the blood flow.

A less specific mechanism is seen when the blood infection fulminates to such an extent that the oxygen-carrying capacity of the corpuscles is reduced (though Maegraith, 1977, minimizes the extent of anoxemic anoxia), and the products of their destruction have a toxic effect. Anemia may proceed more slowly but eventually will result in the death of the host, sometimes by exhaustion of the blood-forming cells in the bone marrow, as occurs in avian and saurian malaria. Specialized effects of an indirect type are discussed in Section IV,G.

The three main causes of death are thus obstruction of the circulation of blood in vital organs, fulminant blood infections, and anemia. The brunt of the disease falls largely on the blood, and it is interesting to note that the so-called malaria parasites, now placed in the genus *Hepatocystis* and confined to multiplication in exoerythrocytic schizogony in the liver, are nonpathogenic, as the blood infection is limited to gametocytes. Moreover, the antigenicity of gametocytes and of the merocysts from which they arise in the liver is so low that immunity is absent, e.g., in *H. kochi* infections.

It is often stated that malaria lowers the resistance of the individual to other diseases, and this opinion is supported by the vital statistics on infant mortality, which is remarkably lessened after successful antimalarial campaigns; not only is there a decline in deaths from malaria but from respiratory and gastrointestinal diseases also.

The presence of malaria parasites in the blood does not necessarily indicate that the principal disease from which the patient is suffering is malaria; it is equally fallacious to assume that the cause of death is malaria because parasites have been found in the blood. In some parts of the tropics 50% or more of the population may exhibit parasitemia, and clearly it would be a mistake to give undue weight to this finding as necessarily having diagnostic significance. Yet the evidence is often misinterpreted, and such figures should be critically examined in community medicine, for the practitioner may possibly miss a hidden bronchopneumonia or mistake meningitis for cerebral malaria because malaria parasites have been found in the blood—it is a trap for the unwary.

E. Sensitization

Certain immunopathological effects are well known in human malaria, particularly blackwater fever and quartan nephrosis, while the anemia often accompanying the disease is now known to be partly an autoantigen antibody reaction in both the human and animal forms of the malady. These subjects are discussed in relation to species, but it would be interesting to seek models among the animal malarias for blackwater and the nephrotic syndrome. Some attempts have been made to demonstrate the latter condition in the quartan parasite (*P. inui*) of monkeys but have met with little success; blackwater was produced in splenectomized chimpanzees infected with piroplasms (Garnham and Bray, 1959) but not with *P. falciparum*. See also Section VI,C.

F. Host Factors

Apart from immunity and various genetic effects, the host–parasite relationship is much influenced by more general factors.

The susceptibility of the host is usually greatest in the youngest animals, provided that no passive immunity has been transmitted from the mother; however, the latter protection fades in less than 3 months after birth. Various other influences are then in operation. If the infant's diet is restricted to milk, which contains no *p*-aminobenzoic acid, the progress of a malaria infection will be inhibited, as the organism requires this metabolite for the synthesis of folic acid (Hawking, 1953); other more artificial circumstances may reduce the baneful effects of malaria in the human child who may be less exposed to mosquito bites by the use of nets or even because there is less skin surface on which the mosquitoes can feed. As the animal grows older, in many instances, it becomes naturally less susceptible; thus *P. gallinaceum* undergoes a rapid and prolific course of development in 1-day-old chicks, whereas the adult bird is only feebly susceptible. On the other hand, an infection of *P. berghei* is equally virulent and lethal both in baby and adult mice.

The nutritional status of the host is an important factor in the progress of a malaria infection; starvation of the host or marasmus induced by another disease such as tuberculosis interferes with normal development of the parasite. Under conditions of severe famine the severity of malaria epidemics may be lessened because the parasite shares the malnutrition of the host, while badly kept animals in a laboratory make poor models of the disease.

The presence or absence of a spleen is of supreme importance in malaria (Garnham, 1970b) and, though the absence of a spleen is rarely a factor in human malaria (but see Section II,A,1), splenectomy is much used in experimental malaria of other mammals. The removal, either before or after infection, of the largest source of immunologically active cells (particularly B and T lymphocytes) renders the animal much more susceptible. Splenectomy of an abnormal host may render it completely susceptible, while removal of the spleen can convert a subpatent chronic infection into one of rampancy. Thereafter the parasites decline in numbers but often persist for the remainder of the life of the host. These revivified infections are usually accompanied by a good crop of viable gametocytes and are thus of much value in studies on the life cycle of the parasite.

G. Species of Malaria Parasites

Each species of *Plasmodium* is of course a zoological entity and causes a specific disease with its own particular characters. Thus human malaria is no more a single disease than is typhus. Strains of the parasite vary in many directions—clinical, response to drugs, behavior in mosquitoes, and behavior in the vertebrate host. Such variations may become so fixed that immunological differences become established, and eventually minor morphological changes become visible. In the last transformations, it is useful to regard the strain as a subspecies. Although differences have often been described in the human species, most workers have been loathe to give them separate taxonomic status (Wenyon, 1926). Various strains of *P. falciparum* have been given subspecific or even specific names such as *P. tenue* (Stephens, 1914), but none has survived except perhaps *P. vivax hibernans* (Nicolaev, 1949) with its clearly described clinical course and constant long prepatency.

II. MALARIA IN MAN

A. Specific Types

Four diseases occur in man; they are due, respectively, to *P. falciparum, P. vivax, P. malariae, and P. ovale. Plasmodium malariae* is also found in the chimpanzee, while species closely allied to *P. falciparum* (namely, *P. reichenowi*) and *P. vivax* (namely, *P. schwetzi*) occur in both the chimpanzee and gorilla. Man is rarely infected in nature with certain simian species and has been shown to be susceptible to others in the laboratory. The clinical features had been described earlier in greater or lesser detail in various textbooks of tropical medicine, but the advent of malaria therapy (see Section II,B) in the treatment of general paresis provided an opportunity for studying the infections under controlled conditions (see, for example, the excellent accounts given by Boyd, Stratman-Thomas, and Kitchen in a symposium on human malaria in 1941 based on this technique).

1. Plasmodium falciparum

This parasite was once the supreme killer of mankind and is still of great importance; the disease it produces is the well-named malignant tertian malaria. The remarks about the protean manifestation of malaria apply particularly to *P. falciparum,* which is peculiar in that it retreats to the capillaries and sinuses of the internal organs for completion of schizogony. This behavior makes malignant tertian malaria the arch simulator; there are innumerable conditions which have been rightly or wrongly attributed to it, from appendicitis, cholecystitis, hyperpyrexia, and myocardial infections to impotence and mental deficiency, to name but a small fraction. Castellani and Chalmers (1919) referred to malignant tertian malaria as the great "mimic," and its differential diagnosis from other diseases may be puzzling unless a blood film is examined.

Although *P. falciparum* malaria is the greatest killer, it is the most easily cured. In the tropics, most cases present no difficulty in diagnosis, and the disease is relatively mild if promptly treated; it is then less severe and less dangerous than an attack of influenza. This statement presupposes the existence of competent medical services; thick and thin blood films should be taken immediately and stained and examined by an experienced person. The following points are essential:

1. The stain must be of proved quality, and the distilled water must be at a pH of 7.0–7.4. If these requirements are not satisfied, the parasites may remain invisible or the species unidentifiable.

2. The films should be made before the patient receives any antimalarial treatment.

3. Repeated slides should be taken if results are negative.

4. If the diagnosis remains in doubt, the patient should be given antimalarial treatment.

It is seldom necessary to resort to serological examination which in the earliest stages of the disease may well give a negative result; however, the titer of immunofluorescence rises quickly (after the first week), and this technique can be useful in some circumstances.

Outside the tropics, the situation is quite different because of the absence today in most places of the indigenous disease. Yet travelers from abroad may well contract malaria which is suppressed by prophylactic drugs and becomes manifest when their administration is suspended. Then the danger arises; a person from abroad develops an acute febrile disease which is mistaken for influenza or some other infection; no blood slides are taken, the patient receives no specific treatment, and his or her condition steadily deteriorates until eventually hospital admission is sought; then the diagnosis of malaria is at last made—not infrequently too late. Table II illustrates the occurrence of imported malaria in England and Wales in 1970–1979 and shows that there were over 50 fatalities; in the preceding 15 years, there were at least 58 deaths. In 1978, the Center for

TABLE II

Malaria Cases and Deaths in England and Wales, 1970–1979

Year	Cases	Deaths (*P. falciparum*)
1970	101	5
1971	261	9
1972	337	7
1973	541	3
1974	662	2
1975	749	5
1976	1220	3
1977	1527	7
1978	1681	8
1979	2503	5

Shute (1970) reported the occurrence of over 2000 imported cases in the previous 15 years with a mortality rate of 4%.

Disease Control, Atlanta, reported the occurrence of 616 cases of malaria in the United States with six deaths.

Pernicious malaria may be divided into various categories of which the most important is cerebral malaria. This syndrome occurs in two clinical forms, true and false. The latter is seen when there is a generalized fulminating septicemic infection with delirium, toxemia, high fever, and early death, but there is no particular localization in the brain. True cerebral malaria occurs when there is extensive blockage of the cerebral capillaries. The pathological changes which follow are described in detail in Volume 2, Chapter 2. The vessels are blocked most commonly throughout both the gray and white matter of the cerebrum and cerebellum, and the patient sinks into a gradually deepening coma. Breathing becomes stertorous, the pupils are contracted, knee jerks may be absent, and the plantar response is extensor; incontinence is not uncommon. Marsden and Bruce-Chwatt (1975) refer to the alterations in the level of consciousness, beginning with a disturbance in normal behavior and mental confusion and progressing to delirium and eventual loss of consciousness. Such conditions may not be recognized as malarial in origin, and the victim may be thought to be suffering from acute alcoholism and confined to a prison cell.

Less often the impact is felt in particular regions of the brain, and different varieties of cerebral malaria were described by Marchiafava and Bignami (1892) and by numerous clinicians in subsequent years. If the motor area is particularly affected, hemiplegia or Jacksonian epilepsy ensues; localization in Broca's area is followed by aphasia; if the heat centers in the pons are affected, there is hyperpyrexia; in the hindbrain symptoms of bulbar paralysis develop, and in the basal ganglia choreiform movements ensue; involvement of the meninges presents as meningismus. Localizing signs are, however, rare and, when present, are often transitory (Marsden and Bruce-Chwatt, 1975). The pathogenesis of these focal forms of cerebral malaria is uncertain.

The diagnosis of cerebral malaria may be difficult, both ante- and postmortem, and especially in fatal cases when death has been delayed by the effects of drug treatment: Malarial granulomata persist in the brain, but most of the parasites have been destroyed. Such cases may be misdiagnosed as uremia, cerebral hemorrhage, alcoholism, or various tropical encephalitides or meningitis.

In young children, the first paroxysms of *P. falciparum* malaria may pass unnoticed, and the disease not recognized until the child has convulsions which are soon replaced by coma.

Algid malaria was once thought to be the result of blockage of blood vessels in the pituitary gland, but the condition is now (Maegraith, 1970) thought to be an end result of the general pathophysiology, ending in "medical shock." The eyes are sunken, the skin cold and clammy, breathing is shallow and fast, and the blood pressure sinks rapidly. Antishock therapy (by blocking agents) is now thought to be even more important than antimalarial drugs.

Other forms of pernicious malaria are much less common, though, curiously enough, they sometimes occur in the form of small epidemics. Thus the intestinal variety in which the capillaries of the large and small intestines are blocked gives rise to symptoms of acute dysentery, and treatment may be disastrously delayed. Choleraic symptoms have been described in children in whom dehydration is quickly fatal. Sir John Boyd (personal communication) encountered a peculiar form of intestinal malaria in soldiers in the Macedonian campaign of 1916; the disease appeared as acute appendicitis, and the capillaries in the submucosa of the organ were found to be blocked with schizonts of *P. falciparum*. Cardiac forms are usually fatal following blockage of the capillaries in the myocardium; a pulmonary type is due to blockage of the alveolar vessels, giving rise to a secondary pneumonia. Barbier (1978) calls attention to the almost certain mortality produced by acute edema of the lung, which sometimes supervenes in pernicious malaria.

The classic theories of Maegraith (expressed originally in his book "Pathological Processes in Malaria," 1948, expanded in subsequent writings, e.g., 1970, and finally summarized in the Craig Lecture, 1977) give the clue to the clinical phenomena of pernicious malaria: The presence in the blood of a chemical factor (as yet undetermined, but with a molecular weight of less than 1000) excites the sympathetic nervous system, with increasing disturbance of the blood circulation by constriction of the smaller vessels; there is a chain reaction, eventually reaching the mitochondria, and the end result is a condition of "shock." (See also Volume 2, Chapter 2.)

Two other fatal effects of *P. falciparum* infections are attributed to sensitization phenomena, well known as potential dangers but still incompletely explained. They are blackwater fever and acute hemolytic anemia in children. Blackwater fever was shown by Stephens and Christophers as long ago as 1901 to be associated with irregular and inadequate treatment of attacks of malignant tertian malaria with quinine. Discovery of the exact mechanism seemed to be on the point of discovery when the use of this drug was superseded by quinacrine and 4-aminoquinoline therapy; the opportunity was thus lost. The apparent explanation of the phenomenon may be as follows. The quininized and parasitized erythrocyte acts as an antigen against which are formed hemolysins; when a dose of quinine is next administered, intravascular hemolysis takes place, methemoglobin is produced, and the kidney is damaged first in the cortex and later, as a result of ischemia and blockage of the capillaries, in the tubules. The excretory function of the organ is lessened, and eventually anuria occurs; at the same time, a very severe anemia is produced. Hemoglobinuria is the prominent and terrifying symptom; the presence of methemoglobin renders the color of the urine dark brown or black. The mortality rate varies in different countries but sometimes reached 50%. It used to be said that it was disastrous to move a patient and that a shelter should be built around him rather than transporting him to a hospital. Many peculiarities of blackwater fever remain unexplained, e.g., its localization to particular areas, even to groups of houses or individual valleys; a special strain of the parasite was thought to be responsible, but no morphological differences were observed on closer investigation.

The signs of blackwater fever are characteristic. The patient was usually a person who had led a rough existence in a holoendemic area and had taken a tablet or two of quinine when he felt off-color. After a few months, or more often years, of such a life the swallowing of the drug was almost immediately followed by malaise, apprehension, pyrexia, and the sudden passage of black (or occasionally red) urine. Within a day, the patient became jaundiced and prostrated. The spleen and liver were enlarged, and anemia pronounced. Even if blood films were taken early, no, or only very scanty, malaria parasites were demonstrable. This dreaded sequela of *P. falciparum* malaria is now extremely rare, but a few cases have been reported after the administration of chloroquine (Maegraith, 1970) and even in association with *P. vivax* infections. Even in the worst blackwater areas, the disease was thought to be confined to Europeans or Indians, though a few cases were seen in black troops who returned to West Africa in War II after a long spell in Burma where they were exposed to different strains of the parasite (Maegraith, 1970).

Hemolytic anemia is a cause of death in African infants in areas of holoendemic malaria. In a series of 22 infantile deaths from this disease, 2 were found to be due to hemolytic anemia of *P. falciparum* origin (Garnham, 1949). The course of this syndrome is very rapid and is usually fatal.

The drugs used in the treatment of malaria are occasionally responsible for toxic signs or symptoms in the recipient. When mepacrine (quinacrine) was in common use for the treatment of malignant tertian malaria, apart from the pronounced yellow discoloration of the skin (rarely followed by lichen planus), transient mania or delusional insanity arose, frightening at first but quickly disappearing when the drug was stopped. Quinine used to be given in rather high doses (e.g., 2 g/day for possibly 2 or 3 weeks) and inevitably caused deafness, but sometimes amblyopia followed and the patient remained blind for months. Prolonged treatment with chloroquine can cause extensive macular degeneration which may be irreversible. Recently, overdosage of the latter drug has been shown by Edwards *et al.* (1978) to cause almost complete heart block with a ventricular rate of 15 beats/minute.

True relapses probably do not occur in malignant tertian malaria, but recrudescences are common in spite of full courses of chloroquine or other schizontocides. Recrudescences are brought about by a variety of stresses, excessive exercise, pregnancy, exposure to cold (e.g., swimming in the sea in temperate climates after a return from the tropics), etc. The parasite is comparatively short-lived, though there are rare and apparently true records that it may have a life of 4 years. The longevity of *P. falciparum* and of the other human species is shown in detail in Table III.

The schizogonic cycle of *P. falciparum* in the blood is 48 hours; shorter intervals have been reported (see above) but are probably due to a partial collapse of synchronicity, perhaps as a result of sequestration of the maturing schizonts in a variety of internal organs. The prepatent period (the cycle in the liver) was shown by Fairley (1947), Shortt *et al.* (1951), and Jeffery *et al.* (1952) to occupy $5\frac{1}{2}$–6 days in human volunteers, and this duration was confirmed by Bray (1958) who inoculated sporozoites of a Liberian strain of *P. falciparum* into chimpanzees. In the latter case mature schizonts were not found until 6 days, possibly because the chimpanzee is not a natural host of the parasite.

The severity of malignant tertian malaria is much affected by different factors

TABLE III

Longevity of Untreated Human Malaria[a]

Species	Approximate average duration (years)	Maximum duration (years)
P. falciparum	1	4
P. vivax	2	8
P. ovale	1	5
P. malariae	4	53

[a] From Garnham (1970a).

of which two are of special interest; one is genetic, and the other is the partial protection afforded by the spleen.

The clinical response and mortality are definitely lowered in heterozygotes for the hemaglobin S. gene (Allison and Clark, 1977). The evidence for this has been analyzed in great detail by Allison (1961) who has shown that a state of balanced polymorphism occurs in populations in which *P. falciparum* is endemic and the gene for this trait is frequent; a biological advantage operates for the heterozygotes, and mortality from this type of malaria is much lower than usual. Evidence for the protective effect of a genetic deficiency of the enzyme glucose-6-phosphate dehydrogenase was at first less convincing. Eventually Luzzato (1977), from studies in the field in tropical Africa and biochemical analysis of the chain of events in the blood, was able to prove the selective advantage of this genetic defect in survival of the possessors of the trait. Multiplication of the parasites in the blood is reduced, parasitemia is low, and symptoms are relatively mild.

The role of the spleen in all forms of mammalian malaria is of great importance (Garnham, 1970b), and the absence of the organ in a person infected with *P. falciparum* is striking, as the following example (Adams, 1968) illustrates. A West African seaman underwent a splenectomy in Rotterdam in 1956; 4 years later he walked into the Tropical Diseases Clinic in Liverpool, complaining of fever and malaise. He had suffered from mild attacks in 1958 and 1959, but now his temperature was 41°C and a blood film showed a 25% invasion rate of all stages of *P. falciparum,* including large numbers of solid forms with heavy pigmentation, many schizonts with 12 merozoites, and immature crescents in the typical cigar- and spindle-shaped forms. However, he did not appear to be very ill, and cerebral symptoms were absent. Chloroquine was given, and within 48 hours the parasitemia had disappeared. His later history is unknown.

2. *Plasmodium vivax*

The common name of the disease (benign tertian malaria) denotes its milder character as contrasted with malignant tertian malaria. However, its greater persistence in the body (see Table III) is accompanied by a gradual deterioration in health, and the long-term effects may be severe; malaria cachexia is probably due more to *P. vivax* than to *P. falciparum*. The course of the disease is more predictable, though the initial fever may be irregular and usually remains quotidian for the first week. The 48-hour periodicity is then established, but the presence of two broods of schizonts may still lead to daily paroxysms. The extra brood may be abolished by the intramuscular administration of 0.2 g of Thiobismol (sodium bismuth thioglycolate), as determined in patients undergoing malaria therapy with this parasite at Horton Hospital (Whelen and Shute, 1943). If chemoprophylaxis is used, the primary attack may be delayed for a variable period (see below) and is then often tertian from the start.

The patient usually exhibits prodromal symptoms before the attack proper begins; lassitude, headache, loss of appetite, and shivering are common. The classic pattern of the paroxysm then follows: The cold stage with severe shivering lasts about an hour; the temperature begins to rise, eventually reaching 40°–41°C, and the hot stage lasts about 4 hours; profuse sweating follows, and after about 3 hours the episode is over, the headache and other symptoms lessening until the next attack begins after the tertian interval. Successive paroxysms occur, and the patient becomes weaker and anemic, and the spleen and liver increase in size; this degree of severity disappears after five or six paroxysms, and the illness is then over temporarily. In untreated patients splenomegaly may be very prominent and the organ becomes hard. Rupture of the spleen is a not infrequent complication, either early in the disease or later after blows on the abdominal wall or unusual exertion. Splenic puncture is inadvisable in the differential diagnosis of kala azar and chronic malaria owing to the possibility of bleeding; if considered essential, the patient should be confined to bed for at least 24 hours and an abdominal bandage placed in position before the puncture and tightened after it. The duration of the paroxysm varies slightly from strain to strain, and according to whether it is early or late in the attack; Coatney and Young (1942) found that the average length of paroxysms in the St. Elizabeth strain was 9 hours.

The normal prepatent period of *P. vivax* is 8 days and ends with a discharge of merozoites from the mature liver schizonts into the blood. Symptoms will arise when sufficient cycles of schizogony have been repeated in the blood, probably at least twice to give an incubation period of $8 + 4 = 12$ days.

Different strains of *P. vivax* exist and are characterized by special relapse patterns and a varying incidence of prolonged prepatency. The so-called normal, tropical, or Chesson pattern always exhibits an 8-day prepatency, and the primary attack is followed by short-term relapses at about 2 month intervals. At the other extreme is the subspecies *P. vivax hibernans* with which prepatency is invariably prolonged to about 350 days and is never less than 250 days; relapses then ensue at shorter intervals. In between these limits occur a number of strains, often with lengthy prepatency and found chiefly in the temperate regions of the world. These curious phenomena (Garnham *et al.,* 1975; Ungureanu *et al.,* 1976; Shute *et al.,* 1976) are thought to be due to the presence in *P. vivax* of two types of sporozoites in differing proportions—one giving rise to prolonged and the other to short prepatency. In some experimental cases, the primary parasitemia was delayed for as long as 637 days and the disease was then asymptomatic.

An interesting genetic factor in its vertebrate host affects the zoogeography of *P. vivax*. This parasite, although almost cosmopolitan in distribution, is absent among West African blacks; the immunity persists even when members of this race are transferred elsewhere, e.g., in the descendants of slaves taken to the New World (Young *et al.*, 1955). There is a tendency today to assign all vivax-like parasites in tropical Africa to *P. ovale* whose home is essentially the territories in West Africa in which *P. vivax* is truly absent; some infections in East Africa and Ethiopia, in particular, are now being wrongly identified as *P. ovale*, a species which certainly occurs on that side of Africa, but where *P. vivax* also undoubtedly occurs. The phenomenon was shown by Miller *et al.* (1976) to be due to the absence in West African blacks of the Duffy factor on the surface membrane of their erythrocytes; this factor is an essential receptor necessary for penetration of the corpuscle by *P. vivax*, but not of other species (except for certain vivax-like species in other primates).

3. *Plasmodium ovale*

This least common species of human malaria parasites is also the least pathogenic. The symptomatology is like that of *P. vivax*. The paroxysms, however, may sometimes be accompanied by severe headache, high fever, and occasionally jaundice. Splenomegaly is slight and becomes evident only after several weeks of infection.

Plasmodium ovale has a tertian periodicity in the blood, although the actual duration of erythrocytic schizogony is between 49 and 50 hours. Exoerythrocytic schizogony in the parenchyma cells of the liver takes 9 days, when the blood becomes invaded by the merozoites. Symptoms do not arise until about 6 days later.

Relapses and prolonged prepatent periods in this parasite are frequent. The latter are often noticed in people returning from endemic regions of the tropics (Africa and the East Indies) about 7 months after they have stopped chemoprophylaxis. Relapses then occur after intervals of about 3 months; the blood is free of parasites in between, and thus they are of the true variety. A peculiarity of the schizonts in the blood in relapses is the doubling of the number of merozoites—16 instead of 8; this unexplained phenomenon has been reported several times in human infections and also in splenectomized chimpanzees (Garnham, 1966).

The separate identity of *P. ovale* was not recognized for many years, yet today there is much confirmatory evidence. Most African blacks have been shown (Coatney *et al.*, 1971) to be fully susceptible to *P. ovale*, unlike *P. vivax* to which they are immune. There is no cross-immunity between the two species, while the morphology and behavior of the exoerythrocytic and sporogonic stages are highly distinctive.

In spite of the infrequency of congenital malaria as a whole, a definite instance of the condition in *P. ovale* malaria has been described. It occurred after a Caesarean section (Jenkins, 1957). A day before the operation, the mother became ill with *P. ovale* malaria, but the baby remained well until 3 weeks later when its temperature rose to 40°C and parasites were found in its blood. The infection of the child presumably took place during the course of the operation.

4. Plasmodium malariae

Quartan malaria was recognized in antiquity, and historical references to this disease are many; James I and Cromwell are said to have died, both in their sixtieth year, from this infection. Quartan malaria presents several unusual features; there is still no explanation for its curiously patchy distribution to which Marchoux (1926) drew attention over 50 years ago in the following words: "Il existe en sujet de la fièvre quarte une sorte de mystère non encore pénétré."

Although quartan malaria has been reported in all continents (except Antarctica), it nearly always takes third place in incidence as compared with the other common species. However, it occasionally appears in localized epidemics, e.g., on the eastern slopes of the Peruvian Amazon region and in villages in the rain forest; in one survey Sulzer *et al.* (1978) found that 83% of the population of Mission Cutiverin were suffering from the disease. The Caribbean Islands have long been known as a focus of quartan malaria, and there has been the same high incidence on the adjoining mainland in Guiana, as described by Giglioli (1930). An even clearer example of localized quartan malaria occurred in 1978 in Granada (C. C. Draper, personal communication). Malaria was eradicated from this Caribbean island in 1962; in March 1978, an old woman was found to be suffering from a chronic fever which was eventually diagnosed as an infection of *P. malariae*. Other cases followed as a result of spread of the disease by *Anopheles aquasalis*. The symptoms were mild, and splenomegaly was minimal; serological examination of the inhabitants revealed that a considerable number of inapparent infections had occurred, even in children.

In all stages of its life cycle, *P. malariae* grows more slowly than the other human species. A classic case exhibits diagnostic periodicity at intervals of 72 hours, corresponding to the maturation and rupture of the schizonts in the blood, accompanied by paroxysms of pyrexia. Sometimes the parasitemia may be so low that parasites cannot be found; yet the characteristic fever pattern indicates the nature of the disease and, eventually, if treatment is withheld, parasites will at last be found in recrudescences. Just as two broods of schizonts give rise to a double tertian fever in some *P. vivax* infections (with a rise in temperature every day), so will two broods of *P. malariae* produce fever on two successive days, leaving the third day free (i.e., a double quartan), or three broods of *P. malariae* will produce fever every day (i.e., a triple quartan).

Plasmodium malariae may persist in the blood for a much longer period than the other species and probably for the lifetime of the infected person; at least, authoritative records of up to 50 years exist (Garnham, 1966). It was once thought that this chronicity was due to the presence of recurring cycles of exoerythrocytic schizogony in the liver, but experimental work (Lupaşcu *et al.*, 1967) with a Rumanian strain (VS) indicates that the liver cycle is limited to the single initial development of the sporozoite and that subsequent recrudescences at however late a date are due to a persistent low-grade cycle in the blood. For this reason, sporozoite-induced *P. malariae* is exceptionally easy to cure with schizontocidal drugs. Some people have found it difficult to accept that true relapses do not occur in quartan malaria and continue to recommend the use of primaquine for radical cure of the infection. The following facts strongly support the contention that relapses (which by definition are of exoerythrocytic origin) are absent in quartan malaria. The late recurrences are thus recrudescences (defined as being due to persisting erythrocytic parasites).

1. *Plasmodium malariae* can be eradicated by blood schizontocides (e.g., chloroquine) alone.
2. After the primary cycle in the liver no exoerythrocytic schizonts have been found (in chimpanzees after very heavy sporozoite dosage, and in one man).
3. Parasites persist in the blood for very long periods; there are no negative periods (see also, blood transfusion malaria, p. 114, Section II.A).
4. Similar behavior is exhibited by the quartan parasites (*P. inui* and *P. brasilianum*) of monkeys.

The liver stage of *P. malariae* is also prolonged, i.e., 15 days, almost double that of *P. vivax* and three times as long as that of *P. falciparum*. The incubation period is thus always more than a fortnight and is usually 3 weeks or longer.

The prodromal symptoms are more marked in quartan than in other forms of malaria; the patient feels exceptionally tired and has pains in the back and a severe headache. The shivering that initiates the first paroxysm (usually in the morning) is often violent and lasts about $\frac{1}{2}$ hour; it is accompanied by a rise in temperature. Shivering is followed by the hot phase during which the patient immediately feels more comfortable; vomiting is uncommon, and the headache lessens. After 3 or 4 hours, heavy sweating brings the paroxysm to an end; it lasts about 3 hours, and the patient then lapses into sleep. After repeated attacks, the spleen becomes greatly enlarged and may extend as an "ague cake" to below the level of the umbilicus; on the other hand, early in the attack, the enlargement of the spleen is often too slight to be palpable, though the organ may be painful.

"Big-spleen disease" or "tropical splenomegaly syndrome" was at first thought by Marsden *et al.* (1965) to be significantly associated with low-grade chronic infections of *P. malariae*, and certainly this species figures in the parasitological picture in subsequent accounts of the syndrome. More recently, Hutt and Hamilton (1972) have discounted the specific effect of *P. malariae* alone and ascribe the condition to malaria in general and to a particular immunological response. The latter is probably manifested by the constant presence of hepatic sinusoidal lymphocytosis and with excessive IgM hyperimmuno-globulinemia (Woods, 1970).

The syndrome has been particularly studied in Uganda, Nigeria, and New Guinea (Crane and Pryor, 1971; Crane *et al.*, 1972), and the clinical features are similar in these regions. The spleen increases enormously in size and extends into the left iliac fossa and across the midline of the abdomen. The organ is firm, smooth, and not tender to the touch, though the huge mass gives rise to a dragging pain. The liver is invariably enlarged; patients are cachectic, anemic, and often edematous and respond poorly to treatment. However, prolonged antimalarial therapy reduces the size of the spleen in some cases; in others, splenectomy may produce a dramatic, but often temporary, improvement in the general condition.

Plasmodium malariae shares with *P. falciparum* a degree of pathogenicity which leads to death in numerous cases, though the cause of death is totally different in the two infections. *Plasmodium malariae* has a peculiar effect on the kidneys; the association was probably first appreciated by Giglioli (1930) in his investigation in Guyana. The following year, Surtek (1931) named the condition "quartana-nephrosis infantum" which he had studied in children in Sumatra. In 1934, Carothers demonstrated the probable role of this parasite in the etiology of the condition in East Africa where, at that time, it was a common sight to see a whole children's ward entirely occupied by edematous patients with albumen and casts in the urine and often *P. malariae* in the blood films; many of these cases died in uremia. Ascites, anemia, and splenomegaly were regularly found. Dropsy was often mentioned in historical times as a clinical entity in malaria. Linnaeus, for instance, described it in detail in his thesis on "intermittent fever" in Sweden (see Garnham, 1980).

The nephrotic syndrome is now widely recognized, particularly in tropical Africa, where Hendrikse *et al.* (1972) finally confirmed the etiology and clarified the pathology. The condition briefly comprises the deposition of immunoglobulins (produced in response to the *P. malariae* antigen) on the capillary walls of the renal glomeruli, leading to glomerular sclerosis and tubular atrophy. It is thus an immunopathological phenomenon and probably involves an autoimmune mechanism.

Response to antimalarial treatment in patients with quartan nephrosis is generally poor, except in the young children with a short history of infection. Anti-inflammatory drugs are of little use, while in general the prognosis is unfavorable.

It is necessary to emphasize today the danger of the contraction of malaria by the transfusion of blood unknowingly containing parasites; such an origin is confined in Europe to quartan malaria. *Plasmodium malariae* may remain for years in the human host without producing symptoms, and in places where the species used to be common indigenous cases of the disease arise. This has been particularly studied in Rumania (Lupaşcu *et al.*, 1963), where malaria control has completely eradicated the other species but has left a residuum of quartan malaria responsible for a number of cases of transfusion malaria. The situation in 1977 was investigated in the adjacent Soviet Republic of Moldavia, where Lysenko *et al.* detected six old infections of quartan malaria by the immuno-fluorescence reaction in 735 inhabitants. The same phenomenon occurs repeatedly in many countries, and a case of unexplained fever after a blood transfusion should always be investigated for malaria. A recent example in Tennessee is described by Najune and Sulzer (1976) in which the blood donor (a Nigerian) was eventually traced and, although no parasites were detected in his blood, titers of 1:1024 against *P. malariae* were repeatedly found in immunofluorescence tests. Of course, blood transfusions may sometimes result in infection with other species, and this is particularly dangerous if *P. falciparum* is present.

5. *Simian Malaria in Man*

The following species are known to infect man either naturally or experimentally (including accidental laboratory infections and therapeutic use):

Natural infections
  P. knowlesi (three cases of Malaysian origin)
  P. simium (one case in Brazil)
Experimental infections in volunteers
  P. malariae (of chimpanzee origin, synonymous with *P. rodhaini*)
  P. schwetzi
  P. brasilianum
  P. knowlesi
  P. cynomolgi cynomolgi
  P. cynomolgi bastianellii
  P. inui
  P. inui shortti
Accidental (laboratory) infections
  P. cynomolgi cynomolgi
  P. cynomolgi bastianellii
Therapeutic infections
  P. knowlesi

The clinical interest of these zoonoses lies in the likelihood of misdiagnosis. Their apparent rarity in nature is confirmed, at least in Malaysia, by the results of an extensive survey carried out in that country by Warren *et al.* (1970) who inoculated the blood of over a thousand inhabitants of an enzootic area into rhesus monkeys without obtaining a single infection in the recipients.

When cases, either naturally or accidentally transmitted, occur, the correct

diagnosis is usually not established for some time; the symptoms are comparatively mild, resemble those of influenza, and arise in an inhabitant of a nonen-
demic region. The clinical features of the infections due to the various species are
briefly discussed below.

Plasmodium knowlesi has long been known to give rise to mild infections in
man after blood inoculation, but the first naturally transmitted case was not
identified until 1965 (Chin *et al.*, 1965). The patient was an American surveyor
who had worked at night in the forests of Pahang; on his return journey home a
week later, he developed prodromal symptoms (fatigue, anorexia, and nausea)
and, on arrival in California, became ill with respiratory symptoms plus rigors,
fever, and sweating; malaria parasites (thought to be rings of *P. falciparum*)
were found in his blood 2 days later, and he was sent to the Clinical Center of the
National Institutes of Health where the infection was first identified as *P.
malariae*. Subsequently, after inoculation into volunteers and rhesus monkeys,
the diagnosis was changed to *P. knowlesi*. The characteristic clinical feature was
quotidian periodicity; the pyrexia reached 40°C, and the parasitemia increased to
20,000/mm^3.

Even without treatment, the infection of *P. knowlesi* disappears after a fortnight. The incubation period after sporozoite inoculation was found by Coatney
et al. (1971) to extend from 9 to 12 days (through the true *prepatent* period is
$5^1/_2$ days; Garnham, 1966). First passages in volunteers remained relatively non-
virulent or even declined in intensity (Nicol, 1935), but this was a temporary
phenomenon, for within a year Ciuča *et al.* (1955) showed that the average
parasitemia had begun to increase (to a maximum of over $1/_2$ million), and the
temperature rose in some patients to over 41°C, with the paroxysms lasting for
8–12 hours (see Section IV,E).

Only a single natural infection of *P. simium* has been reported by Deane *et al.*
(1966, also personal communication) in a small forest on the edge of the city of
Saõ Paulo in Brazil where no human malaria had occurred for years before this
episode. The patient was an entomological assistant employed in collecting
mosquitoes on a tree platform; he developed a fever with tertian periodicity and,
suspecting that it was of simian origin, refrained from taking any antimalarial
treatment. A light infection of *P. simium* was identified in his blood. The patient
suffered from headache, fever (up to nearly 40°C), and sweating. A specimen of
his blood was inoculated into a *Saimiri* monkey, and *P. simium* appeared in its
blood in large numbers a few days later. (The *Saimiri* had been splenectomized
at least a month previously and, as no parasitemia followed, the animal was
assumed to be free of any malarial infection).

Plasmodium schwetzi is infective to man as first shown by Rodhain and
Dellaert (1955). The course of the disease was fairly mild with a maximum of 14
paroxysms of tertian fever rising to 41°C but with no palpable splenomegaly.
Coatney *et al.* (1971) studied sporozoite-induced infections in volunteers and
later blood infections with similar results except that they detected enlargement

of the spleen in a few patients. Two interesting clinical points were observed: Black volunteers proved to be nonsusceptible (with a similar racial immunity to *P. vivax*; see Section II,A,2), and a delayed prepatent period of 104 days occurred after the inoculation of sporozoites into a Caucasian.

Plasmodium brasilianum was transmitted to human volunteers by Coatney and Contacos (1963), and a mild infection of less than 1 month's duration followed, with an irregular periodicity which only occasionally showed a quartan pattern. Headache, loss of appetite, and a temperature not exceeding 40°C were noted. The spleen became enlarged in some of the patients.

The subspecies of *Plasmodium cynomolgi* (*P. cynomolgi cynomolgi*, *P. cynomolgi bastianellii*, and the Cambodian variety) have all proved to be infective to man, either accidentally or deliberately in volunteers. Twenty-six patients infected with *P. cynomolgi cynomolgi* were studied by Coatney *et al.* (1971). Blacks proved to be insusceptible to this parasite which is closely allied to *P. vixax* (see Section II,A,2), but Caucasians developed malaria after an incubation period of 16–37 days (the prepatent period is 8 days). The tertian periodicity was not constant, and the temperature rose to a maximum of 40°C. Headache, anorexia, muscle pains, and nausea were the symptoms, and enlargement of both the spleen and liver was observed. *Plasmodium cynomolgi bastianellii* is highly infectious to man and laboratory infections readily occur (Garnham *et al.*, 1962). The striking feature of these cases is the low parasitemia and the severity of the disease; patients usually have influenza-like symptoms, and parasites may remain undetectable for 6 days—there is a low threshold level of parasitemia. This feature may be useful in the differential diagnosis of the zoonosis from *P. vivax* in the field in places where *P. cynomolgi* is enzootic; exact identification may be obtained by inoculating the patient's blood into rhesus monkeys, which are insusceptible to *P. vivax* but which are highly susceptible to *P. cynomolgi*. The average incubation period is 13 days, though prepatency terminates on the eighth day after the mosquito bite.

Plasmodium inui was found to be infectious to man by inoculating blood from infected monkeys (Dasgupta, 1938); 23 days later a few parasites were found in the volunteer's blood, and he became ill for 3 days with daily peaks of fever up to 39 °C. The subspecies, *P. inui shortti*, was tested for its infectivity to man (vide Coatney *et al.*, 1971) by allowing infected anopheline species to feed on volunteers; a quartan fever was produced with a maximum temperature of 39.5°C. The usual mild symptoms of short duration occurred and were followed by spontaneous recovery.

B. Malaria Therapy

Fever therapy for neurological disorders had been used occasionally since classic times, but it was not applied on a systematic scale until Wagner-Jauregg introduced it at his clinic for nervous diseases in Vienna in 1922 for the cure of general paralysis of the insane (GPI), although he had been testing its efficiency since 1917. The method was applied on a large scale at Horton Hospital in England from 1923, and over 13,000 patients with neurosyphilis were treated with one or other of the four human species of plasmodia during the next 45 years. In 1926 Ciucă established another large center at Socola, Rumania, where an equal number of cases were treated in the next 40 years; even today the Hospital for Mental Diseases in Jassy still continues the practice of malaria therapy. In 1925, Walter Reed Hospital initiated the treatment of cerebrospinal syphilis with *P. vivax* malaria in the United States (St. John, 1927); and a few years later, the centers in Milledgeville and Columbia began using the technique on large number of psychiatric patients.

It is not our intention in this chapter to evaluate malaria therapy in GPI, but there is no doubt that many permanent cures were effected and the condition of other patients greatly improved; even today it probably still has a use, e.g., in drug-resistant cases.

The progress of malaria research was much accelerated by the facilities that became available for study of the subject under controlled conditions. It is important, however, to realize that the disease—even if induced by the natural route of mosquito bites—was being observed in abnormal hosts, i.e., in patients suffering from chronic syphilis. The mental symptoms of these patients were not necessarily malarial in origin, and the course of the infection presented some differences from that seen under natural conditions. The longevity, even of completely untreated cases, was less than the maximum duration reported in natural infections of the different species (see Table III).

Plasmodium vivax was the favored species for use in malaria therapy; if immunity to this species developed and the patient still required treatment, *P. falciparum* was sometimes employed with special care in the management of the ensuing attack. If available, *P. malariae* might be substituted, and in Rumania, in particular, *P. knowlesi* was used. The quotidian fever of the last-mentioned parasite was particularly valuable, but repeated passage enhanced the virulence to such a degree that Ciucă *et al.* (1955) finally found the infections almost unmanageable.

The purely clinical results which emerged from observations in these centers are summarized as follows:

1. Precise incubation time and prepatent periods after infection with sporozoites of the different species.
2. The fever pattern throughout the course of the untreated disease.
3. The progress of the various signs and symptoms.
4. The recurrence and duration of recrudescences and relapses, respectively.
5. The pattern of the disease in these renewed manifestations.
6. The clinical pathology.

7. The effect on the disease of the developing immunity.
8. Response to a variety of old and new chemical compounds.

No mention is made here of the invaluable contributions malaria therapy has provided on the nonclinical side of malaria, e.g., elucidation of the tissue cycles, gametocytogenesis, sporogony, and immunity.

III. MALARIA IN APES

It is practically impossible to study malaria or indeed any disease in animals living in their natural environment. At most, one may observe the last moments of a moribund creature, e.g., a monkey dying of yellow fever in a South American forest or a bird in the last stages of a severe malaria infection. Under exceptional circumstances it is possible to watch apes which have been confiscated from illegal owners and then set free at rehabilitation centers in special forest reserves; such animals return for food for several months or longer. Their illnesses may then be recognized and appropriately treated (see Section III,B). Records, however, are rare and incomplete. The problem was discussed by Baker (1969) in a symposium on diseases in free-living wild animals, where a few examples were described, e.g., malaise, weakness, drooping wings in wild birds suffering from relapses of malaria.

Practically all the information we possess about diseases of wild animals emanates from laboratory studies either on natural infections or on infections induced in captivity and often in highly abnormal hosts. The main purpose of most investigations is to use the animals as models of a comparable human disease, and extremely useful data have been obtained. It must be emphasized that fallacies in the interpretation and application of the results are, however, liable to occur (see Section I,2,A and VI,A).

A. Chimpanzees and Gorillas

Chimpanzees contract forms of malaria closely resembling those caused by the three common human species of *Plasmodium*. *Plasmodium schwetzi* is the ape equivalent of *P. vivax,* and *P. reichenowi* of *P. falciparum; P. rodhaini* is so indistinguishable from *P. malariae* that the former name is now regarded as a synonym. Only the first two species have been found in gorillas.

Animals acquire the infections at an early age, but the morbidity and mortality are unknown. Symptoms are apparently minimal, and *P. reichenowi* has less of a tendency than *P. falciparum* to migrate into the deeper tissues to undergo schizogony. Schizonts are often seen in the blood, and after splenectomy they are very frequent. Pathogenicity due to obstruction by schizonts of the capillaries in the organs is therefore absent, and pernicious malaria has never been reported in the chimpanzee. A second difference between the ape parasite and its human counterpart relates to relapses. These appear to be absent in *P. falciparum* infections, but Schwetz (1934) noted that *P. reichenowi* lasted a long time in chimpanzees, and Garnham *et al.* (1956) observed "relapses" of this parasite 3 years after the blood infection had been sterilized by drug therapy.

There is little information about the clinical course of *P. schwetzi* infections in the chimpanzee or gorilla. Splenomegaly occurs in the former animal, and the periodicity of the fever is tertian. The behavior of the parasite has been more closely observed in human volunteers (see Section II,A,5). Although the spleen becomes enlarged in natural infections in the ape, the enormous hypertrophy of the organ (the ague cake) of chronic malaria in man has never been reported in the chimpanzee, in spite of the fact that, in some West African forests, it must be exposed to almost constant infection.

B. Orangutan

Two species of malaria parasites are found in these animals, often as double infections: *P. pitheci* and *P. silvaticum*. The former parasite was first seen by Laveran in 1905 and has been studied on few occasions since its mild pathogenicity was noted. Dobb (1913), however, ascribed the death of one animal in an Australian zoo to a severe infection of this parasite.

Malaria in these animals was studied in considerable detail by Peters *et al.* (1976). The Sepilok Forest Reserve in Sabah has been set aside for the conservation of this threatened species, and confiscated orangutans are rehabilitated at the center. Records are kept of the fate of the animals and show that mortality, especially of young apes, is high. The malaria infection rate was found to be 55% in a single survey and 85% after repeated examination of the blood, but no deaths could be attributed directly to the disease. Little pyrexia accompanied the resurgence of malaria observed in animals admitted from the forest to a veterinary clinic for other conditions. Splenomegaly was slight or absent. One juvenile female was found to be suffering from a typical paroxysm; she was ill with the cold phase occurring at 09.45 and the hot phase ensuing $2\frac{1}{2}$ hours later when the rectal temperature rose to 38°C.

Probably malaria reduces the resistance of the animals to other infections, particularly dysentery caused by *Entamoeba histolytica* or *Balantidium coli*.

Malaria infections appear to remain chronic for a long time in orangutans, at least up to 7 years.

C. Gibbons

Four species (*P. hylobati*, *P. jefferyi*, *P. youngi*, and *P. eylesi*) have been described in different species of *Hylobates* (Coatney *et al.*, 1971). Natural infections appear to cause little illness but, if the spleen of an infected gibbon is removed, parasitemia reaches a high level, and the animal becomes very weak and lethargic and will die in the absence of antimalarial treatment. American workers commented on the unusual severity of *P. youngi* infections in laboratory-infected gibbons, which became listless, ill, and anemic, and exhibited a fever of over 41°C.

D. Susceptibility of Higher Apes to Human Malaria Parasites

Perhaps the best model for the study of human malaria is the chimpanzee. The liver of this animal is able to support natural growth of the human parasites, although the erythrocytes are only feebly susceptible to *P. vivax, P. falciparum,* and *P. ovale;* the quartan parasite, however, is common to man and chimpanzees. If the animal is splenectomized, the human parasites undergo fulminant multiplication in the blood, and the infection may need to be damped with a suitable drug if the animal is to survive.

Apart from the cost of chimpanzees and the undesirability of using fairly rare animals for experimentation, the chimpanzee may not be as suitable as its close phylogenetic relationship to man suggests. Thus, at least three important questions cannot be investigated in the chimpanzee: cerebral malaria, blackwater fever, and quartan nephrosis, for none of these conditions can apparently be provoked in this animal. Moreover, immunological observations cannot be directly made on an animal whose spleen has been extirpated and whose natural immunity mechanisms have been shattered.

Splenectomized gibbons were infected with *P. falciparum* and *P. vivax* (Cadigan *et al.,* 1969) but, although the parasitemia reached 8% and lasted for over a year, no clinical symptoms were found. The prolonged parasitemia of *P. falciparum* in gibbons suggests that such infections could provide useful models for study of the action of drugs.

IV. MALARIA IN LOWER PRIMATES

Fourteen species or subspecies of *Plasmodium* occur in monkeys, and many of them have proved of immense value in malaria research during the past 50 years. Six examples have been taken to illustrate the clinical picture of simian malaria, of which two (*P. cynomolgi* and *P. simium*) are tertian and vivaxlike, two (*P. inui* and *P. brasilianum*) are quartan, one (*P. knowlesi*) is uniquely quotidian, and one (*P. coatneyi*) is tertian but with doubtful affinities.

Practically nothing is known about the diseases caused by the remaining simian parasites and still less about the malaria parasites of lemurs. The latter are of some interest, in that in nature the infections of *P. girardi* and *P. foleyi* are cryptic and can only be detected after splenectomy.

A. *Plasmodium cynomolgi* and Subspecies *Plasmodium cynomolgi bastianellii*

This species complex is widely distributed in southern Asia from India and Sri Lanka to Burma, Cambodia, Viet Nam, Thailand, Malaysia (West and East), and through the East Indian archipelago to Taiwan and southern China. There is evidence that speciation has taken place from the probable original home in Malaysia (*P. cynomolgi cynomolgi*) westward to Sri Lanka (*P. cynomolgi ceylonensis*) and eastward to Taiwan (*P. cynomolgi cyclopis*).

The natural hosts of *P. cynomolgi cynomolgi* are kra monkeys (*Macaca fascicularis* and subspecies), the pigtailed macaque (*M. nemestrina*), the rhesus (*M. mulatta*), the stump-tailed macaque (*M. speciosa*), and various species of langurs (*Presbytis* spp.). Parasites from the last group should probably be given separate subspecific status. *Plasmodium cynomolgi bastianellii* was isolated from *M. fascicularis* in Malaya.

The clinical course of *P. cynomolgi* runs as follows. The prepatent period of *P. cynomolgi cynomolgi* is 8 days and of *P. cynomolgi bastianellii,* 7 days; the paroxysms occur synchronously in both subspecies, but the former usually starts at about 0700 hours and the latter at midday. The infection reaches its height about 14 days after sporozoite induction and subsequently declines slowly, disappearing from the blood after 4 or 5 weeks. A true relapse follows about $3\frac{1}{2}$ months after the date of infection, although relapses probably occur also at earlier intervals and may continue to break out up to 2 years later in chloroquine-suppressed infections (see Warren *et al.*, 1973).

Signs of disease are few or absent. The spleen increases in size, particularly after relapses, and the organ may become quite prominent in the abdomen; its consistency eventually becomes very hard. The temperature of monkeys is difficult to ascertain, because it may rise considerably when the animal is handled; however, Aberle (1945) states that the rectal temperature rises from the normal figure of 39°–40°C to 41°–42°C during the acute attack. A degree of anemia is indicated by the pallor of the skin and the mucous membranes, and the animal loses its appetite.

B. *Plasmodium simium*

This tertian species is confined to three states in southern Brazil, where Deane studied it in two subspecies of *Alouatta fusca* and in *Brachyteles arachnoides,* the woolly spider monkey. The general appearance of this parasite is similar to that of *P. vivax,* and it has been suggested that, like *P. brasilianum,* it may represent a zoonosis of the human parasite in reverse (see Section IV,D). Coatney *et al.* (1971) studied the parasite in two splenectomized *Saimiri* after sporozoite inoculation and stated that the "prepatent periods" were 24 and 38 days, respectively. The true prepatent period (i.e., duration of exoerythrocytic schizogony) is likely to be much shorter.

Natural infections in howler monkeys are usually light and asymptomatic; after splenectomy, however, the animal appears cachectic and anemic, while it suffers from diarrhea, its hair drops out, and pyrexia may reach about 41°C (Deane, 1976).

C. *Plasmodium inui*

This quartan parasite of Asian monkeys probably includes a complex of related species, which differ in species of host, geographic distribution, length of exoerythrocytic schizogony (varying between 10 and 12 days with comparable prepatent periods), and morphology. The form which occurs in India is *P. inui shortti.* In spite of its 72-hour periodicity, it differs from *P. malariae* or *P. brasilianum* in many major characters, and thus it makes a poor (and deceptive) model for the human parasite.

Like the other quartan parasites, however, it runs a chronic course, persisting probably for the life of the host. Symptoms of disease in the monkey are slight or nil, though in human volunteers Coatney *et al.* (1971) noted that typical malarial symptoms occurred with quartan periodicity.

D. *Plasmodium brasilianum*

This quartan parasite is widely distributed in New World monkeys in Central and South America. In most features *P. brasilianum* bears a striking resemblance to the human *P. malariae,* and there is a growing feeling that the simian species originated from man, perhaps at the time of the arrival of the conquistadores or later during the importation of African slaves. It was suggested (Garnham, 1967, 1973) that the human infection spread into the monkey population, thus representing a zoonosis in reverse; Coatney (1968) thought that *P. malariae* became adapted to New World monkeys sometime in the early seventeenth century. The simplest way of confirming these speculations would be to investigate the closeness in identity of the respective isoenzymes.

The exact duration of the prepatent period is not precisely known, but it is probably about 14 days (Coatney *et al.,* 1971). The course of the natural infection is protracted, and the parasitemia may last at least as long as 16 months. Synchronicity of schizogony in the blood is usually marked with schizonts rupturing at about midday every 72 hours. Recrudescences occur at frequent intervals, and the parasites appear to remain in the blood in larger or smaller numbers, or they may be subpatent, just as in the quartan malaria of man. American investigators (W. E. Collins and P. G. Contacos, personal communication) stress the absence of true relapses in *P. brasilianum*.

The clinical course varies in severity according to the species of monkey but is rarely fatal. Dr. and Mrs. Taliaferro (1934b) have observed that there is a marked correlation between the height of parasitemia and the fever pattern. Splenomegaly is also greatest at the time of the crisis. Anemia is most marked in chronic infections and, as in infections of *P. simium* (Section IV,B), hair is likely to be lost, particularly from the distal part of the tail and the legs; new growth of hair is characterized by loss of pigment (Aberle, 1945).

The chronicity of *P. brasilianum* in monkeys suggested that these animals might exhibit the nephrotic syndrome well known as a sequela in human quartan malaria. Voller (1971) studied the immunopathology caused by the simian parasite after a 10-week infection and demonstrated the presence of immune complexes in the glomeruli of the kidneys of animals which had suffered from a very severe illness accompanied by facial edema and albuminuria.

E. *Plasmodium knowlesi*

This parasite of macaques and leaf monkeys in Southeast Asia is remarkable for its unique quotidian periodicity in the blood and its almost 100% lethality in *M. malatta*. For these reasons, it has been widely studied, particularly in relation to chemotherapy. The frequent occurrence of hemoglobinuria in subterminal stages at first suggested that *P. knowlesi* would be a good model for elucidation of the pathogenesis of blackwater fever in man, but the mechanisms of the two conditions appear to be quite different. The severity of the infection in natural hosts, such as *M. fascicularis,* is much less, and these animals almost always survive; if splenectomized however, they die after a fulminating infection. *Macaca fascicularis* was shown (Schmidt *et al.*, 1977) to respond differently from the normal according to the origin of the monkey; Philippine kra monkeys were much less affected than those of Malayan origin which usually died of the infection. These observations illustrate the need for specifying both strain of animal and strain of parasite in descriptions of experiments.

The prepatent period is just under 6 days. The rapid course of schizogony in the blood (24 hours) results in equally rapid multiplication, and the animal soon becomes profoundly ill. For 2 days before death, it is very weak and lies on the floor of the cage; it refuses all food, and there is marked pallor of the skin and conjunctiva. These signs are accompanied by high fever until shortly before death when the temperature becomes subnormal.

Intravascular hemolysis is often present and is accompanied by hemoglobinuria. If the disease is temporarily arrested by the administration of quinine, the parasitemia declines, but a few weeks later a very severe hemolytic anemia ensues and the animal dies within a day or two. This condition seems to be similar to the fatal hemolytic anemia in children in *P. falciparum* infections (see Section II,A,1). The work of Avivah Zuckerman (1966) and of Kretschmar (1964) (both now prematurely dead), has demonstrated that the phenomenon of excessive blood destruction is the result of autoimmunization. It has been studied experimentally also in *P. berghei* (e.g., Kreier *et al.*, 1966; Kreier and Leste, 1968) and in other infections (see Volume 2, Chapters 2 and 3).

F. *Plasmodium coatneyi*

Plasmodium coatneyi is another lethal malaria parasite of Malaysian macaques *(M. fascicularis)* and is thought by some workers to offer a useful model for the study of *P. falciparum,* because of the similarity in morphology of the "ring forms" and their tendency to become sequestrated in the internal organs. However, *P. falciparum* belongs to another subgenus (*Laverania*), and it seems unlikely that there is any real affinity between the two parasites.

Plasmodium coatneyi often kills rhesus monkeys which when intact have a 40% mortality rate and, when splenectomized, a 100% mortality rate. The natural host exhibits a mild, low-grade, chronic infection (Coatney *et al.*, 1971).

Few observations on the clinical course of the disease have been made. The prepatent period is 10 days or less, after which the infection reaches a peak parasitemia 9 days later (Collins *et al.*, 1967). Garnham (1965) studied the pathology of the acute and chronic disease in rhesus monkeys. After a week of parasitemia, the animal becomes markedly pale as the result of a severe hemolytic anemia. The spleen becomes enlarged, and in the chronic disease there is great hypertrophy of the Malpighian corpuscles of the organ. The brunt of the infection falls on the smaller capillaries of the heart, which become blocked by the schizonts, and this condition, together with the anemia, is probably the cause of death. There are no cerebral symptoms or obstruction of the vessels of the brain.

G. Human Parasites

The routine use of chimpanzees as experimental models of human malaria has been shown (Section III, D) to be impracticable, while until quite recently, the susceptibility of monkeys to human species was thought to be too low for them to be of any value in research. Then, in 1966, Young *et al.* succeeded in establishing *P. vivax* in *Aotus* monkeys by blood and mosquito passage; in 1967, Geiman and Meagher infected *Aotus* with *P. falciparum,* while in 1969, Geiman and Siddiqui transferred *P. malariae* to the same species of monkey. In the following decade, large numbers of *Aotus* were used for malaria research—to such an extent that the continued existence of these animals was threatened, and their export from Latin America was prohibited.

In a series of papers, Leon Schmidt (1978) described the useful results of this research and included his own observations on the course of malaria infections in the monkey. The susceptibility of *Aotus* varies according to the subspecies of *A. trivirgatus; A. trivirgatus trivirgatus* (with orange fur) is a poor host, while *A. trivirgatus griseimembra* (with gray fur) is excellent. Leon Schmidt used nearly 2000 *Aotus* in his experiments which he supervised himself and conducted under highly controlled conditions. He was thus able to produce a detailed account of the behavior of *Aotus* suffering from infections of eight strains of *P. falciparum* and two strains of *P. vivax*. There was a considerable difference in the response of intact (i.e., unsplenectomized) animals to the different strains after adaptation by rapid blood passage. Most strains of *P. falciparum* soon became highly virulent, but the Cambodian strain remained comparatively mild; the more recently isolated strain of *P. vivax* from Vietnam was more virulent than the Chesson strain isolated from a New Guinea infection more than 20 years earlier.

The course of untreated infections of most strains of *P. falciparum* terminated fatally in 70–90% of the animals, the lethality being roughly proportional to the height of the parasitemia. The overt reactions included anorexia, anemia, and loss of muscle tone, followed by prostration and coma; hematuria and jaundice were often present. Such signs were not apparent in acute infections until 3 days before death, but in more chronic but still fatal infections the critical state lasted for about 2 weeks. Recrudescences in animals which eventually recovered, were largely asymptomatic. An interesting feature was the frequent presence of pleural effusion and ascites in the more acute cases; such conditions are rarely present in human malignant malaria. Pulmonary edema was often present, as it sometimes is in children (see Section II,A,1). The abdominal organs were much enlarged, the spleen often being hypertrophied to three times its normal size.

Plasmodium vivax infections were directly fatal in 26% of animals in the Viet Nam strain and 5% in the Chesson. The more severe infections exhibited the following signs: cyanosis, anorexia, loss of weight, and rigidity and tenderness of the abdomen; the majority of monkeys which survived the infection were asymptomatic. Splenomegaly was much greater in *P. vivax* than in *P. falciparum* infections, the spleens in some animals extending from the diaphragm to the brim of the pelvis. Recrudescences were remarkable in that the intervals between them tended to be of a constant duration; unfortunately, these experiments of Leon Schmidt were limited to blood-induced infections in which the relapse phenomenon is, of course (Section I,C) absent. Now that *P. vivax* has been well adapted to nonsplenectomized animals, it should be possible to investigate some of the still unexplained features of prolonged prepatency in certain strains of the parasite.

Fortunately other investigators (Young *et al.*, 1966; Ward *et al.*, 1969) have shown that mosquito transmission of various strains of *P. vivax* is relatively easy using *Aotus*. Moreover, other species of monkeys can be used, e.g., *Saimiri* spp., *Saguinus* sp., *Ateles* spp., and *Cebus* sp., though in most of these examples splenectomized animals were used and this condition makes them unsuitable for observations on the relapse phenomenon, etc.

The mild susceptibility of a variety of both New and Old World monkeys to both *P. vivax* and *P. falciparum* has been known for a considerable time. Dr. and Mrs. Taliaferro in 1934 (1934a) reported their success in infecting howler monkeys with *P. falciparum*, but in most of these experiments the infections were transient.

Some recent work in China (Jingbo Jiang *et al.*, 1978) describes a new technique for studying human malaria parasites in monkeys (*M. mulatta* and *M. assamensis*). The blood of these animals was largely replaced by human blood just before inoculation with *P. falciparum*, and repeated passage (11 times) in monkeys, similarly transfused, resulted in heavy infections in the animals. The greatest density was 46% invasion of erythrocytes. Two animals died, and their intestines showed pathological features exactly comparable to those of pernicious intestinal malaria of man. This technique allows the collection of considerable numbers of merozoites for antigen production.

V. RODENT MALARIA

Rodent malaria comprises a complex of closely related species confined to a rather restricted area in West and Central Africa. The subject is discussed in great detail in the book edited by Killick-Kendrick and Peters (1978) and by Carter and Diggs (1977). The species fall into three groups as shown in Table IV.

A very large amount of work has been done on rodent malaria since the original discovery of *P. berghei* by Vincke and Lips in 1948. It is curious how little attention has been devoted to the purely clinical aspects, except for a few isolated examples in relation to pyrexia, anemia, and splenomegaly.

The duration of the prepatent period is as important in rodent as in primate malaria for the identification of species or subspecies. The development of the exoerythrocytic schizonts was found to be unexpectedly rapid, less than one-half that of the primate parasites. The criteria of identification plus data on sporogony and host response confirm the evidence from biochemical analysis (isoenzymes, etc.) that this species complex represents genetically distinct organisms.

While the duration of the prepatent period has clinical significance, most of the other diagnostic features (morphological or biochemical) are outside the scope of this chapter. The mortality and susceptibility of different rodents are, however, of relevance. As in other animals, the effect of the parasite is very different on laboratory animals than on the natural host. The latter comprises a variety of

TABLE IV

Rodent Malaria Parasites and Distribution[a]

	Species	Distribution[b]
I.	*P. berghei*	Zaire (eastern districts)
	P. yoelii yoelii	C.A.R.
	P. y. killicki	D.R.C.
	P. y. nigeriensis	Nigeria
II.	*P. vinckei vinckei*	Zaire (eastern district)
	P. v. petteri	C.A.R.
	P. v. lentum	D.R.C.
	P. v. bruce-chwatti	Nigeria
III.	*P. chabaudi chabaudi*	C.A.R.
	P. c. adami	D.R.C.

[a] Unnamed subspecies in the three groups have been described from Cameroun by Bafort (1977).

[b] C.A.R., Central African Republic; D.R.C., Democratic Republic of Congo.

thicket rats (*Thamnomys* spp., *Grammomys*, and others), some of which can easily be bred in the laboratory, and in certain work they should be used in preference to the various breeds of white mouse or of other laboratory rodents.

Each of the three species of rodent malaria parasites and to a lesser extent their subspecies exhibit a different degree of virulence in unnatural hosts. Certain strains of white mice in general prove to be the most susceptible and, as in other types of malaria, the youngest animals show higher degrees of infection than adults. The main susceptibilities are as follows.

Plasmodium berghei berghei causes practically 100% mortality in many strains of white mice; in the NMRI strain (developed at the National Medical Research Institute at Bethesda, Maryland), on the other hand, the death rate may be as low as 25%. In the former, the curve of mortality is bimodal (Carrescia and Arcoles, 1958): During the first 6 days of infection, mature erythrocytes are invaded; there is thrombocytopenia, hemoglobinuria, and anemia, and the mouse dies in a condition of shock. If the mouse survives the first phase, the blood contains many reticulocytes which are preferentially attacked, anemia becomes profound, and the animal dies about the third week in a condition of anoxia. The anemia is due both to destruction of parasitized corpuscles and to the operation of autoantibodies (see Kreier and Leste, 1968). In general, the high fulminating parasitemia of rodent malaria is accompanied by an extreme pallor, which is tinged with brown as a result of the deposition of malaria pigment in the skin and mucous membranes. The animals are extremely ill in the developed disease, cachectic, and with staring hair, both in *P. berghei* infections and in virulent mutants of the other species. Mercado and Coatney (1951) comment on the inactivity, labored breathing, and somnolence of mice in the terminal stages.

Kretschmar (1962) showed that a greater number of animals survived infections of the less virulent strains if they were not subjected to stress, e.g., repeated handling or the taking of blood specimens.

The periodicity of the blood stages is difficult to assess, because no species in the groups shows much synchronicity. However, a quotidian cycle is thought to be normal for schizogony in the blood (22–25 hours for *P. berghei* and *P. yoelii*, and 24 hours for *P. vinckei* and *P. yoelii*, Landau, 1978).

Sergent and Poncet (1961) studied the temperature of mice suffering from berghei malaria. They first recorded the rectal temperature of normal mice and showed that it fluctuated between 35° and 39°C. After infection, the curve was little affected during the first 4 days and no rise was noticed; but on the fifth day the temperature suddenly fell and remained at 28°C or below until the mice died. If the infected mice were left in an incubator at 37°C, they were found to die even more quickly.

Kretschmar (1961) confirmed this unusual phenomenon of hypothermia but showed that in NMRI mice there was a steady decline in temperature from the fourth day (37°C) to 32°C on the eighteenth day and 26°C on the twenty-eighth day (at death). There was a close inverse relationship between the declining body temperature and the rising parasitemia. He stressed the striking degree of hemolytic anemia and the loss of weight of the animals, in which death was due to hypoxia.

The other clinical feature that has received some attention is splenomegaly. Sergent and Poncet (1955) found that enlargement of the spleen in *P. berghei* infections was less than in human or avian malaria, probably because the course was rapidly fatal. They found that the average weight of the spleen of mice rose from the normal 200 to 300 mg at death; the spleen of rats rose from 500 to over 900 mg (in one rat to 5000 mg).

Suntherasamai and Marsden (1969–1972) specifically investigated splenomegaly in mice (TO strain) infected with *P. yoelii yoelii*. They showed that the spleen became enlarged to six times the normal size; the organ reached its peak weight about 12 days after infection and thereafter declined with the fall in parasitemia, eventually reverting to nearly normal size on recovery about a month later. The degree of splenomegaly was uninfluenced by the concomitant presence of *Eperythrozoon coccoides*. On the other hand, a low protein diet reduced the impact of malaria on the host, by reducing the parasitemia and by causing only slight enlargement of the spleen. Nevertheless, these mice failed to get rid of the infection and suffered from severe anemia.

Plasmodium yoelii yoelii normally differs greatly from *P. berghei* in that it causes a mild disease in mice and young rats, and it is not often fatal. However, Yoeli (1976) accidentally discovered that a strain which had been cryopreserved for 110 days, had undergone a great enhancement of virulence and produced massive invasion of the cerebral capillaries. He thought that this virulent strain would provide an excellent model for human cerebral malaria, but this is only partially true because many of the major pathological lesions, e.g., ring hemorrhages and pseudogranulomata (vide Edington and Gilles, 1969), of the human disease are absent.

Mercado (1965) described an interesting neurological syndrome in weanling rats infected with *P. berghei* (KBG 173): The hindlegs and less often the forelegs became paralyzed, and the animals died in coma. The symptoms began between the sixth and eleventh days after infection when the parasitemia had reached 10%. There were extensive hemorrhages in the brain, but no blockage of capillaries by parasites. It is possible that a virus was involved, but none was identified.

VI. AVIAN MALARIA

Over 30 valid species of malaria parasites have been described from about 500 species of birds, of which 6 have been selected here because of their use in malaria research or their importance in veterinary medicine. The related genus, *Leucocytozoon*, is beyond the scope of this chapter, though some of the species are of considerable veterinary interest or throw light on the relapse phenomenon in avian malaria (see Desser *et al.*, 1968; Akiba, 1964).

The avian parasites were classified into four subgenera by Corradetti *et al.* (1963) on the basis of biological and morphological characters. Two examples of the subgenera *Haemamoeba* and *Giovannolaia*, and one each of the subgenera *Novyella* and *Huffia*, are discussed in relation to their clinical features.

There are fundamental differences between avian and mammalian parasites, which are shown in Table V. Some of these directly affect the clinical picture, e.g., the length of the prepatent period and the extent of mortality. The immune reaction of the host is usually different, in that mammalian malaria is often followed by the complete disappearance of parasites from the blood and a sterile immunity, while avian malaria is typically characterized by the persistence of parasites in the blood and premunition.

Seed and Manwell (1977) in a discussion on the clinical aspects of malaria in birds stress that there are often no "visible symptoms" and that the fever and paroxysms of the human disease are absent except in infections of *P. pinottii* in pigeons. The same authors state that "clinically there is a dramatic increase in blood urea nitrogen" in gallinaceum malaria of chickens, but this is in the domain of pathology and is considered elsewhere in this volume, Chapter 5.

TABLE V

Differential Characters of Mammalian and Avian Species of Malaria Parasites

Character	Mammalian species	Avian species
Invertebrate host	Invariably *Anopheles* sp.	Most often culicine mosquito
Cristate mitochondrion in asexual erythrocytic stages	Absent	Present
Number of generations of preerythrocytic schizogony	One	Two
Length of preerythrocytic schizogony	5 days or more[a]	3 days
Site of preerythrocytic schizogony	Liver parenchyma	Mesodermal cells
Number of preerythrocytic merozoites	2000 or more per schizont	Less than 100
Origin of exoerythrocytic schizogony	Invariably sporozoites	Sporozoites, exoerythrocytic and erythrocytic merozoites
Important cause of death	Blockage of capillaries by erythrocytic schizonts[b]	Blockage of capillaries by exoerythrocytic schizonts

[a] Except in rodent malaria.
[b] *Plasmodium falciparum.*

It was emphasized earlier in this chapter that malaria in the wild or natural host is frequently unaccompanied by much obvious pathogenicity. In birds, however, this generalization is less applicable, because it is not uncommon to find moribund or dead birds which have dropped to the ground from their nests. Gabaldon (1980) describes the frequency with which dead nestlings are found below the "heronries" in the llanos of Venezuela and suggests that malaria is a powerful factor in regulating the size of the population (of pigeons and ducks). In the laboratory, where the course of the Venezuelan infection was watched in inoculated ducklings, the birds showed few or no signs of illness until about 3 hours before death; during this short interval, they lay on the floor of the cage and exhibited slight convulsive movements of the head and limbs.

Epizootics of malaria can cause havoc among domestic birds, such as turkeys with *P. durae,* or chickens with *P. gallinaceum* and *P. juxtanucleare.* These are examples of "veterinary zoonoses" (Garnham, 1969): in *P. durae* acquired from a reservoir in francolins and in *P. gallinaceum* and *P. juxtanucleare* from jungle fowl, partridges, and other wild birds. Migration of wild birds into localities where enzootic avian malaria is present may result in the acquisition by the former of infections which may be accompanied by a mortality much heightened by the stress of long flights (Markus, 1974); or migrant birds may themselves bring a pathogenic species to islands (e.g., the Hawaiian islands, Warner, 1961) where malaria is absent and actually decimate certain of the avian fauna to the point of extinction. The allied hemosporidian parasite *Leucocytozoon* is exceptionally virulent when it is introduced into populations of birds which have not been exposed previously to the infection; a "lightning" devastation is the result—as Levine (1975) relates, a flock of ducklings may appear to be in normal health in the morning, ill in the afternoon, and dead the following morning. This disease is characterized by convulsions, drowsiness, and coma, or when less acute, by excessive anemia, emaciation, and stunted growth.

A. *Plasmodium (Haemamoeba) relictum*

Plasmodium relictum is the commonest malaria parasite found in birds and is the most well-known component of a complex of several closely related species (*P. cathemerium, P. subpraecox, P. matutinum, P. lutzi,* and *P. giovannolai*) and subspecies (e.g., *P. relictum biziurae*). Many of the earlier descriptions (e.g., Manwell, 1938) of these parasites referred to one or other of these members of the complex but were identified as *P. relictum,* and for this reason the figures for periodicity of schizogony in the blood and the maturation time of erythrocytic and exoerythrocytic schizonts show wide variations, as do the morphological descriptions, nature of vectors, etc. Except where stated otherwise, the following account applies to *P. relictum sensu stricto.*

Various passeriform birds act as hosts for *P. relictum,* of which Grassi and Feletti's type host was a sparrow (*Passer hispaniolensis*) together with a Sicilian lark and a chaffinch. The canary is readily susceptible to all strains and is the bird most commonly employed in experimental work; the behavior of the parasite in this host provides the best practical criterion for the identification of species. Sergent and Sergent (1952) studied *P. relictum* in more than 6000 canaries over a course of 47 years, and their observations are referred to repeatedly below.

The periodicity of the asexual stages in the blood is probably 36 hours, though asynchronous development makes this figure difficult to estimate; the schizonts rupture in the morning. *Plasmodium matutinum* differs from *P. relictum* in being highly synchronous in a 24-hour cycle, with the schizonts maturing at a regular hour (8 A.M.). Preerythrocytic development of the sporozoite occurs in two steps, the cryptozoic stage occupying about 36 hours and the metacryptozoic 30 hours, so that the prepatent period is approximately 65 hours (Raffaele, 1936), and the blood becomes infective when inoculated into canaries after this interval. However, invasion of erythrocytes was not actually seen at such a time, and the infectivity of the blood may have been due to circulating cryptozoic merozoites before their invasion of new tissue cells; much greater metacryptozoic production occurs on the fourth day.

The mortality in canaries is high and may reach 63%. Birds at the peak of the illness (usually during the second week) look ill, with ruffled plumage, drooping head, and anemia. The spleen becomes greatly enlarged and may attain a volume 20 times that of the normal organ. Huff (1939) attempted to study the course of pyrexia in canaries, by means of thermocouples inserted deep into the pectoral muscles, and at the same time observed the maturation of schizonts in the blood. The experiments were carefully controlled in uninfected birds and, to Huff's surprise, while he found striking differences (up to 6 °C) in the temperatures taken at day and at night, these occurred both in normal and infected canaries and bore no relationship at all to the schizogony of the parasite. The mean temperature (42.8 °C) in the canaries infected with *P. relictum* was practically identical with that (42.7 °C) in the controls.

B. *Plasmodium (Haemamoeba) gallinaceum*

This pathogenic malaria parasite of chickens has been used very widely in malaria research since its discovery by Brumpt in 1935, though when *P. berghei* was isolated in mice by Vincke and Lips in 1948, the rodent parasite largely replaced the former in experimental work. The use of these two parasites as models for the human disease has been strongly defended by Bruce-Chwatt (1978) in relation to mass screening programs of new compounds, the biochemistry of the parasite, the drug resistance problem, and immunity in the host; however, the comparison must always be interpreted with care and it must be noted that "extrapolations have their limits" (Huff, 1963).

Very little is known about the infection in the natural hosts which are three species of the jungle fowl in Sri Lanka, India, and Malaysia where epizootics of the disease occur in imported chickens.

The mortality is high in imported breeds of chickens, and epizootics can seriously affect chicken farms in Asia. The turnover of the population is so rapid that there is not enough time for immunity to control the disease. Fortunately the reservoir is often distant from settled areas, and infection in the domestic fowl may die out when the epizootic is over (Garnham, 1977b).

The mortality rate of *P. gallinaceum* in the domestic hen depends upon three equally important factors. The breed, the age of the host, and the source of infection, i.e., blood or sporozoite-induced. The local chickens ("country fowl") suffer mild infections, and they seldom die, whereas imported breeds are highly susceptible and the death rate is high. The mortality rate in experimental chickens (of European origin) depends upon the age—1-day-old chicks die very frequently, but by 6 weeks they are less affected, and in adults death is rare. In experiments on 3-week-old birds, the death rate after the inoculation of blood stages of the parasites was about 25%, whereas after sporozoite induction almost all the birds succumbed during the second week. These observations were made by Dhanapala (1969) on the second strain of the parasite which he, like Brumpt with the first, had isolated in Colombo. It is difficult to make direct comparisons, because different techniques have been employed by various workers who have rarely given the exact number of parasites in the inoculum. Thus Al-Dabagh (1966), using the original strain, states that the death rate is 88% in blood-inoculated chicks and 85% after sporozoite induction.

In epizootics, the disease runs a rapid course; the bird is unable to stand, its face and comb become much congested, though the mucous membranes are pale from the intense anemia, the feathers are ruffled, and diarrhea is often present (Crawford, 1945). Death is due to secondary shock as a result of anoxemic anoxia. If, for any reason the chick survives the first onslaught, the massive exoerythrocytic development of the parasite blocks the vessels of the brain, and the bird dies during the second or third week with cerebral signs. This picture is often seen in chicks treated with quinine which suppresses the erythrocytic infection but entirely fails to affect the exoerythrocytic stages.

Both the liver and spleen become enlarged, but in the acute disease these organs are soft in consistency and may not be easily palpable. If the infection becomes chronic, fibrosis and hypertrophy occur, and splenomegaly is very obvious.

A peculiar sign of the disease was described in detail by Al-Dabagh (1961a). In 17% of 1-day-old chicks infected by blood stages, eyelid lesions developed during the first week. Photophobia and lachrymation initiate the process, and these are quickly followed by reddening of the conjunctivae; eventually there is necrosis of the tissues accompanied by a thick exudate. A similar syndrome has been seen in *P. lophurae* malaria (see Section VI, D), and an allied condition is common in rabbits infected with *Trypanosoma brucei*. Al-Dabagh suggests that the condition is the result of a deficiency in pantothenic acid.

Soni and Cox (1975) described an acute nephrotic syndrome in gallinaceum malaria, probably due to an antigen antibody reaction.

C. *Plasmodium (Giovannolaia) durae*

Plasmodium durae was first described by Herman (1941) in epizootics of domestic turkeys in a farm near Nairobi in Kenya. In more recent years it, or a closely allied species, has been isolated in West Africa by Barnes (1974), while finally and most surprisingly, a durae–like parasite has been found in wild turkeys by Telford and Forrester (1975) in Florida—the region where the bird originated. After much consideration, this species in the New World was given a new name (*P. hermani*). Small morphological differences exist between the various strains of the turkey parasites, and it is possible that the species has undergone mutation in the course of the three centuries since its arrival in Africa (see Garnham, 1977b). The periodicity of schizogony in the blood was found to be 24 hours (de Jong, 1971).

The epizootics in domestic turkeys in Africa were accompanied by considerable mortality, although the flocks were not exterminated. The birds become ill and weak and have ruffled feathers; they rest with their heads on the ground, and their legs become edematous. Eventually cerebral symptoms ensue, and they may die with convulsions or become paralyzed (the vessels in the brain are found to be blocked by the large exoerythrocytic schizonts). However, the infection usually follows a more chronic course, and Purchase (1942) states that a high blood pressure is characteristic of this type of infection, although this syndrome was not confirmed by de Jong (1971). She studied the course of the infection in 172 turkeys and found that the mortality varied according to the size of the inoculum and the age of the host: birds 3 weeks old or less and infected with 2 million parasites or more all died of the disease; the mortality was reduced to 25% in birds between 3 and 6 weeks in age, while those over this age usually recovered. The virulence increased with serial passage. Signs of the disease were first noted about 11 days after infection; these included lethargy, ruffling of feathers, drooping of eyelids, loss of appetite, and red or green, watery diarrhea. A gradual weakness in the legs developed, and toward the end in the younger birds convulsions occurred with muscular rigidity and hyperextension of the neck. Anemia was a constant feature, as well as enlargement of the spleen. In older birds, the infection became chronic, and the signs of disease gradually disappeared. No significant differences in the blood pressure were found in normal and infected birds, in both of which the blood pressure was found to increase with age.

D. *Plasmodium (Giovannolaia) lophurae*

This malaria parasite was isolated on a single occasion by Coggeshall (1938) from a fire-backed pheasant in the New York Zoological Gardens. It is included here because at one time it was extensively used in malaria research, as ducklings and, to a lesser extent, chicks proved to be highly susceptible to the infection. Unfortunately, although the strain still exists, it has long lost its capacity to produce gametocytes. *Plasmodium lophurae* is probably most interesting in that McGhee (1951) adapted it to mice, a most remarkable and probably unique feat—the breaking of the class barrier in malaria parasites.

The clinical features of the disease have been described in ducklings, chicks, and other birds; the mortality is highest in ducklings. The latter become lethargic and unsteady with ruffled feathers; they appear to stare at imaginary objects, and finally cerebral signs develop; they usually die in convulsions (due to blockage of the capillaries of the brain). Aaemia is a marked feature and may be a primary cause of death in some infections. The temperature is said to rise by as much as 3°C, though such records may merely represent the result of handling (see Section V). The spleen may reach nine times the size of the uninfected organ (Rigdon, 1944).

The schizogonic cycle in the blood of unnatural hosts tends to be asynochronous, but has been variously estimated as 24 hours (with segmentation in the evening) or 36 hours.

E. *Plasmodium (Novyella) juxtanucleare*

This widely distributed avian parasite probably originated in tropical Asia from which it may have traveled to Japan and the New World where it occurs in various countries of Latin America. *Plasmodium juxtanucleare* produces epizootics in the domestic hen and causes a heavy mortality in American though less in Asian infections. The disease is much less acute than malaria due to *P. gallinaceum*. In its natural home, the infection represents a veterinary zoonosis in which the reservoir is the jungle fowl.

The duration of the asexual cycle in the blood is thought to be 24 hours, with the schizonts rupturing in the early morning.

Laboratory infections of American strains give rise to a mortality rate varying between 38 and nearly 100%. The birds usually die in about 2 months, but some survive for a year. In the Sri Lankan strain, the mortality rate even in 1-week-old chicks was only 16%.

Chronic infections of *P. juxtanucleare* are unaccompanied by pyrexia even during recrudescences, but anemia becomes severe, while extensive exoerythrocytic infection of the organs, particularly of the brain, heart, kidneys, and testes, leads to characteristic signs of the disease. Pallor of the comb and mucous membranes is intense, movement is restricted, and diarrhea is common. A characteristic paralytic syndrome was reported by Al-Dabagh (1961b). The chronic myocarditis is probably responsible for the sudden death of some birds.

Splenomegaly became apparent in the second week of infection and increases during the course of the long illness. The spleen reaches a size 13 times that of normal.

Plasmodium juxtanucleare is such a small parasite and is so often embedded in the host cell nucleus that its presence may easily be overlooked and the nature of the chronic debilitating illness missed. Diagnosis may present difficulties in Asian infections which are often accompanied by the equally small *Aegyptianella,* but the presence of a small dot of pigment in the malaria parasite should confirm the identification.

F. *Plasmodium (Huffia) elongatum*

This cosmopolitan parasite differs from those present in the other three subgenera in that exoerythrocytic schizogony occurs exclusively in the hemopoietic system, so naturally the predominant sign of the disease is anemia. *Plasmodium elongatum* is found in over 30 species of mainly passeriform birds. The canary is easily infected in the laboratory, and the mortality rate is very high; the duckling is almost equally susceptible. Fruma Wolfson (1946) noted that 50% of the latter died during the 10-day period after inoculation as a result of anemia, sometimes having as low as 300,000 red blood cells per cubic millimeter. The effect of *P. elongatum* infections on the wild bird population is unknown, though in my experience no nestlings have been found moribund or dead as a result of this type of malaria.

The periodicity of asexual schizogony in the blood is 24 hours, and the schizonts rupture between 8 and 10 A.M. The duration of the prepatent period was originally thought to be about 12 days, but Corradetti *et al.* (1968) showed by inoculating sporozoites (derived from a strain in an owl bitten by *Culex pipiens*) into canaries that it was much shorter, 5 days or less.

A grave anemia quickly develops as a result of the invasion of the stem cells in the bone marrow, and hemopoiesis is almost obliterated; parasitemia in the peripheral blood may be quite low, in contrast to massive development of *P. elongatum* in the bone marrow. Hemopoiesis of course also takes place in various organs including the spleen and liver, but no great changes in size of these organs are usually reported in infections with *P. elongatum*.

VIII. REPTILIAN MALARIA

A very large number of species of malaria parasites from lizards have been described, and difficulties have arisen with regard to their classification, because of (1) the absence of pigment in some species and (2) their transmission by insects other than mosquitoes. For these reasons they cannot belong to the genus *Plasmodium;* phylogenetically it is probable that they are precursors of the true malaria parasite. Details of the clinical features of these animals are very limited, and therefore they are not considered here. A good description of reptilian malaria parasites has been provided by Ayala (1977) and in numerous papers by Telford up to 1980.

REFERENCES

Aberle, S. D. (1945). "Primate Malaria." Natl. Res. Counc., Div. Med. Sci., Off. Med. Inf., New York.

Adams, A. R. D. (1980). Remarkable malignant tertian parasitaemia. *Trans. R. Soc. Trop. Med. Hyg.* **54**, 2.

Akiba, K. (1964). Leucocytozoonosis in Japan. *Bull. Off. Int. Epizoot.* **62**, 1017–1022.

Al-Dabagh, M. A. (1961a). Eyelid lesions in chicks infected with *Plasmodium gallinaceum. Trans. R. Soc. Trop. Med. Hyg.* **55**, 351–354.

Al-Dabagh, M. A. (1961b). Symptomatic partial paralysis in chicks infected with *Plasmodium juxtanucleare. J. Comp. Pathol.* **72**, 217–221.

Al-Dabagh, M. A. (1966). "Mechanisms of Death and Tissue Injury in Malaria with Special Reference to Five Species of Avian Malaria." Shafik Press, Baghdad.

Allison, A. C. (1961). The distribution of the sickle cell gene. *Ann. N.Y. Acad. Sci.* **91,** 710–715.

Allison, A. C., and Clark, I. A. (1977). Specific and non-specific immunity in malaria. *Am. J. Trop. Med. Hyg.* **26,** 216–222.

Ayala, S. C. (1977). Plasmodia of reptiles. *In* "Parasitic Protozoa" (J. P. Kreier, ed.), Vol. 3, Chapter 6, pp. 267–309. Academic Press, New York.

Barbier, M. (1978). Le paludisme. *Horus. Rev. Med. Chir. Panafr.* **3,** 10–48.

Bafort, J. (1977). New isolations of murine malaria in Africa, Cameroun. *Proc.* 5th *Internat. Cong. Protozool.* New York. No. 343.

Baker, J. R. (1969). Trypanosomes of wild mammals in the neighborhood of the Serengeti National Park. *In* "Diseases in Free-living Wild Animals" (A. McDiarmid, ed.), Symp. Zool. Soc. London No. 24, pp. 147–158. Academic Press, New York.

Barnes, H. J. (1974). *Plasmodium* sp. infecting turkeys in northern Nigeria. *Vet. Rec.* 218–219.

Boyd, M. F., Stratman-Thomas, W. F., and Kitchen, S. F. "A Symposium on Human Malaria," No. 15. Am. Assoc. Adv. Sci., Washington, D.C.

Bray, R. S. (1958). *Laverania falciparum. Am. J. Trop. Med. Hyg.* **7,** 20–24.

Bruce-Chwatt, L. J. (1978). Introduction. *In* "Rodent Malaria" (R. Killick-Kendrick and W. Peters, eds.), pp. xi–xxv. Academic Press, New York.

Brumpt, E. (1935). *Plasmodium gallinaceum* n. sp. de la poule domestique, *C. R. Acad. Sci.* **200,** 783–785.

Cadigan, F. C., Ward, R. A., and Chaicumpa, V. (1969). Further studies on the biology of human malarial parasites in gibbons from Thailand. *Mil. Med.* **134,** 757–766.

Carothers, J. C. (1934). An investigation of the etiology of subacute nephritis as seen among children in north Kavirondo. *East Afr. Med. J.* **10,** 335–336.

Carrescia, P. M., and Arcoles, G. (1958). Ulteriori ricerche con ceppi virulenti di *Plasmodium berghei* nei topi albini. *Riv. Malariol.* **37,** 57–68.

Carter, R., and Diggs, C. L. (1977). Plasmodia of rodents. *In* "Parasitic Protozoa" (J. P. Kreier, ed.), Vol. 3, Chapter 8, pp. 359–465. Academic Press, New York.

Castellani, A., and Chalmers, H. J. (1919). "Manual of Tropical Medicine," 3rd ed. Baillière, London.

Chin, W., Contacos, P. J., Coatney, G. R. and Kimball, H. R. (1965). A naturally acquired quotidian type malaria in man transferable to monkeys. *Science* **149,** 865.

Ciucă, M., Chelarescu, M., Sofletea, A., Constantinescu, P., Tenteanu, E., Cortez, P., Balanovschi, G., and Ilies, M. (1955). "Contribution expérimentale à l'étude de l'immunité dans le paludisme," Sect. 204. Editions Acad. Repub. Pop. Români, Bucharest.

Coatney, G. R. (1968). Simian malaria in man: Facts, implications and predictions. *Am. J. Trop. Med. Hyg.* **17,** 147–155.

Coatney, G. R. (1976). Relapse in malaria—An enigma. *J. Parasitol.* **62,** 3–9.

Coatney, G. R., and Contacos, P. G. (1963). Experimental adaptation of simian malarias to abnormal hosts. *J. Parasitol.* **49,** 912–918.

Coatney, G. R., and Young, M. D. (1942). A study of the paroxysms resulting from induced infections of *Plasmodium vivax. Am. J. Hyg.* **35,** 138–141.

Coatney, G. R., Collins, W. E., Warren, M., and Contacos, P. G. (1971). "The Primate Malarias." US Department of Health, Education and Welfare, Bethesda, Maryland.

Coggeshall, L. J. (1938). *Plasmodium lophurae:* A new species of malaria parasite pathogenic for the domestic fowl. *Am. J. Hyg.* **27,** 615–618.

Collins, W. E., Contacos, P. G., Guinn, E. G., and Held, J. R. (1967). Infections and transmission of *Plasmodium coatneyi* into *Anopheles freeborni* and *A. balabacensis balabacensis* mosquitoes. *J. Parasitol.* **53,** 1130–1134.

Corradetti, A., Garnham, P. C. C., and Laird, M. (1963). New classification of the avian malaria parasite. *Parassitologia* **5**, 1–4.

Corradetti, A., Neri, I., Scanga, M., and Cavallini, C. (1968). I cicli pre-eritrocitico e sporogonico di *Plasmodium (Huffia) elongatum. Parassitologia* **10**, 133–143.

Crane, G. G., and Pryor, D. S. (1971). Malaria and the tropical splenomegaly syndrome in New Guinea. *Trans. R. Soc. Trop. Med. Hyg.* **65**, 315–324.

Crane, G. G., Wells, J. V., and Hudson, P. (1972). Tropical splenomegaly syndrome in New Guinea. I. Natural history. *Trans. R. Soc. Trop. Med. Hyg.* **66**, 724–732.

Crawford, M. (1945). *Plasmodium gallinaceum,* a malaria parasite of the domestic fowl. *Vet. Rec.* **7**, 386–397.

Dasgupta, B. M. (1938) Transmission of *Plasmodium inui* to man. *Proc. Natn. Inst. Sci. India,* **4**, 241–244.

Deane, L. M. (1976). Epidemiology of simian malaria on the American continent. Sci. Publ., Pan. Am. Health Organ. **317**, 144–163.

Deane, L. M., Deane, N. T., and Ferreira-Neto, J. (1966). Studies on transmission of simian malaria and on a natural infection of man with *Plasmodium simium* in Brazil. *Bull. W. H. O.* **35**, 805–808.

de Jong, A. C. (1971). Some haemosporidian parasites of parakeets and francolins. Ph.D. Thesis, University of London.

Demina, N. A. (1959). Contribution à l'étude de l'influence de régime nycthémeral de l'hôte sur l'évolution de la multiplication de *Plasmodium relictum. Riv. Malariol.* **38**, 27–44.

de Sanctis Monaldi, T. (1953). Sulla fase negative del sangue e nell' infezione da *P. vivax. Riv. Malariol.* **14**, 344–351.

Desser, S. S., Fallis, A. M., and Garnham, P. C. C. (1968). Relapses in ducks chronically infected with *Leucocytozoon simondi* and *Parahaemoproteus nettionis. Can. J. Zool.* **45**, 1061–1065.

Dhanapala, S. B. (1962). The occurrence of *Plasmodium juxtanucleare* in domestic fowls. *Riv. Malariol.* **41**, 3–10.

Dodd, S. (1913). Anaplasms or Jolly bodies? *J. Comp. Path. Ther.* **26**, 97–110.

Edington, G. M., and Gilles, H. M. (1969). "Pathology in the Tropics." Arnold, London.

Edwards, A. C., Meredith, T. J., and Sowton, E. (1978). Complete heart block due to chronic chloroquine toxicity managed with permanent pacemaker. *Br. Med. J.* **1**, 1109–1110.

Fairley, N. H. (1947). Sidelights on malaria in man obtained by subinoculation experiments. *Trans. R. Soc. Trop. Med. Hyg.* **40**, 621–676.

Gabaldon, A. (1980). Holoendemicity in avian malaria. *Trans. R. Soc. Trop. Med. Hyg.* **74**, Part 4.

Garnham, P. C. C. (1949). Malarial immunity in Africa: Effects in infancy and early childhood. *Ann. Trop. Med. Parasitol.* **43**, 47–61.

Garnham, P. C. C. (1965). The pathology of *Plasmodium coatneyi* malaria. *In* "Omagiu lui Prof. Dr. M. Ciuča," pp. 191–203. Acad. Repub. Soc. România, Bucharest.

Garnham, P. C. C. (1966). "Malaria Parasites and Other Haemosporidia." Blackwell, Oxford.

Garnham, P. C. C. (1967). Malaria in mammals excluding man. *Adv. Parasitol.* **5**, 156–159.

Garnham, P. C. C. (1969). Malaria as a medical and veterinary zoonosis. *Bull. Soc. Pathol. Exotique* **2**, 325–332.

Garnham, P. C. C. (1970a). Longevity of malaria parasites in man and its epidemiological significance. *In* "Festschrift for Maruashvilli," pp. 65–71. Tbilisi, Georgia S.S.R.

Garnham, P. C. C. (1970b). The role of the spleen in protozoal infections with special reference to splenectomy. *Acta Trop.* **27**, 1–14.

Garnham, P. C. C. (1973). Recent research on malaria in mammals excluding man. *Adv. Parasitol.* **11**, 620–621.

Garnham, P. C. C. (1977a). The continuing mystery of relapses in malaria. *Protozool. Abstr.* **1**, 1–12.

Garnham, P. C. C. (1977b). The origins, evolutionary significance and dispersal of haemosporidian parasites of domestic birds. *In* "Origins of Pests, Parasites, Disease and Weed Problems" (J. M. Charrett and G. R. Sagar, eds.), pp. 57–70. Blackwell, Oxford.

Garnham, P. C. C. (1980). Notes and comments on Linnaeus' thesis: "A new theory on the cause of intermittent fevers," with the first complete translation into English. *J. Linn. Soc. London* (in press).

Garnham, P. C. C., and Bray, R. S. (1959). The susceptibility of the higher primates to piroplasms. *J. Protozool.* **6**, 352–355.

Garnham, P. C. C., Lainson, R., and Gunders, A. E. (1956). Some observations on malaria parasites in chimpanzees with particular reference to the persistence of *Plasmodium reichenowi* and *Plasmodium vivax*. *Ann. Soc. Belge Med. Trop.* **36**, 811–822.

Garnham, P. C. C., Molinari, V., and Shute, P. G. (1962). Differential diagnosis of bastianellii and vivax malaria. *Bull. W. H. O.* **27**, 197–202.

Garnham, P. C. C., Bray, R. S., Bruce-Chwatt, L. J., Draper, C. C., Killick-Kendrick, R., Šergiev, P. G., Tiburskaya, N. A., Shute, P. G., and Maryon, M. (1975). A strain of *Plasmodium vivax* characterised by prolonged incubation: Morphological and biological characteristics. *Bull. W. H. O.* **52**, 21–30.

Geiman, Q. M., and Meagher, M. J. (1967). Susceptibility of a New World monkey to *Plasmodium falciparum* from man. *Nature (London)* **215**, 437–439.

Geiman, Q. M., and Siddiqui, W. A. (1969). Susceptibility of a New World monkey to *Plasmodium malariae* from man. *Am. J. Trop. Med. Hyg.* **18**, 351–354.

Giglioli, G. (1930). "Malarial Nephritis." Churchill, London.

Hawking, F. (1953). Milk diet, *p*-aminobenzoic acid and malaria (*P. berghei*). *Br. Med. J.* **1**, 1201–1203.

Hawking, F., Worms, J., and Gamage, K. (1968). 24- and 48-hour cycles of malaria parasites in the blood: Their purpose, production and control *Trans. R. Soc. Trop. Med. Hyg.* **42**, 731–776.

Hendrikse, R. G., Adeniye, A., Edington, G. M., Glasgow, E. F., White, R. H. R., and Houba, V. (1972). Quartan malarial syndrome. *Lancet*, **2**, 1143–1149.

Herman, C. M. (1941). *Plasmodium durae*, a new species of malaria parasite from the common turkey. *Am. J. Hyg.* **34**, 22–27.

Huff, C. G. (1939). Relations between malarial infections and body temperatures in canaries. *Am. J. Hyg.* **29**, 149–154.

Huff, C. G. (1963). Experimental research on avian malaria. *Adv. Parasitol.* **1**, 1–65.

Hutt, M. S. R., and Hamilton, P. J. S. (1972). Tropical splenomegaly syndrome. *In* "Medicine in a Tropical Environment" (A. G. Shafer, J. W. Kibukomusoke, and M. S. R. Hutt, eds.), pp. 35–51. Br. Med. Assoc., London.

Jeffery, G., Wolcott, G. B., Young, M. D., and Williams, D. (1952). Exoerythrocytic stages of *Plasmodium falciparum*. *Am. J. Trop. Med. Hyg.* **1**, 917–926.

Jenkins, H. G. (1957). Congenital malaria in England—*Plasmodium ovale*. *Br. Med. J.* **1**, 88–89.

Jingbo Jiang, Zupei Long, and Jiexian Zou (1978). The successive passages and heavy infections of *Plasmodium falciparum* in two species of macaques, the blood of which being partly replaced by human blood. *Acta Sci. Nat. Univ. Sunyatsen* No. 4, p. 52 (in Chinese with English summary).

Killick-Kendrick, R., and Peters, W., eds. (1978). "Rodent Malaria." Academic Press, New York.

Kreier, J. P., and Leste, J. (1968). Parasitaemia and erythrocyte destruction in *Plasmodium berghei*-infected rats. II. Effect of infected host globulin. *Exp. Parasitol.* **23**, 198–204.

Kreier, J. P., Shapiro, H., Dilley, D. A., Szilvassy, I., and Ristic, M. (1966). Autoimmune reactions in rats with *Plasmodium berghei* infection. *Exp. Parasitol.* **19**, 155–162.

Kretschmar, M. (1961). Infektionsverlauf und Krankheitsbild bei mit *Plasmodium berghei* infezier-ten Mäusen des Stammes NMRI. *Z. Tropenmed. Parasitol.* **12**, 346–367.

Kretschmar, W. (1962). Resistenz und Immunitat bei mit *Plasmodium berghei* infurzieten Mäusen. *Z. Tropenmed. Parasitol.* **13**, 159–175.

Kretschmar, W. (1964). Parasitendichte und Erythrocytenverlust bei der Malaria (*P. berghei*) in der Maus. *Z. Tropenmed. Parasitol.* **15**, 386–399.

Krotoski, W. A., Krostoski, D. M., Garnham, P. C. C., Bray, R. S., Killick-Kendrick, R., Draper, C. C., Targett, G. A. T., and Guy, M. W. (1980). Replapses in primate malaria: discovery of two populations of exoerythrocytic stages. Preliminary note. *Br. Med. J.* **1**, 103.

Landau, I. (1978). *In* "Rodent Malaria" (R. Killick-Kendrick and W. Peters, eds.), Chapter 2. Academic Press, New York.

Levine, N. D. (1975). "Protozoan Parasites of Domestic Animals and of Man," 2nd ed. Burgess, Minneapolis, Minnesota.

Lupaşcu, G., Bossie, A., Smolinski, M., Balif, E., Constantinescu, P., Isfan, T., Petrea, D., Mazilu, V., and Roman, V. (1963). Le problème des infections à *P. malariae* et les programmes d'éradication du paludisme. *Arch. Roum. Pathol. Exp. Microbiol.* **22**, 333–348.

Lupaşcu, G., Constantinescu, P., Negulici, E., Garnham, P. C. C., Bray, R. S., Killick-Kendrick, R., Shute, P. G., and Maryon, M. (1967). The late primary exoerythrocytic stages of *Plasmodium malariae*. *Trans. R. Soc. Trop. Med. Hyg.* **61**, 482–489.

Luzzatto, L. (1974). Genetic factors in malaria. *Bull. W.H.O.* **50**, 195–202.

Lysenko, A. J., Alekseeva, M. I., Glazunova, Z. I., Gorbunova, U. P., Kulish, E. A., Ermolin, G. A., Efremov, E. E., Panomareuva, A. M. and Chumak, M. P. (1977). "Serological Profile of a Population in Former Foci of *Plasmodium malariae* in the Moldavian Soviet Socialist Republic," WHO/MAL/77.888, pp. 1–4. WHO, Geneva.

McGhee, R. B. (1951). The adaptation of the avian malaria parasite *Plasmodium lophurae* to a continuous existence in baby mice. *J. Infect. Dis.* **88**, 86–97.

Maegraith, B. G. (1948). "Pathological Processes in Malaria and Blackwater Fever." Blackwell, Oxford.

Maegraith, B. G. (1970). Malaria. *In* "Medicine in the Tropics" (A. W. Woodruff, ed.), Chapter 3, pp. 51 et seq. Churchill-Livingstone, Edinburgh and London.

Maegraith, B. G. (1977). Interdependence. The Craig Lecture. *Am. J. Trop. Med. Hyg.* **26**, 344–355.

Manwell, R. D. (1938). The identification of the avian malarias. *Am. J. Trop. Med.* **18**, 563–575.

Marchiafava, E., and Bignami, A. (1892). "Sulle febbri malariche estivo-autumnale." Loescher, Roma.

Marchoux, E. (1926). "Paludisme." Baillière et Fils, Paris.

Markus, M. B. (1974). Arthropod-borne disease as a possible factor limiting the distribution of birds. *Int. J. Parasitol.* **4**, 609–612.

Marsden, P. D., and Bruce-Chwatt, L. J. (1975). *In* "Topics on Tropical Morphology" (Hornibrook ed.), Chapter 3. Cerebral Malaria. Davis, Philadelphia, Pennsylvania.

Marsden, P. D., Hutt, M. S., Wicks, N. E., Voller, A., Blackman, V., Shah, K. K., Connor, D. H., Hamilton, P. J. S., Cranwell, J. G. and Lunn, H. F. (1965). An investigation of tropical splenomegaly at Mulago Hospital, Kampala, Uganda. *Br. Med. J.* **1**, 89–93.

Mercado, T. (1965). Paralysis associated with *Plasmodium berghei* malaria in the rat. *J. Infect. Dis.* **26**, 115 and 465–472.

Mercado, T., and Coatney, G. R. (1951). The course of the blood induced *Plasmodium berghei* infection in white mice. *J. Parasitol.* **37**, 479–482.

Miller, L. H., Mason, S. J., Clyde, D. F., and McGinniss, M. A. (1976). The resistance factor to *Plasmodium vivax* in blacks. The Duffy blood group genotype, Fy Fy. *N. Engl. J. Med.* **295**, 302–304.

Most, H. (1940). Malaria in drug addicts. *Trans. R. Soc. Trop. Med. Hyg.* **34**, 139–172.

Najune, G. R., and Sulzer, A. J. (1976). Transfusion-induced malaria from an asymptomatic carrier. *Transfusion* **16**, 473–476.

Nicol, W. D. (1935). Monkey malaria in G.P.I. *Br. Med. J.* **2**, 760.

Nicolaev, B. P.)1949). Subspecies of the parasite of tertian malaria (*Plasmodium vovax*). *Dokl. Akad. Nauk SSSR* **67**, 201–210.

Peters, W., Garnham, P. C. C., Killick-Kendrick, R., Rajapaksa, N., Cheong, W. H., and Cadigan, F. C. (1976). Malaria of the orang-utan (*Pongo pygmaeus*) in Borneo. *Phil. Trans. R. Soc. London, Ser. B* **275**, 439–482.

Purchase, H. S. (1942). Turkey malaria. *Parasitology* **34**, 278–283.

Raffaele, G. (1936) Potere infettante del sangue durante l'incubazione della malaria aviaria. *Riv. Malariol.* **15**, 1–11.

Rigdon, R. H. (1944). A consideration of the mechanism of splenic infarcts in malaria. *Am. J. Trop. Med.* **24**, 349–354.

Rodhain, J.)1956). Les formes pré-érythrocytaires du *Plasmodium vivax* chez le chimpanzée. *Ann. Soc. Belge Méd. Trop.* **26**, 99–103.

Rodhain, J., and Dellaert, R. (1955). Contribution à l'étude de *Plasmodium schwetzi* E. Brumpt: Transmission du *Plasmodium schwetzi* à l'homme. *Ann. Soc. Belge Med. Trop.* **35**, 73–76 and 757–777.

St. John, J. H. (1927). Observations on the use of *Plasmodium vivax* in the treatment of cerebrospinal syphilis. *Am. J. Syph.* **11**, 3–11.

Schmidt, L. H. (1978). *Plasmodium falciparum* and *Plasmodium vivax* infections in the owl monkey (*Aotus trivirgatus*). I. The courses of untreated infections. II. Responses to chloroquine, quinine and pyrimethamine. III. Methods employed in the search for new blood schizontocidal drugs. *Am. J. Trop. Med. Hyg.* **27**, 671–732.

Schmidt, L. H., Fradkin, R., Harrison, J., and Bossen, R. N. (1977). Differences in the virulence of *Plasmodium knowlesi* for *Macaca irus (fascicularis)* of Philippine and Malayan origins. *Am. J. Trop. Med. Hyg.* **26**, 612–622.

Schwetz, J. (1934). Contribution à l'étude des parasites malariens des singes supérieurs africains. *Riv. Malariol.* **13**, 143–147.

Seed, T. M., and Manwell, R. D. (1977). Plasmodia of birds. *In* "Parasitic Protozoa" (J. P. Kreier, ed.), Vol. 3, Chapter 7. Academic Press, New York.

Sergent, E. (1963). *In* "Immunity to Protozoa" (P. C. C. Garnham, A. E. Pierce, and I. Roitt, eds.), Chapter 3, p. 40. Blackwell, Oxford.

Sergent, E., and Poncet, A. (1955). Etude expérimentale du paludisme des rongeurs à *Plasmodium pergsei*. *Arch. Inst. Pasteur d'Algér* **33**, 287–306.

Sergent, E., and Poncet, A. (1961). De la température des souris blanches pendant l'accès parasitaire de paludisme. *Arch. Inst. Pasteur Algér.* **39**, 133–134.

Sergent, Ed., and Sergent, Et. (1952). Recherches expérimentales sur l'infection latente et la prémunition dans le paludisme. *Arch. Inst. Pasteur Algér.* **30**, 203–239.

Shortt, H. E., Fairley, N. H., Covell, G., Shute, P. G., and Garnham, P. C. C. (1951). The pre-erythrocytic stage of *Plasmodium falciparum*. *Trans. R. Soc. Trop. Med. Hyg.* **44**, 405–419.

Shortt, H. E., and Garnham, P. C. C. (1948). Demonstration of a persisting exoerythrocytic cycle of *Plasmodium cynomologi* and its bearing on the production of relapses. *Br. Med. J.* **1**, 1225–1228.

Shute, P. G. (1970). Malaria, *Trans. R. Soc. Trop. Med. Hyg.* **64**, 210–216.

Shute, P. G., Lupaşcu, G., Branzei, P., Maryon, M., Constantinescu, P., Bruce-Chwatt, L. J., Draper, C. C., Killick-Kendrick, R., and Garnham, P. C. C. (1976). A strain of *Plasmodium vivax* characterised by predominantly prolonged incubation: The effect of numbers of sporozoites on the length of the prepatent period. *Trans. R. Soc. Trop. Med. Hyg.* **70,** 474–481.

Stephens, J. W. W. (1914). A new malaria parasite of man. *Ann. Trop. Med. Parasitol.* **8,** 119–124.

Stephens, J. W. W., and Christophers, S. R. (1901). "Blackwater Fever Cases 9–16," Reports to the Malaria Committee of the Royal Society, 5th ser., pp. 12–27. Harrison, London.

Sulzer, A. J., Sulzer, K. R., Cantella, R. A., Colichon, H., Latorre, C. R., and Welch, M. (1978). Study of coinciding foci of malaria and leptospirosis in the Peruvian Amazon area. *Trans. R. Soc. Trop. Med. Hyg.* **72,** 76–82.

Suntherasamai, P., and Marsden, P. D. (1969). Studies of splenomegaly in rodent malaria. 1. The course of splenomegaly in mice infected with *Eperythrozoon coccoides, Plasmodium berghei yoelii* and the two infections combined. *Trans. R. Soc. Trop. Med. Hyg.* **63,** 64–70.

Suntherasamai, P., and Marsden, P. D. (1972). 3. Protein calorie malnutrition and splenomegaly in mice infected with *Plasmodium berghei yoelii. Trans. R. Soc. Trop. Med. Hyg.* **66,** 214–221.

Surtek, K. E. (1931). A striking case of quartana-nephrosis. *Trans. R. Soc. Trop. Med. Hyg.* **25,** 201–205.

Taliaferro, W. H., and Taliaferro, L. G. (1934a). The transmission of *Plasmodium falciparum* to the howler monkey, *Alouatta* sp. *Am. J. Hyg.* **19,** 318–324.

Taliaferro, W. H., and Taliaferro, L. G. (1934b). Alteration in the time of sporulation of *Plasmodium brasilianum* in monkeys by reversal of light and dark. *Am. J. Hyg.* **20,** 50–59.

Telford, S. R., and Forrester, D. J. (1975). *Plasmodium hermani* sp.n. from wild turkeys (*Meleagris gallipavo*) in Florida. *J. Protozool.* **22,** 324–348.

Ungureanu, E., Killick-Kendrick, R., Garnham, P. C. C., Branzei, P., and Shute, P. G. (1976). Prepatent periods of a tropical strain of *Plasmodium vivax* after inoculations of tenfold dilutions of sporozoites. *Trans. R. Soc. Trop. Med. Hyg.* **70,** 482–483.

Vincke, I. H., and Lips, M. (1948). Un nouveau *Plasmodium* d'un rongeur sauvage du Congo, *Plasmodium berghei* n.sp. *Ann. Soc. Belge Méd. Trop.* **28,** 97–104.

Voller, A., Draper, C. C., Tin Sheve, and Hutt, M. S. R. (1971). Nephrotic syndrome in monkey infected with human quartan malaria. *Br. Med. J.* **4,** 208–210.

Wagner-Jauregg, J. (1922). The treatment of general paralysis by inoculation of malaria. *J. Nerv. Ment. Dis.* **55,** 369–375.

Ward, R. A., Rutledge, L. C., and Hickman, R. L. (1969). Cyclical transmission of Chesson-vivax malaria in subhuman primates. *Nature (London)* **224,** 1126–1127.

Warner, R. E. (1961). Susceptibility of the endemic Hawaiian avifauna to mosquito-dome malaria and bird-pox. *Proc. X Pacific Sci. Compr., Honolulu.* pp. 242–243.

Warren, M., Cheong, W. H., Fredericks, H. K., and Coatney, G. R. (1970). Cycles of jungle malaria in West Malaysia. *Am. J. Trop. Med. Hyg.* **19,** 383–393.

Warren, M., Powers, K. G., Garnham, P. C. C., and Shiroishi, T. (1973). *Plasmodium cynomolgi:* Influence of X-irradiation and sporozoite dilution on relapse patterns in infected rhesus monkeys. *Exp. Parasitol.* **35,** 266–271.

Wenyon, C. M. (1926). "Protozoology," Vol. 2. Baillière, London.

Whelen, M., and Shute, P. G. (1943). Thiobismol in therapeutic malaria. *J. Trop. Med. Hyg.* **46,** 1–5.

Wolfson, F. (1946). *Plasmodium elongatum* in the Pekin duck. *Am. J. Hyg.* **44,** 268–272.

Woods, J. V. (1970). Immunological studies in tropical splenomegaly syndrome. *Trans. R. Soc. Trop. Med. Hyg.* **64,** 537–546.

World Health Organization (1963). "Terminology of Malaria and of Malaria Eradication." WHO, Geneva.

Yoeli, M. (1976). Chadwick lecture: The quest for suitable experimental models in parasitic diseases in man. *Trans. R. Soc. Trop. Med. Hyg.* **70,** 24–35.

Young, M. D. Eyles, D. E., Burgess, R. W., and Jeffery, G. M. (1955). Experimental testing of the immunity of negroes to *Plasmodium vivax*. *J. Parasitol.* **41**, 315–318.

Young, M. D., Porter, J. A., and Johnson, C. M. (1966). *Plasmodium vivax* transmitted from man to monkey to man. *Science* **153**, 1006–1007.

Zuckerman, A. (1966). Recent studies on factors involved in malarial anaemia. *Mil. Med.* **131**, 1201–1216.

Chemotherapy of Malaria

Wallace Peters

I. HISTORICAL REVIEW

Chemotherapy has been defined as the "administration of a substance with a systemic anti-microbic action" (Garrod and O'Grady, 1971). Hawking (1963)

Malaria, Vol. 1
Copyright © 1980 by Academic Press, Inc.
All rights of reproduction in any form reserved.
ISBN 0-12-426101-9

interpreted the term as "the search for chemical compounds which will destroy infective parasites or organisms without destroying their animal host," and referred to Ehrlich as the founder of this science. He and his associate (Guttman and Ehrlich, 1891) were the first to attempt to treat patients suffering from malaria with a synthetic dyestuff, methylene blue. We prefer, however, the first definition, if only for the reason that *quinine* then becomes the first true chemotherapeutic agent, having been recognized for centuries by the Amerindians of Peru to have potent activity against fever. Although the date of the first use of the bark of the cinchona tree by the Spanish conquistadores for the treatment of malaria, then of course a disease of unknown etiology, has been lost in the mists of time, a number of conflicting views are held (Guerra, 1977a,b). It is claimed traditionally that powdered "fever tree" bark was used by Don Juan de Vega to treat the Countess of Chinchon, wife of the Viceroy of Peru, in 1638 and that his subsequent importation of a supply of the powder into Spain in 1641 was its first introduction to European medicine. It was indeed known for many years thereafter as *Pulvis comitissae* or "countess's powder." Probably, however, it was introduced into Spain as early as 1632 by Jesuit priests, since there is a record of its use in that country in 1639 (Anonymous, 1927). Certainly to the countess's use of it must be attributed the introduction of the term cinchona bark. Depending upon one's loyalties to the Church, as distinct from the nobility, it was also called Jesuits' powder or Cardinal's powder, since it was mainly due to the efforts of the Jesuit order in Spain and Italy that larger quantities of the powder were imported, and its use for the treatment of fevers was critically studied (Guerra, 1977a,b).

Cinchona bark is reputed to have formed the secret basis of a patent fever remedy in England at the end of the seventeenth century. The potency of this substance for curing malarial fevers led to its rapid increase in popularity, and numerous prescriptions for its employment were published (Fig. 1). Not only was the genuine bark prescribed, but also various fake remedies purporting to contain cinchona bark. It undoubtedly formed the basis of numerous patent remedies of that period, such as that sold by R. James (1749). His descriptions of various fevers against which his "powder" was highly successful ranged from what undoubtedly was one or another form of malaria to smallpox and even yellow fever. It was, however, in times of war that quinine, as was to happen in recent years with synthetic antimalarials, really came into its own. From the Napoleonic wars onward to World War I malaria and its remedy took on increasing importance. With the increasing and uncontrolled exploitation of natural sources of bark in South America steps clearly had to be taken to cultivate the cinchona tree elsewhere. In the face of obstruction by those countries in the forests of which the tree was native, seeds were taken to Ceylon and India and then to Java in the Dutch East Indies where plantations were established in the latter half of the nineteenth century. It was partly the threat to these supplies

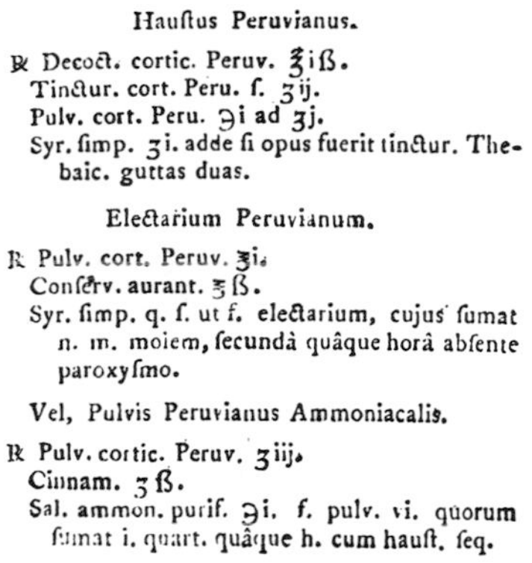

Hauſtus Peruvianus.

℞ Decoct. cortic. Peruv. ℥iß.
Tinctur. cort. Peru. f. ℨij.
Pulv. cort. Peru. ℈i ad ℨj.
Syr. ſimp. ℨi. adde ſi opus fuerit tinctur. The-
baic. guttas duas.

Electarium Peruvianum.

℞ Pulv. cort. Peruv. ℥i.
Conſerv. aurant. ℥ß.
Syr. ſimp. q. f. ut f. electarium, cujus ſumat
n. m. moiem, ſecundà quâque horà abſente
paroxyſmo.

Vel, Pulvis Peruvianus Ammoniacalis.

℞ Pulv. cortic. Peruv. ℨiij.
Cinnam. ℨß.
Sal. ammon. purif. ℈i. f. pulv. vi. quorum
ſumat i. quart. quâque h. cum hauſt. ſeq.

FIG. 1. Prescriptions containing quinine (in the crude form of ''Pulv. cortic. Peruv.'') in an old English pharmacopoeia (Anonymous, 1778). Peruvian bark was first officially recorded in the London Pharmacopoeia of 1677.

during World War I that triggered intensive research to find synthetic drugs with which to replace quinine, and the renewed threat during World War II that resulted in a revival of this effort. The most extensive search of all time for new antimalarials resulted from a combination of two threats, first, the advent of a major war in the Far East in the 1960s and second, the recognition of drug-resistant strains of falciparum malaria that responded only to quinine, supplies of which suddenly began to dry up.

About two centuries after its introduction into Europe, the French chemists Pelletier and Caventou (1820) separated a number of alkaloids from cinchona bark, among them quinine itself and cinchonine. From then on quinine, the constitutent with the most potent antimalarial properties, was employed almost exclusively. It was, unfortunately, a substance that could not readily be synthesized and, indeed, it took an additional century before Woodward and Doering (1944) were able to do so. Subsequently, synthetic analogs have been described, a number of which are far more active than quinine itself (Brossi et al., 1971).

Findlay (1951) has provided the best account of the history of antimalarial chemotherapy up to the 1950s, starting with the classic researches by German investigators following the lead of Paul Ehrlich. Robert Koch was the first to recognize the potential value of quinine for the control of malaria among the indigenous populations of endemic areas (Fig. 2), and Dempwolff's (1904) report from the then German New Guinea must be considered a description of the birth of malaria control by mass chemoprophylaxis. This experience undoubtedly helped to form the basis of quinine prophylaxis as applied to the armies of both Germany and her opponents during the Macedonian campaigns of World War I, and it was during this period in particular that it came to be recognized that there was a marked difference in response to quinine therapy in people with *Plas-*

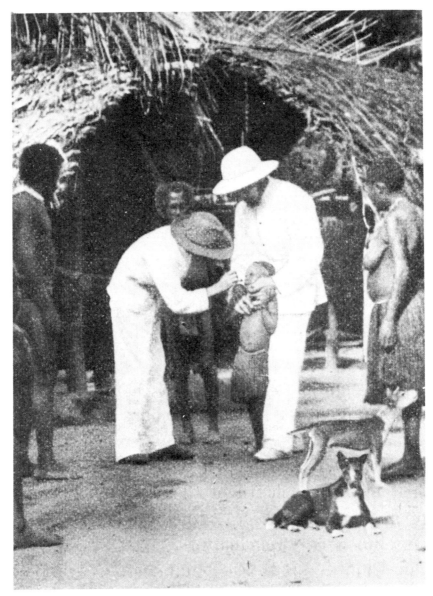

FIG. 2. Distribution of quinine to villagers in a holoendemic area of New Guinea; probably the first trial of quinine by mass drug administration. A marked but temporary reduction was achieved in the level of parasitemia (Dempwolff, 1904).

modium falciparum and in others suffering from *P. vivax* or *P. malariae* infection. This difference and, later, the special curative action of 8-aminoquinolines on sporozoite-induced vivax malaria, were to point the way finally to the existence of the exoerythrocytic cycles of mammalian malaria and the origin of malarial relapses.

The first model for the study of antimalarial drugs was living *P. falciparum* in human blood (Laveran, 1893) (of which details are given later in this chapter), and it is curious to note how the pendulum has swung back with recent descriptions of *in vitro* tests of drug response in the same model (Rieckmann *et al.*, 1968b) over 70 years later. Laveran noted that the gametocytes of *P. falciparum*, unlike the asexual stages, survived treatment with quinine which, however, he believed caused the ''flagella'' (microgametes he saw in wet preparations at room temperature, formed by what we now recognize as exflagellation) to disappear. (Laveran believed, incidentally, that the ''crescents'' were responsible for continuation of the infection and subsequent ''relapse'' of fever.) Some years later, Wasiliewski (1908) examined the effect of quinine on the avian species *P. praecox* (probably a race of *P. relictum*) in canaries, and Kopanaris (1911) used the same parasite *in vivo*. Early searches for new, synthetic antimalarials utilized the same model in a standardized screening technique established by Roehl, working with the Bayer Company in Germany in the 1920s (Peters, 1970a). In this model, pamaquine, the first successful synthetic antimalarial, was identified. Roehl's successor, Kikuth, later employed Java rice birds infected with *Haemoproteus orizivorae* to distinguish between the gametocytocidal effects of 8-aminoquinolines and schizontocidal action, a technique that eventually led to the development of mepacrine and 4-aminoquinolines. *Plasmodium cathemerium,* which could be used to infect ducklings, proved popular for a while but was shortly replaced by *P. gallinaceum* which formed the mainstay of large-scale drug screening at the U.S. National Institutes of Health and elsewhere during World War II. Mepacrine, developed in Germany shortly before the outbreak of hostilities, and pamaquine suffered from a number of limitations including some measure of toxicity, and superior drugs were sought, particularly in England and the United States. These investigations culminated in the synthesis of two radically new antimalarials, the dihydrofolate antagonists proguanil and pyrimethamine, and of a new 8-aminoquinoline, primaquine, that was better tolerated than its predecessor, in the recognition (and rejection) of the potential antimalarial action of sulfonamides, and in resurrection of the 4-aminoquinoline chloroquine, which had been dismissed shortly after its synthesis in 1934 in Germany as being too toxic for clinical use (Coatney, 1963).

Following its release in about 1946, chloroquine became the drug of choice for the treatment of malaria and shared with proguanil and pyrimethamine the major role in antimalarial prophylaxis. Primaquine gained sole place in the radical cure of infection with the relapsing malarias, *P. vivax, P. ovale,* and *P. malariae,* by virtue of its destructive action on secondary tissue schizonts (although in the light of current ideas on the origin of relapses in malariae infection the rationale of its continuing use is open to doubt). This happy state of affairs was not to last long since, within a year or two of the drugs' introduction, proguanil- and pyrimethamine-resistant strains of human malaria parasites were being recognized. Chloroquine, however, retained its reputation, and it was not until 1959 that the first undoubted cases of *P. falciparum* infection resistant to chloroquine were reported in South America (see review in Peters, 1970a). This unfortunate event, coinciding as it did with the outbreak of hostilities in Indochina, and the involvement of the U.S. Army, led to the buildup of a massive search for further new antimalarials and the exploration of new ways of using some of the older drugs, particularly to prevent or treat infection with chloroquine-resistant and multiple drug-resistant *P. falciparum*. Drug screening was intensified, and well over a quarter million compounds, old and new, were evaluated by the U.S. Army in a simple test using the parasite of African thicket rats, *P. berghei,* in albino mice. Laboratory and clinical studies revealed also the value of combining drugs such as sulfonamides and pyrimethamine to overcome the problem of resistance to the latter drug, and such combinations were found to be generally effective for the treatment of chloroquine-resistant *P. falciparum* infections which frequently exhibited resistance also to pyrimethamine when this compound was administered alone.

From the current antimalarial screen has emerged a handful of potent drugs such as the 4-quinolinemethanol mefloquine, the full potential of which is still being explored in the laboratory and in humans. Most recently a new phase of antimalarial chemotherapy has been opened with the recognition that all the weapons we hold with which to combat malaria are still inadequate to remove the disease from its hard-core areas of endemicity. In addition to the problem of drug resistance are the ever present logistic problems of mass drug distribution and of the limited value of existing blood and tissue schizontocidal drugs for this purpose. More effective and safer tissue schizontocidal agents are urgently needed to replace primaquine, and the direction of the U.S. Army program has recently been modified to identify such compounds. The World Health Organization in its new Special Programme for Research and Training in Tropical Diseases (1976a) has stressed the need for antimalarials with a very prolonged action, preferably administerable by injection and capable of being deployed on a large scale. In such a country, for example, as India where, in 1976, 6.4 million cases of malaria were officially admitted, and where the number is still high, the problem is essentially that of a resurgence of *P. vivax* (Fig. 3) against which primaquine has proved less than successful, except in courses of too long a duration to be of universal value.

Thus, today, in the presence of a global increase in malaria transmission, we

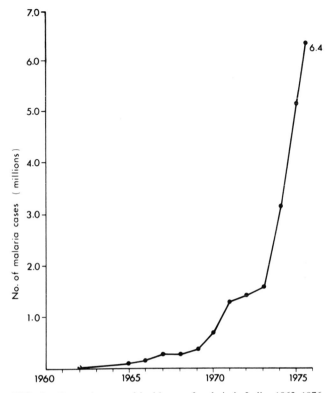

FIG. 3.   Increasing annual incidence of malaria in India, 1962–1976.

find ourselves searching as urgently for new antimalarial drugs as we were in the first decades of this century, with the difference that we now recognize the uncanny ability of the malaria parasite to combat all our efforts to eliminate it. Furthermore, the best drug our research has yielded is one that, ironically, appears to work in much the same way as the 350-year-old quinine (albeit dose-for-dose more efficiently) and which is, in a sense, not much more than a synthetic analog of the quinine molecule. Perhaps then, this chapter is relevant to the problems not only of malaria today but also of tomorrow. I find it hard to believe that the best drugs we have now will survive more than a decade of usage, so that, unless other ways are found to eliminate malaria from humans, we will still need reliable models with which to identify in the laboratory new antimalarial drugs, or better ways of deploying those we already have. With this in mind I have given an account of models I believe are of current use, leaving those interested in more historic techniques to read about them elsewhere (Findlay, 1951; Peters, 1970a; Thompson and Werbel, 1972).

II. PRINCIPLES OF ANTIMALARIAL DRUG SCREENING

Hawking (1963) listed the phases of chemotherapeutic research as follows (1) identification of the organism causing a disease; (2) study of its biology and, in particular, a search for ways of keeping it in culture *in vitro* or *in vivo;* (3) testing (screening) of chemicals against the organism; and (4) study of the mechanisms of action of compounds that prove active.

In malaria chemotherapy research it is in one way fortunate that, while only four species of *Plasmodium* cause the disease in man, there is a large choice of species of *Plasmodium* that infect other animal species, and some of these form convenient laboratory models. Unfortunately, on the other hand, the first of these on which extensive chemotherapeutic studies were based were malaria parasites of birds. In retrospect we now see that many biological features of avian plasmodia are radically different from those of mammalian parasites and, in particular, those of man and other primates. A number of lessons learned on avian models have to be unlearned. In spite of this certain avian host–parasite systems are still of value.

The principles of antimalarial drug screening were examined in detail by Peters (1970a), and those considered of maximum value were summarized in the report of a WHO scientific group (1973). This group has stressed that drug screening is a complex process that must be carried out in a sequence of logical steps, no single one of which can give more than one piece of information. The steps and their interaction, with feedback of information at each stage, start with primary screening and end with the safe administration of a new drug to man.

A large choice of laboratory models is available for most stages of the screening process. Table I includes only those that appear at the present time to be the most valuable and relevant.

III. EXPERIMENTAL MODELS AND PROCEDURES

In this section detailed procedures are given for a number of the most widely used models listed in Table I. Further details of procedures not described here will be found in Schnitzer and Hawking (1963), Peters (1970a, 1974a), and WHO (1973). Certain general points need first to be stressed. Irrespective of the species of host or parasite, or whether a test is being carried out *in vivo* or *in vitro,* standardization is all-important if potential antimalarial compounds are to be discovered and, once discovered, evaluated in depth. The experimental conditions that govern the response to any compound with potential antimalarial activity are summarized in the following outline.

TABLE I

Stages and Models of the Antimalarial Screening Process

Stage I   Primary Screening
  In vivo models
    i. To select blood schizontocides (using drug-sensitive lines)
        P. berghei—mouse, 4-day test (Peters, 1965a)
        P. berghei—mouse, Rane test (Peters, 1970a)
        P. vinckei—mouse, single-dose test (Fink and Kretschmar, 1970)
    ii. To select tissue schizontocides
        P. yoelii nigeriensis—mouse (Gregory and Peters, 1970; Hill, 1975)
        P. berghei—mouse (Most and Montuori, 1975)
        P. gallinaceum—chick (Davey, 1946a,b; Rane and Rane, 1972)
        P. cathemerium—canary (Fink *et al.,* 1970)
    iii. To select sporontocides
        P. gallinaceum—*Aedes aegypti* (Gerberg, 1971)
        P. cynomolgi—*Anopheles stephensi* (Gerberg, 1971)
        P. yoelii spp.—*Anopheles stephensi* (Ramkaran and Peters, 1969a)
  In vitro models
    i. Direct techniques
      a. For blood schizontocides
        P. falciparum (from *Aotus trivirgatus* or culture) (Rieckmann *et al.,* 1968b, 1978; Richards and Williams, 1975; Richards and Maples, 1979)
        P. berghei (Richards and Williams, 1973)
        P. knowlesi (Canfield *et al.,* 1970)
      b. For tissue schizontocides
        P. fallax—tissue culture (Beaudoin *et al.,* 1969)
    ii. Indirect techniques (use of surrogate models)
        Tetrahymena pyriformis
Stage II   Secondary Screening
  Antiparasitic studies
    i. Quantify dose–activity relationship
    ii. Qualify type of action
        By different routes of administration
        Preliminary studies of mode of action
        Analysis of dose–activity regression line
        Action of metabolites, e.g., *p*-aminobenzoic acid
        Morphological changes in parasites
    iii. Spectrum of activity against different stages
    iv. Spectrum of activity against different laboratory models
    v. Spectrum of action against drug-resistant lines
  Preliminary toxicity studies
  Chemical studies—study of analogs
Stage III   Tertiary Screening
  Antiparasitic action in nonhuman primates
    i. Simian malarias—blood schizontocidal action (Schmidt *et al.,* 1977b)
        P. knowlesi—*Macaca mulatta*
        P. knowlesi—*Cercopithecus aethiops*

(continued)

TABLE I—*Continued*

---

    ii. Simian malarias—blood and tissue schizontocidal action
        P. cynomolgi bastianellii—*M. mulatta* (Davidson *et al.*, 1976; Schmidt *et al.*, 1966, 1977a)
   iii. Human malarias in nonhuman primates (Schmidt, 1973)
        P. falciparum—*Aotus trivirgatus* (drug-sensitive and drug-resistant parasites)
        P. vivax—*A. trivirgatus* (drug-sensitive and drug-resistant parasites)
  Preclinical pharmacological studies
    i. *In vivo* procedures with same formulation
   ii. Pharmacokinetic observations (if techniques available)
  iii. Classic *in vitro* studies
Stage IV Clinical Screening
  Phase 1. Clinical pharmacology
  Phase 2. Preliminary clinical trials in infected volunteers
      Causal prophylaxis—*P. falciparum, P. vivax*
      Blood schizontocidal action—*P. falciparum, P. vivax*
      Antirelapse activity—*P. vivax*
      Gametocytocidal and sporontocidal action—*P. falciparum, P. vivax*
  Phase 3. Pilot field trials in partially immune subjects
  Phase 4. Treatment of hospital patients
  Phase 5. Extended field trials
  Phase 6. Observations on mass drug administration

---

1. Parasite-dependent factors
  1.1. Variation within a single *Plasmodium* species
    1.1.1. Sensitivity variation among different clones
    1.1.2. Geographic races
    1.1.3. Time since isolation of "wild" strain
  1.2. Variation among different *Plasmodium* species
  1.3. Mode and intensity of infection
2. Host-dependent factors
  2.1. Innate factors
    2.1.1. Host species
      i. Peculiarities in pharmacodynamics relating to the drug
      ii. Innate immunity
    2.1.2. Variations among individuals of the same species
      i. Strain
      ii. Age and sex
      iii. Immune status
    2.1.3. Intercurrent infections
  2.2. Environmental factors
    2.2.1. Temperature and stress
    2.2.2. Nutrition

3. Drug-dependent factors
   3.1. Mode of formulation
   3.2. Route of administration
   3.3. Drug dosage regimen
4. Parameters for determining activity

A description of the individual rodent malarias is given in Killick-Kendrick and Peters (1978), of simian species in Coatney *et al.* (1971), and of avian species in Garnham (1966). Rodent malaria provides a good illustration of the experimental conditions that need to be controlled.

   4.1.   Parasite and rodent species or strain (Fig. 4)

A given parasite species may behave quite differently in different host species or host strains. For example *P. berghei* Keyberg 173, runs an acute, fulminating course in random-bred Swiss mice but a much slower course in NMRI mice, whereas *P. vinckei vinckei* runs an equally acute course in either line. The

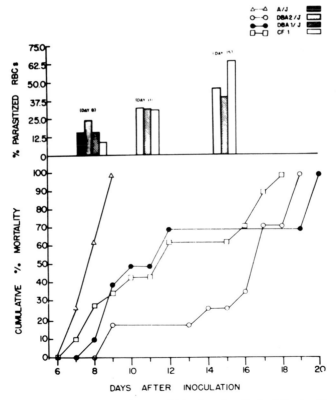

FIG 4.   Parasitemia and mortality in several inbred strains of mice following blood-induced *P. berghei* infection (2×10^5 parasitized red blood cells) (Most *et al.*, 1966).

difference is particularly marked in the case of sporozoite-induced infections, some mouse lines proving highly refractory while others are highly susceptible.

4.2. Age, weight, and sex of the host

These should be standardized, since rodents tend to become relatively less susceptible to malaria infection with increasing age. This is particularly true of rats. The role of sex as a variable factor in chemotherapy studies has not been accurately determined. Early reports on this point ignored the importance of other variables such as the existence of concomitant infections. The pharmacokinetics and metabolism of a drug may also differ according to the age and sex of the animal. Male mice of approximately 20 g weight are optimal for most drug experiments. (They also require less drug than larger animals.)

4.3. Environment

Ambient temperature (Fig. 5) and humidity and especially stress can play an important role in determining the course of malaria infection in rodents. A controlled environment of about 20°C and 40% R. H. is generally satisfactory. Not more than five animals should be kept in one cage. A normal diurnal cycle of night and day should be maintained.

4.4 Diet

The most important single dietary factor in relation to malaria infection is p-aminobenzoic acid. The diet should be well balanced, and most standard proprietary rodent pellets are satisfactory, except for their p-aminobenzoic acid content. Not only is this often present in inadequate amounts, but the content may also vary from batch to batch. The influence this can have on the subsequent

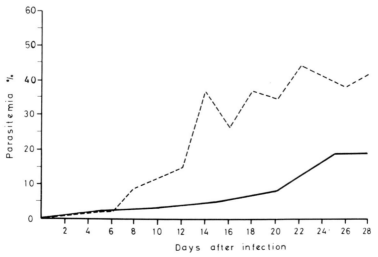

FIG. 5.   Influence of temperature on course of infection of *P. berghei* in NMRI mice. Solid line, Mean of 24 animals held at 12 °C; broken line, mean of 45 animals held at 22 °C (Kretschmar, 1965).

TABLE II

Rate of Spontaneous Recoveries of NMRI Mice Left Undisturbed by Repeated Examinations after Infection with *Plasmodium berghei*[a]

Diet	Addition of PAB[b] or water	Number of mice tested	Rate of spontaneous recoveries (%)
Standard diets			
Altromin	Water	114	17.5
Ssniff	Water	54	48.2
Murilan	Water	60	50.0
Latz	Water	110	71.8
Latz	PAB 1:100,000	60	28.3
Latz	PAB 1:10,000	60	8.3
Milk diets			
Whole milk		107	78.4
Nestle milk powder	Water	72	80.6
Nestle milk powder	PAB 1:10,000	60	11.7
Nestle milk powder	PAB 1:1,000	60	0.0
Nestle milk powder	PAB 1:10	64	20.3

[a] Maintained on diet from the fifth day before to the thirty-fifth day after infection (from Kretschmar, 1965).

[b] PAB, *p*-Aminobenzoic acid.

course of a malaria infection in rodents is most striking. Unfortunately it is difficult to assay the *p*-aminobenzoic acid content of animal feed. The malaria infection itself is as good a bioassay as can be obtained. Too high a content will have the effect of antagonizing the action of drugs such as sulfonamides and sulfones, so that a reasonable and happy median must be found. I have found Oxoid modified mouse diet 41B to be a generally satisfactory preparation in England. Kretschmar (1965) observed that Altromin rodent food pellets gave good results in Germany (Tab. II).

4.5. Contaminating infections

Most commercially available rodents are notoriously prone to infection with a variety of agents, viral, bacterial, protozoal, and helminthic. Of all that are important for malaria chemotherapy two are outstanding, *Eperythrozoon coccoides* in mice and *Haemobartonella muris* in rats. Both may occur in mice, although the latter species is uncommon. The influence they may have on the course of a malaria infection is illustrated in Fig. 6.

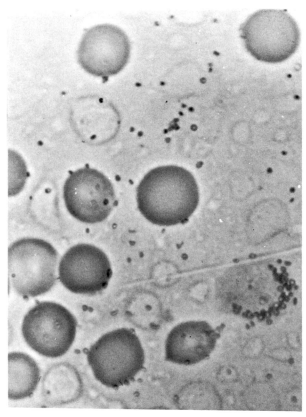

FIG. 6. *Eperythrozoon coccoides* in mouse blood. (Giemsa stain. Photographed with phase-contrast optics. Original negative ×1300.) The organisms attached to the surface of a hemolyzed polychromatic erythrocyte (lower right) are particularly clear.

Whenever the level of parasitemia appears to fluctuate unexpectedly in a group of otherwise identically handled mice, particularly if the infection appears to have been slowed up more than anticipated, the presence of *E. coccoides* should be suspected. In rats the opposite is likely to occur when they are infected with *H. muris*. This organism rapidly causes hemolytic anemia. This in turn is followed by a rapid erythropoetic response. The reticulocytes that arise are more favorable to invasion by *P. berghei* than normocytes, and the malaria infection consequently becomes fulminating.

It is important to remember that such contaminants may arise in association with (a) primary isolates from wild rodents, (b) a laboratory colony of rodents, and (c) a contaminated parasite strain—even after cryopreservation.

The parasite strain must be cleaned up (decontaminated) before passaging into clean rodents. An organic arsenical such as neoarsphenamine (NAB) or oxophenarsine can be used, since these compounds, unlike antibiotics such as tetracyclines, remove the contaminants but depress the plasmodia only temporarily. A total of two subcutaneous doses, each of 125 mg/kg body weight of NAB given on two consecutive days (or 5–10 mg/kg of oxophenarsine daily for 7 days), should clean up infection with these contaminants. If necessary, the course can be repeated in two or three consecutive passages. The presence of latent infection in new hosts can be revealed by splenectomizing random animals from a batch and making a daily inspection of Giemsa-stained thin blood films in which the presence of *E. coccoides* or *H. muris* will be seen within a few days.

4.6 Size and route of inoculations

The course of malaria infection is dependent on the size of the inoculum and the route. A 10-fold decrease in inoculum size of *P. berghei* Keyberg 173 in mice is associated with approximately 1 day's delay in the buildup of parasitemia (Fig. 7). Variations in the course of infection among animals in a single group can be avoided by using the intravenous route of inoculation rather than the intraperitoneal route which is so often employed. With practice it becomes as rapid to inoculate infected blood via the tail vein of a mouse as to give the inoculum intraperitoneally. The use of an infrared lamp to warm the animals gently and a simple device for fixing the tail greatly facilitate the procedure which should certainly be used when sporozoite inoculation is called for.

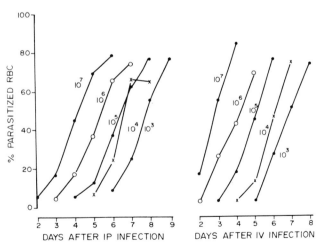

FIG. 7. Course of parasitemias in mice inoculated intraperitoneally and intravenously with various dosages of *P. berghei* (Wellde *et al.*, 1966).

A. Rodent Malaria

1. The "4-Day Suppressive Test" of Blood Schizontocidal Action against Plasmodium berghei in Mice

Although a wide range of malaria parasites of rodents is now available (Killick-Kendrick and Peters, 1978), few have been used in chemotherapy investigations. The most widely employed is the original strain of *P. berghei* Keyberg 173, isolated by Vincke and Lips in Katanga in 1948 and since passaged thousands of times in many laboratories throughout the world. The Keyberg 173 strain has long since lost its ability to produce gametocytes and has probably changed in many of its biological characters since its original isolation. One peculiarity, however, is the strong likelihood that what has always been thought of as a single parasite has in fact all these years consisted of a mixture of two species, the dominant one being the true *P. berghei* with which has been mixed a parasite of the *P. yoelii* complex, cryptic because of its very small proportion in the mixture (Peters *et al.,* 1978).

In spite of this the "*P. berghei*" old laboratory strain has been much utilized in malaria chemotherapy. It is highly sensitive to most antimalarial drugs in acute studies, hence the designation "N strain" (for normal drug sensitivity) in our laboratory. Only chronic exposure to chloroquine has exposed the presence of the second organism (the "NS line") which is both mildly resistant to chloroquine as well as capable of producing biologically active gametocytes.

The 4-day test is convenient for use as a routine procedure in most laboratories, since it can be started on a Monday and finished on a Friday, i.e., a normal working week in many countries. The procedure is summarized as follows:

A suitable line of mice (e.g., random-bred Swiss albino CF1) is chosen, and males of 20 ± 2 g are selected for use. A donor mouse with rising parasitemia of 20% infected red blood cells is killed with chloroform, and the blood collected in a lightly heparinized syringe from the axillary vessels. The blood is diluted with TC medium 199 so that each 0.2 ml contains approximately 10^7 infected red cells. Recipient mice receive a single inoculum of 0.2 ml, preferably intravenously via the tail vein, or intraperitoneally. The former route produces less scatter of parasite levels among individual mice. The day of infection is termed D0, and succeeding days D+1, D+2, etc.

Compounds to be tested are made up to suitable dose levels (e.g., 3, 10, and 30 mg/kg) in solution or suspension, the latter often requiring the addition of a small quantity of a 0.2% solution of Tween 80 or 0.5% carboxymethycellulose and the application of an ultrasonicator (simple homogenization with Tween 80 in a pestle and mortar will suffice if no more sophisticated means are available). The drugs are administered once daily starting from D0 for 4 days, subcutaneously or orally. On D+4 thin blood films are made from tail blood and stained with a Romanowsky stain such as that of Giemsa at pH 7.2; parasitized red cells are recorded as a percentage of the total. Individual percentages may be recorded, or they can be scored on a simple arbitrary scale, say from 0 to 5. A mean group level of about 90% or less that of mock-treated control animals usually indicates that the test compound is active. The dose levels can be increased or decreased according to the preliminary findings, up to the maximum tolerated dose if necessary, in order to obtain a range of values of dose and percentage activity that can be plotted (Fig. 8) in order to obtain a dose–activity curve for calculation of the 50 and 90% effective doses (ED_{50} and ED_{90}). These values can readily be read off if the doses are plotted as logarithms and the activities as probits. Standard deviations too are readily obtained by simple calculation.

This test can be run in simplified form as a large-scale screen, using a single arbitrary dose level, or as a secondary screen with a higher level of sophistication according to need. The drug-sensitive Keyberg 173 strain of *P. berghei* (N line) is suitable for this test, but other parasites can be used (Table III). The test also lends itself readily to the use of drug-resistant lines of *P. berghei* (or other species) for secondary drug evaluation. Further details of the test are given by Peters (1970a).

2. Rane Test of Blood Schizontocidal Activity against Plasmodium berghei

This simple screening procedure (Osdene *et al.*, 1967), used to examine over 265,000 compounds during the last 16 years, relies on the ability of a standard inoculum of *P. berghei* to kill recipient mice within about 6 days, and the extension of their survival beyond twice this figure by a single drug administration. It is thus simple in execution, demanding nothing more than preparation of the compounds to be tested (by solution, or suspension by ultrasonication in arachis oil), the intraperitoneal infection of mice with a virulent *P. berghei* line, the administration of a single drug dose, and the observation of mortality times. The inoculum consists of approximately 10^6 infected donor red cells given intraperitoneally. Drugs are given in an initial range of, e.g., 640, 320, 160, and 80 mg/kg on D+3 subcutaneously. Survival more than twice that of the controls is considered evidence of activity, and above 60 days of "cure." The minimum effective dose (MED) is obtained and compared with the maximum tolerated dose (MTD) that produces no more than one in five toxic deaths. (Dose levels are titrated downward to find the MED and an indication of the therapeutic index.) Intermediate activity may be followed up using the 4-day test or a modification of the Rane test in which parasite counts are made at suitable intervals. A number of other minor modifications of the original procedure, including use of the oral route for some compounds, have now been adopted (A. L. Ager, personal

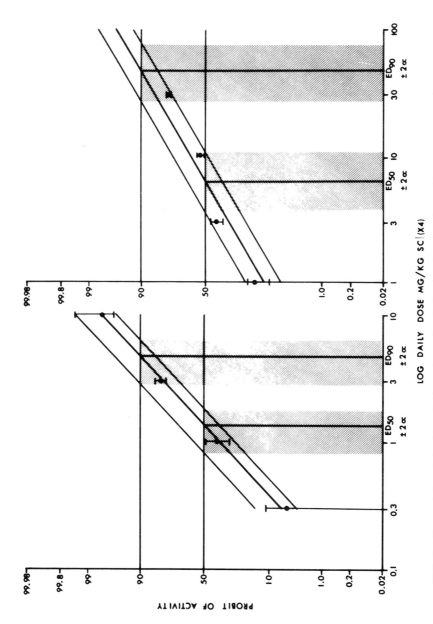

FIG. 8. Dose-activity relationships of chloroquine against *P. berghei* plotted on log-probit graph paper. (Left) Drug-sensitive N. Strain. (Right) Chloroquine-resistant NS line. Note the flattened angle of the dose-activity regression line and higher ED_{50} and ED_{90} levels of the latter. (Figure by B. L. Robinson).

TABLE III

Blood Schizontocidal Activity against Trophozoite-Induced *Plasmodium berghei* Infection in Albino Mice[a]

Compound	\[c\] 1	2[d]	3	4	5	6	7	8	9	10
	Minimum effective doses as base (mg/kg/day)[b]									
	ED(50)	(50)	(50)	(?)	(80)	(~90)	(~90)	(75)	(98)	(99+)
Quinine			38.3	~23	83	80	104	35	>100	133
Chloroquine		1.63	1.52	~1.8	4.95	1–2	2.5	1.65	2.3	5.0
Amodiaquine		1.55	1.97					1.8		18.3
Mepacrine			2.55	~3.0	7.8	2–4	3.93	3.45	3.3	15.7
Pamaquine				~11.5	4.5	3.25	>13.5		37.0	
Primaquine		1.38	1.25				2.85	2.1		
Proguanil			30.0	~5.0	12.3		8.75	12	>10	17.5
Cycloguanil			0.25					2.0		
Pyrimethamine	0.15	0.39	0.10				0.25	0.16	5.0	
Sulfadiazine	0.20		0.01		0.05			0.06	0.3	
Dapsone	0.60		0.09					0.90		0.18
Sulformethoxine	1.0		0.04							0.05
Route	po	po	sc	po	po	sc	sc	sc	ip	po

[a] Peters, 1970a.

[b] Criteria are given in parentheses.

[c] Key to references: 1. Richards (1966); 2. Jacobs *et al.* (1963); 3. Peters (1965b); 4. Goodwin (1949); 5. Thompson *et al.* (1967); 6. Hill (1950); 7. Schneider *et al.* (1949); 8. Schneider (1954); 9. Hawking (1966); 10. Thurston (1950).

[d] All old laboratory strains except no. 2 which is NYU-2.

TABLE IV

Suppressive, Curative, and Toxic Doses of Some Antimalarials against *Plasmodium berghei* in Mice as Reflected in the Rane Test

Compound	Dose (mg/kg) sc × 1	Mean survival time (days in excess of control)	Number "cured"	Toxic deaths[b]	Reference
Chloroquine	640			5/5	Peters, 1970a
phosphate	320	17		2/5	
	160	10			
	80	5.8			
	40	4.6			
	20	3.8			
Mepacrine	640			5/5	Peters, 1970a
methane-	320	23.4			
sulfonate	160	9.4			
	80	8.2			
	40	5.6			
	20	4.6			
Quinine sulfate	1280	7.5		1/5	Peters, 1970a
	640	5.4			
	320	3.2			
	160	2.0			
	80	1.4			
WR 33063	640	?	4/5		Nodiff *et al.*
	320	?	4/5		(1971)
	160	?	3/5		
	80	?	1/5		
	40	6.7			
	20	4.5			
	10	2.1			
WR 122455	640	?	5/5		Nodiff *et al.*
	320	?	5/5		(1971)
	160	?	5/5		
	80	?	5/5		
	40	?	2/5		
	20	18.9			
	10	9.1			
WR 30090	320		5/5	p	Strube (1975)
	160		5/5	p	
	80	22.9[a]	4/5	p	
	40	11.9[a]	3/5		
	20	14.9[a]	1/5		
	10	10.7			
	5	6.1			
	2.5	4.1			

TABLE IV—*Continued*

Compound	Dose (mg/kg) sc × 1	Mean survival time (days in excess of control)	Number "cured"	Toxic deaths[b]	Reference
WR 142490	40	?	5/5		Ohmacht *et al.*
(mefloquine	20	?	4/5		(1971)
hydro-	10	?			
chloride)					
Primaquine	1280			5/5	Peters, 1970a
phosphate	640			5/5	
	320			5/5	
	160	7.0		2/5	
	80	6.4			
	40	4.2			
	20	2.2			
Proguanil hydro-	640			5/5	Peters, 1970a
chloride	160			5/5	
(chloro-	40	~3.5		3/5	
guanide)					
Sulfanilamide	1280	13.3			Peters, 1970a
	640	12.5			
	320	7.5			
	160	4.9			
	80	2.5			
Dapsone	1280			10/10	Peters, 1970a
	640	>60	4/10	6/10	
	320	>60	8/10	2/10	
	160	>60	3/10		
	80	>60	2/10		
	40	11.1			
	20	7.3			
Diformyl	640	>60	10/10		Peters, 1970a
dapsone	320	>60	10/10		
	160	>60	9/10		
	80	>60	5/10		
	40	15.7			
	20	11.6			
Diacetyl	640	>60	5/5		Peters, 1970a
dapsone	160	11.1			
	40	10.7			

[a] Survivors not cured.
[b] p indicates phototoxicity at 50 mg/kg.

communication, 1978). [Rane and Rane (1972) described a similar procedure using *P. gallinaceum* in the chick.]

Although the Rane test as developed by the late Louis Rane and his wife at the University of Miami for the U.S. Army antimalarial drug screening program (Osdene *et al.*, 1967) has proved its value by demonstrating the activity of new compounds such as mefloquine (Table IV), it has been much criticized as being too insensitive a procedure to demonstrate activity in every type of potentially interesting compound. The valuable antimalarial proguanil, for example, shows slight activity only (Peters, 1970a). However, this particular compound is not readily metabolized in the mouse to its active metabolite, cycloguanil, and shows poor activity even in the 4-day test, so that this criticism cannot be taken as a valid argument against the Rane test only.

3. Single-Dose Test of Blood Schizontocidal Activity Using Plasmodium vinckei in NMRI Mice

Fink and Kretschmar (1970) have described a simple procedure whereby *P. vinckei vinckei* is used to infect albino mice of the NMRI line (which is readily obtainable in Europe), which are then treated once only with the test drug. Activity is assessed by prolongation of the survival time. They claim that this test is superior to the 4-day test because *P. vinckei* does not preferentially invade immature red cells as does *P. berghei,* because a single intraperitoneal administration is economical both of time and test compound, and because time is not required to make or examine blood films. An inoculum of 10^7 infected donor cells is given on D0, and this kills mock-treated control animals in 5–6 days. The compound is administered once, within a few hours of infection, at different dose levels. The MED is the dose that produces more than a 20% increase in survival time beyond that of the controls. The ED_{50} and ED_{90} (unlike the MED) have to be calculated by carrying out parasite counts on blood films and plotting them as in the 4-day test.

4. Gregory and Peters Test (1970) for Tissue Schizontocidal Action Using Plasmodium yoelii nigeriensis in Albino Mice

At the time of its meeting in 1972 the WHO Scientific Group on the Chemotherapy of Malaria and Resistance to Antimalarials (1973) had insufficient evidence to recommend this test for routine screening of potential tissue schizontocidal agents, which had, therefore, to depend still on the old avian malaria model, sporozite-induced *P. gallinaceum* in the chick, which is described below, or *P. cathemerium* in the canary. Neither of these are today considered satisfactory, since the biology of the tissue stages of mammalian and avian malarias differs radically and, consequently, the response of mammalian or avian tissue stages to many compounds is also quite different. Fortunately enough evidence has now been acquired to indicate that sporozoite-induced infection with *P. yoelii nigeriensis* in the albino mouse provides an excellent model for tissue schizontocidal agents of potential value against simian and human malaria. It is, if anything, too sensitive, yielding positive compounds in the mouse that fail to give equally good activity in monkey models or in man.

The original procedure as described by Gregory and Peters (1970) has recently been simplified by Peters *et al.* (1975b).

The readily colonized mosquito *Anopheles stephensi* is a suitable vector for this parasite which undergoes sporogonic development in about 8 days at a mean environmental temperature of 25°C. The sporozoites can be harvested between days 11 and 14 by the simple procedure of grinding whole mosquitoes, gland dissection not being required for routine studies. Blood inocula are prepared and administered as described for the 4-day test above, but using the line *P. yoelii nigeriensis* N 67 which has an innate low level of resistance to chloroquine.

Mosquitoes are fed on donor mice that have male and female gametocytes, using the technique described by Ramkaran and Peters (1969b). They are then given sucrose to feed on while being held in the insectarium at 25°C and 75% R.H. until mature sporozoites are present in the salivary glands. Batches are then stunned with carbon dioxide or ether and ground in a Teflon tube with a small quantity of 50% (v/v) calf serum with Grace's insect TC medium or Ringer's solution after removal of the wings and legs. The mixture is lightly centrifuged to remove coarse debris, leaving the sporozoites in the supernatant; the whole operation is carried out on ice and in a refrigerated centrifuge.

Two groups of mice are inoculated with a suspension of sporozoites in 0.2 ml via the tail vein on D0. Each mouse should receive the equivalent of about two mosquitoes' load of sporozoites. A single dose of compound is administered within 1 hour of infection. For primary screening we use a dose of 30 mg/kg. This can be increased or decreased on a logarithmic basis for subsequent tests in the light of experience up to the MTD and down to the minimum fully active dose (MFAD). One group of mice receives only the sporozoite infection. The second receives in addition an intravenous inoculum of 10^7 infected erythrocytes of the same parasite from a suitable donor 48 hours after the sporozoite inoculum. Suitable mock-treated controls are set up for each group. Thin blood films are made and examined daily from D+3 to D+14. A compound is considered (from experience) to be causally prophylactic if all blood films are negative on D+14. The exception to this rule obtains when the group that has received an infected blood inoculum shows a reduced blood infection, thus demonstrating that the compound has a residual action longer than the 48 hours' duration of the preerythrocytic cycle of this parasite.

The mathematical basis of the calculation needed to demonstrate that any activity seen is due to an action on the tissue schizonts is complicated, and the original description should be studied (Gregory and Peters, 1970). In practice,

TABLE V

The Evaluation of Causal Prophylactic Activity to Show the Method of Calculation[a]

Compound	Dose as base (mg/kg)	Group patency			Group mean pre-2% period			Activity[b]		Comment
		C° or T°	XC	C^x or T^x	p^f or p^h	p^b	p^c or p^a	Residual (i)	On EE stages (ii)	
Control		3/3		3/3	5.12	4.39	4.15			
T 1237	300	3/3		3/3	4.80		3.96	−0.21	−0.11	Inactive
Control		4/5	3/3	5/5	6.01	4.75	4.46			
T 1237	600	2/3	3/3	3/3	5.89		4.14	−0.36	+0.24	Inactive
T 1237	1000	3/3		3/3	5.80		3.87	−0.64	+0.43	Inactive
Conclusion: inactive, nontoxic at 1000 mg/kg										
Control		4/5	3/3	3/3	5.26	3.58	4.23			
WR 5990	10	2/3		3/3	5.24		3.98	−0.17	+0.15	Inactive
WR 5990	30	0/3		0/3						LD$_{100}$
Conclusion: inactive at maximum tolerated dose of 30 mg/kg										
Control		3/3	3/3	3/3	5.65	4.33	4.35			
Metachloridine	10	2/3		3/3	8.67		4.41	+0.06	+2.96	Slightly active
Metachloridine	30	1/3		3/3	11.26		4.45	+0.10	+5.51	Active
Metachloridine	100	0/3		3/3	14.00		4.74	+0.39	+7.96	Fully active
Conclusion: fully active, MFAD 30–100 mg/kg, no residual activity										
Control		4/4	3/3	3/3	5.82	4.49	4.15			
ICI 56780	0.3	2/3		3/3	11.26		3.84	−0.36	+5.80	Active
ICI 56780	1.0	1/3		3/3	11.19		4.54	+0.45	+4.98	Active
ICI 56780	3.0	0/3		3/3	14.0		8.56	+5.11	+3.07	Fully active?
Conclusion: fully active, MFAD 1–3 mg/kg, marked residual activity at 3 mg/kg										

[a] All treatments on D0, 2 hours after inoculation. Peters *et al.* (1975b).

[b] (i) Calculated from the formula $\dfrac{(p^b - a)(p^c - a)}{(p^c - a)} - (p^f - a)$, where $a = 2.0$; (ii) Calculated from the formula $(p^h - p^f) - $ (i). (Note that i may be a negative value).

[c] C = control, T = treated mice inoculated with sporozoites (C°, T°), trophozoites (XC), or both (C^x, T^x), p = number of days required to reach a 2% parasitemia level in group C° (p^f), T° (p^h), C^x (p^c), T^x (p^x), or XC (p^b).

however, it is simple. Examples are shown in Tables V and VI. Experience has shown that a figure of less than $+1.0$ for prophylactic activity is insignificant, as is one of less than $+0.5$ for residual activity.

We are currently developing a modification of this procedure that will permit one to differentiate between true tissue schizontocidal action and residual activity against emerging erythrocytic merozoites. Meanwhile use can be made of the following technique.

5. Hill Test (1975) for Tissue Schizontocidal Action of Compounds with Residual Properties against Plasmodium yoelii nigeriensis

This test is similar to the procedure just described but involves the subinoculation of clean mice with blood from treated animals in which merozoites may have emerged from preerythrocytic liver schizonts. Possible residual action of test compounds is checked by treating a group of mice 48 hours before they receive

TABLE VI

A Comparison of Causal Prophylactic Data Obtained by Fink (1974) with Those of Gregory and Peters (1970), and Those of the Present[a]

Compound	P. b. yoelii 17X (NMRI mice) CPD$_{50}$ (95% limits)[b]	P. b. nigeriensis N67 (CFW mice) MFAD[c]
Chloroquine	Inactive at MTD	Inactive at MTD
Quinine	Inactive at MTD	Inactive at MTD
Mepacrine	Inactive at MTD	Inactive at MTD
Primaquine	6.6 (4.5–9.0)	30–60
Dapsone	20 (13–32)	3–10
Sulfadiazine	30 (15–60)	30–60
Sulfadoxine	84 (60–118)	3–10
Proguanil	1.6 (1.0–2.5)	3–10
Cycloguanil	0.3 (0.2–0.4)	1–2
Pyrimethamine	0.1 (0.07–0.14)	0.3–1.0
RC 12	Inactive at MTD (200)	Slight activity at 300
Ni 147/36	4.0 (2.4–6.8)	1–3
Ba. 138/111	23 (16–32)	10–30
Clindamycin		10–30
U-24729A[d]	2.0 (1.4–2.8)	0.3–1

[a] All doses base or salt (milligrams per kilogram) as indicated, administered once on D0, 2–4 hours after inoculation.

[b] As base, intraperitoneally.

[c] As salt except pyrimethamine, dapsone, and sulfonamides; subcutaneously, except pyrimethamine which was intraperitoneal.

[d] U-24729A is N-demethyl-4'-pentylclindamycin.

an inoculum of 10^4 trophozoites in infected donor erythrocytes. The activity is judged by observing the time taken for the parasitemia to reach the 2% level as compared with controls (Warhurst and Folwell, 1968). If the delay to 2% exceeds 7 days, lower doses are employed, or the following modification of the procedure is used. Otherwise the degree of activity is judged simply by the appearance or nonappearance of parasitemia by D+14 following a simple sporozoite inoculum.

If residual activity is shown for a test compound, blood is collected from infected mice between 52 and 53 hours after sporozoite infection, 0.2 ml by heart puncture from each animal, and inoculated intraperitoneally into clean animals, one recipient per donor. The blood of the new recipients is examined daily up to

TABLE VII

Activity against the Tissue Stages of *Plasmodium berghei*: Doses with Little or No Residual Effect[a]

Compound	Dose (mg/g)	Route	Residual effect (days)	Proportion of mice developing parasitemia[b]
Sulfadoxine	0.25	po	2	10/16[c]
Cycloguanil pamoate	0.1	po	0	0/4
	0.004	po		0/6 }
	0.001	po		3/5 }
	0.004	sc	0	0/4 }
	0.001	sc		0/4 }
	0.0005	sc		1/4 }
	0.000125	sc		4/4 }
	0.004	po		2/4)
	0.001	po		4/4 (
	0.001	sc		0/4 (
	0.00025	sc		3/4)
Clindamycin	1.0	po	0	0/4
	0.25	po		0/4
	0.0625	po		0/4 }
	0.08	po		0/4 }
	0.02	po		4/4 }
Doxycycline	0.5	po	0	0/4
	0.25	po		1/4 }
	0.0625	po		3/4 }
Spiramycin	1.0	po	0	0/14[d]
	0.25	po		4/4
Tetracycline	2.0	po	0	0/6 }
	1.0	po		2/4 }

[a] Hill (1975).
[b] Data with brace a direct comparison.
[c] Combined results of four experiments.
[d] Combined results of two experiments.

14 days. If less than half the recipients of blood inocula in these secondarily infected animals develop parasitemia, the test compound is considered active (i.e., against the preerythrocytic tissue infections of the donors), and if more than 75% become infected, it is judged to be negative. Intermediate figures indicate marginal activity (Table VII).

The basic premise upon which this test is based is that most antimalarial compounds require 3–4 hours to produce irreversible changes in intraerythrocytic parasites. To make quite certain that this is so in the case of specific compounds that appear to have both tissue schizontocidal and residual action, a further test is run in which a comparison is made of the "2% time" in mice infected intravenously with untreated parasites (10^4 trophozoites) or parasites that have been exposed *in vivo* to the drug 48 hours previously. Subinoculation is made from these animals to clean recipients 3–4 hours after the intravenous infection. The 2% time from both these recipients and their controls should show no significant difference (Table VIII).

TABLE VIII

Activity against the Tissue Stages of *Plasmodium berghei*: Doses with Prolonged Residual Activity[a]

Compound	Dose (mg/g)	Route	Proportion of mice developing parasitemia	
			Recipients	Controls
Mepacrine hydrochloride	0.25	po	7/8	5/6
Acedapsone	1.0	sc	2/10	
Mepacrine hydrochloride	0.25	po	10/10	5/5
Acedapsone	1.0	sc	1/10	
Control donors			10/10	
Acedapsone	1.0	sc	0/10	
	0.25	sc	0/6	4/4[c]
Control donors			5/6	
Acedapsone	0.1	sc	3/7	
	0.0125	sc	5/7	4/4
Control donors			7/7	
Cycloguanil pamoate	0.1	sc	0/6	
Mepacrine hydrochloride	0.25	po	5/5	6/6
Sulfadoxine	1.0	po	0/10	
Control donors			10/10	4/4
12278 RP	0.5[b]	po	7/8	
Control donors			8/8	4/4

[a] Hill (1975).

[b] Maximum tolerated dose.

[c] One mouse was negative on the fourth day although positive by the seventh day.

6. Procedure of Most, Herman, and Schoenfeld (1967) for Showing Tissue Schizontocidal Activity against *Plasmodium berghei* in Rats (Modified by Most and Montuori, 1975)

In their original technique Most *et al.* (1967) infected A/J Bar Harbor albino mice, hamsters, or rats with an inoculum of between 10,000 and 15,000 sporozoites of *P. berghei* obtained from *A. stephensi* either by trituration or dissection. The inocula were given either intravenously or intraperitoneally. A few animals of both treated and control groups received extra heavy inocula of 200,000–250,000 sporozoites. Compounds to be tested were administered subcutaneously (except quinine which was given orally) on D−1 and D0. Animals in which parasitemia failed to develop were observed for at least 60 days, and a sample were splenectomized. The livers of heavily infected animals were sectioned, stained, and searched for preerythrocytic schizonts.

As this technique failed to distinguish between drug action in tissue schizonts and activity against emerging intraerythrocytic merozoites, the authors infected separate groups of animals with 10,000 sporozoites intravenously and commenced treatment with the same drugs on the third day of patency to see whether a radical cure could be effected. Most and Montuori (1975) have described a simplified procedure in which 19-day-old female Sprague–Dawley rats are infected with *P. berghei* by intravenous inoculation of sporozoites of *P. berghei,* four animals of each group receiving 10,000 and two 250,000. Liver biopsies are made from the latter between 43 and 45 hours after infection. The animals are treated twice daily, subcutaneously on D−1 and D0, starting with a total dose of 640 mg/kg (or less if this is toxic). In a second step lower doses are given to determine the MFAD. Blood films are examined on D+6 or D+10 and D+15. If no parasites are seen, they are killed between D+15 and D+20, and 0.2 ml of their pooled blood is subinoculated into clean CF1 and A/J mice. If these animals show no infection, the preserved livers of the heavily infected pair of rats are sectioned, stained, and examined. The authors claim that this technique is better than their earlier one. While designed primarily to detect causal prophylactic activity, it also reveals a compound's suppressive or therapeutic potential.

These tests do not appear to have any advantage over those described in Sections III,A,4 and 5 and have the disadvantage that very heavy inocula are needed to produce sufficient liver schizonts for practical detection in stained sections.

7. In Vitro Test of Richards and Williams (1973) for Blood Schizontocidal Action against *Plasmodium berghei*

Many attempts have been made to cultivate malaria parasites *in vitro,* and numerous authors have reported on the use of short-term cultures for experimental chemotherapy (see review in Peters, 1970a). In Volume 2, Chapter 6, Trager and Jensen summarize this work which has culminated in the successful *in vitro* maintenance of *P. falciparum* (Trager and Jensen, 1976; Haynes *et al.*, 1976). Trigg (1975) has summarized the reports of attempts to cultivate other *Plasmodium* species, among them *P. berghei*. This organism has been used by Richards and Williams (1973) to screen blood schizontocides *in vitro*, taking the influence of the compounds on the parasites' incorporation of [³H]leucine as the main parameter for drug activity.

An essential prerequisite of this technique is the separation of leukocytes from the infected rat blood, the metabolic activity of which is very high in relation to that of the parasites (Fig. 9). This procedure as described by Williams and Richards (1973) involves passing the infected blood through a cellulose powder column to which the leukocytes adhere, a technique pioneered by Fulton and Grant (1956). To avoid bacterial contamination Williams and Richards designed a special apparatus which permits the addition of drugs to the parasites in culture and the periodic removal of samples for assay of [³H]leucine uptake.

Siliconized glass chromatography columns (1.5 × 25) cm are tightly packed with dry Whatmann CF11 cellulose powder and then sterilized by heat. A drug-sensitive line of *P. berghei* is maintained in Wistar rats from which blood is collected aseptically by heart puncture into lightly heparinized syringes when the parasitemia is between 2 and 3%. The blood is diluted 1:6 with Trigg and Gutteridge's (1971) minimal medium and then passed through the column at the rate of 15 ml/minute under slight positive pressure, with a 5% carbon dioxide-air mixture. All parts of the column and culture vessels are held at 38°C. As the dry powder lyses the red cell, the first few milliliters of eluate are discarded, the rest then being separated in 10-ml fractions using a series of four columns for the leukocyte separation. Leukocyte-free parasitized red cells in the culture medium are finally transferred to culture flasks (Fig. 10).

The cultures are incubated with the addition of [³H]leucine for 24 hours at

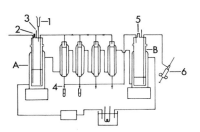

FIG. 9. Apparatus for the routine preparation of leukocyte-free blood dilution cultures. A and B, Graduated glass vessels 200 ml, placed on magnetic glass stirrers; each vessel is enclosed in a water jacket with circulating water at 38°C; 1, Millipore filter; 2 and 5 serum caps; 3, gas outlet; 4 (and other x's), taps; 6, Cornwall syringe. See original paper for further details (Williams and Richards, 1973).

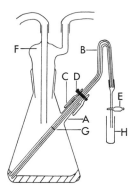

FIG. 10. Culture vessel based on a modified 100-ml Erlenmeyer flask A, side arm; B, swan-neck capillary tube; C, rubber pressure tubing; D, securing clip; E, artery clip to close fine-bore silicone-rubber tubing; F, Dreschel bottle head; G, predetermined level marker; H, sample vial. See original paper for further details (Williams and Richards, 1973).

38.5°C in a shaking water bath under a flow of 5% carbon dioxide in air. (The original description contains fine points of detail to which reference may have to be made.) Drugs are added in appropriate quantities to the incubation mixtures in the culture flasks on sterile pieces of filter paper.

The authors also utilized this procedure to determine the effect of drugs on asexual trophozoites of the Nuri strain of *P. knowlesi*. While developing their technique they compared protein synthesis by uninfected blood of several mammalian species including rat, mouse, hamster, rhesus, and *Aotus* monkey. Rat blood was found to incorporate [³H]leucine to the greatest extent, and rhesus cells the least. Most of this activity was found to be attributable to the leukocytes and the reticulocytes present in the rat blood. Once these were removed, the mature, leukocyte-free red cell suspensions showed little incorporation of the amino acid. They did not find it necessary to remove leukocytes from rhesus blood in order to determine leucine uptake by *P. knowlesi* (nor that by *P. falciparum* in *Aotus* blood (see Section III,D,2).

Over an 18-hour period both chloroquine and pyrimethamine were found to inhibit [³H]leucine incorporation by *P. berghei* in rat blood leukocyte- and reticulocyte-free dilution cultures, the 50% inhibitory concentration (IC) being calculated as 7 and 18 μg/ml, respectively, for the two compounds. The 50% IC for chloroquine against *P. knowlesi* was much lower, namely, 0.01 μg/ml (Fig. 11).

8. Test for Sporontocidal Action against Plasmodium yoelii nigeriensis in Anophetes stephensi (Ramkaran and Peters, 1969b)

These workers developed a simplified version of a technique originally described in 1947 by Terzian who studied the activity of sporontocides against *P. gallinaceum* in *Aedes aegypti*.

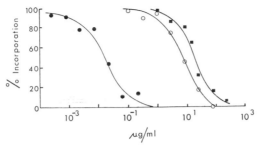

FIG. 11. Dose–response curves for chloroquine versus *P. knowlesi* (●) and versus *P. berghei* (○) and pyrimethamine versus *P. berghei* (■) in leukocyte-free blood dilution cultures. The IC_{50} values derived from these curves by inspection were 0.010, 7.0, and 18 μg/ml, respectively. Each curve indicates the inhibition of leucine uptake after 18 hours relative to the uptake by untreated control cultures at each of seven threefold dilutions of the drug (Richards and Williams, 1973).

On D0 *Eperythrozoon*-free albino mice receive an intraperitoneal inoculum of a cyclically transmissible strain of a *P. yoelii* subspecies such as *P. yoelii nigeriensis*. *Anopheles stephensi* reared in the insectary are allowed to hatch, females then being separated into containers holding about 25 each and given 4% sucrose solution for the next 5 days. They are held at a constant temperature of 24 ± 2°C and 75 ± 10% R.H. After 24 hours' starvation the mosquitoes are allowed to feed on mice in which the infection has reached D+3. Prior to this the mice are examined to ascertain that male and female gametocytes are present and mature. The animals are then anesthetized with a single intraperitoneal dose of 60 mg/kg body weight of sodium pentobarbitone and simply laid on top of the mosquito containers so that the insects can feed through the gauze cover for about 30 minutes. Unfed mosquitoes are removed and destroyed, the remainder then being held in the insectary and given 4% sucrose *as lib* on a cotton wool pad.

On the seventh day following the blood feed a sample of each batch of mosquitoes is removed, and the insects are dissected. The midguts are examined with the aid of semidarkground illumination to detect the presence of oocysts, counts being made on each gut. The mean oocyst count for each batch of insects is determined (including those with no oocysts).

To determine the inhibitory effect of a drug on the development of oocysts it is dissolved in 4% sucrose and fed *ad lib* to the insects subsequent to the blood meal. Usually a batch of 10 *A. stephensi* for each drug dose level and for the control groups is sufficient to provide data from which the drug action can be calculated from a comparison of mean oocyst counts in treated and in control batches (Fig. 12).

A similar technique has been employed by Gerberg (1971) to screen for sporontocidal action against *P. cynomolgi* and *P. falciparum* in *A. stephensi*. There is no reason why other rodent malaria species could not be used instead of *P. yoelii nigeriensis* provided that their cyclic transmission can regularly be accomplished through this insect. It must be remembered that a lower insectary

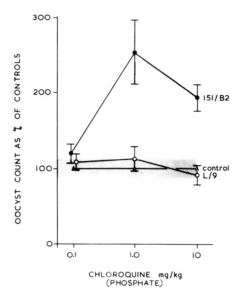

FIG. 12. The effect of chloroquine phosphate given to *P. berghei*-infected mice on the numbers of oocysts developing in *A. stephensi* fed on the mice 12 hours later. Line 151/B2 is a resistant line developed from the chloroquine-sensitive parent L/9 line of *P. berghei* NK65. The control counts and scatter for 151/B2 and L/9 are virtually identical. The scatter is indicated by shading over and above 100%. Bars indicate the extent of the standard error in treated groups (Ramkaran and Peters, 1969a).

temperature (19°–21°C) and a longer development time would be necessary if *P. berghei* is used.

B. Avian Malaria

1. Davey Test for Tissue Schizontocidal Action against Plasmodium gallinaceum in Chicks

Davey (1946a,b) described methods for the detection of blood and tissue schizontocidal action against this avian parasite. Since the blood schizontocidal test against *P. gallinaceum* has been replaced for many years by others employing rodent parasites, only the tissue schizontocidal method is described here. It too is little favored at the present time. *Aedes aegypti* are fed on chicks with a 4- to 6-day infection of *P. gallinaceum* at a time when many gametocytes are present. The mosquitoes are held for 8 days at about 25°C and 80% R.H. They are then killed and triturated with heparinized chicken blood to which is added some Ringer–Locke solution. After light centrifugation to eliminate large particles, the supernatant is diluted with this solution to yield an inoculum containing the equivalent of one-half to one mosquito per 0.2 ml. This is injected intravenously into each chick. Treatment is given twice daily from 2 hours before infection to D+5. Untreated birds usually die from heavy cerebral infection with secondary exoerythrocytic phanerozoites by D+8 to D+10, while parasitemia is usually detected by D+5. Drug activity is shown as a delay in patency of the parasitemia, increased survival time, or complete prevention of the infection (Tables IX and X).

Rane and Rane (1972) described a simplification of this technique along the lines of their rodent screen. Infection is similar to that just described, but the birds are treated once only, subcutaneously immediately after sporozoite inoculation. Activity is judged as a survival time at least double that of the controls. The test does not differentiate the site of action of the test compounds and has failed to show a prophylactic effect in several well-known compounds such as primaquine and dapsone which are both active against rodent tissue schizonts. The value of these models in relation to prophylaxis or radical cure of mammalian malaria is therefore open to doubt.

2. Fink Test for Tissue Schizontocidal Action against Plasmodium cathemerium in the Canary

The Hartman strain of *P. cathemerium,* first described in 1927, was much used for antimalarial drug screening in Germany prior to World War II but was largely replaced elsewhere by *P. gallinaceum* after Brumpt's discovery of this parasite in 1935. Nevertheless the older species, which readily infects canaries,

TABLE IX

Causal Prophylactic Action against Sporozoite-Induced *Plasmodium gallinaceum*[a]

Compound	Dose as base, twice daily, po (mg/kg) and duration (days)		Results
Mepacrine	125	(as long as possible)	No effect on mortality
Pamaquine	20.25	(6 days)	Mortality delayed a few days; no cures
Proguanil	51.5	(5 days)	Cure (toxic to some birds)
	34.3	(5 days)	Some cures
	17.15	(5 days)	Marked delay in infection
	4.3	(6 days)	Death delayed some days
	1.74	(6 days)	Death delayed in some birds
Pyrimethamine	2.0	(3½ days)	Some cured, some delayed mortality
Sulfadiazine	500	(4 days)	Cure
	250	(4 days)	Some cures
	125	(4 days)	Marked delay in infection, no cures
	20	(4 days)	Marked delay in some birds
	10	(4 days)	No effect on mortality

[a] Treatment from day of infection. Peters (1970a), modified from Davey (1946b), except for data on pyrimethamine which are from Falco *et al.* (1951).

TABLE X

Baseline Data on Sensitivity of *Plasmodium gallinaceum* 8A Strain to Blood Schizontocides[a]

Drug	MTD[b]	METD[b]	TI[b]	References
Quinine	449	16	28	
Mepacrine	16.9	1	16.9	Coatney *et al.* (1953)(all drugs in
Chloroquine	30	1	30	terms of mg/kg base)
Amodiaquin	100	2	50	
Primaquine	6	0.2	30	
Pamaquine	8.9	1	8.9	
Pentaquine	5.7	0.1	57	
Isopentaquine	7.3	0.19	38.4	
Proguanil	44	1	44	
Sulfadiazine	1500	62	24	
Dapsone		128		Ramakrishnan *et al.* (1962)
Pyrimethamine		0.03		Falco *et al.* (1951)

[a] Peters (1970a).
[b] MTD, maximum tolerated dose; METD, ED_{75}; TI, MTD/METD.

remained in use in Germany, and in 1970 Fink, who had invested considerable effort in the standardization of sporozoite infection with this species, described his method of screening for tissue schizontocidal action with its aid (Fink *et al.*, 1970).

The salivary glands of infected *Culex pipiens* are dissected out and triturated in a 2:1 mixture of canary serum with physiological saline on ice. Canaries are infected intravenously with an inoculum of 2500 sporozoites, which leads to a patent parasitemia in untreated controls by D+3 to D+5. Test compounds are administered daily from D0 through D+3 by the intravenous route, and blood films are examined daily from D+5 until the parasitemia exceeds 2%. Drug action is judged by the delay produced in reaching the 2% level in treated as compared with control birds, and an ED_{50} can be calculated by determining from a dose–activity graph the dose required to produce a 50% increase in the 2% time (Fig. 13).

This procedure has not been widely adopted, partly because it is technically more difficult to manage than a rodent model and partly because of doubts about the relevance of findings in avian malaria to mammalian tissue schizonts and their response to chemotherapy.

3. Screening for Sporontocidal Action against Plasmodium gallinaceum in Aedes aegypt (Gerberg, 1971)

This is a modification of the procedure first described by Terzian (1947) in which test compounds are fed directly to mosquitoes in which the sporogonic

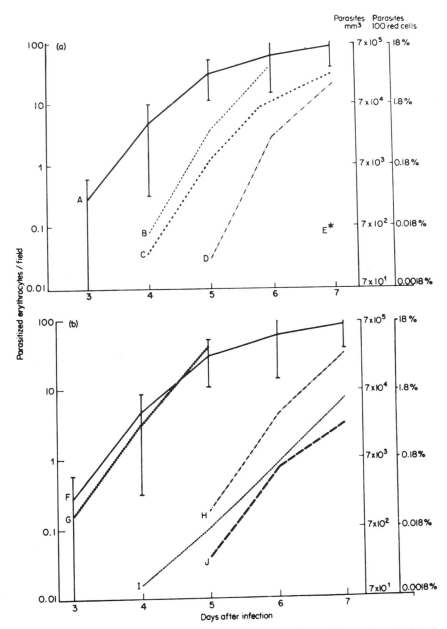

FIG. 13. Response of *P. cathemerium* infection in canaries to blood schizontocides. A, Controls; B, quinine; C, chloroquine; D, pamaquine; E, mepacrine; F, control; G, sulfadiazine; H, primaquine; I, proguanil; J, pyrimethamine. All doses given once intravenously 1–2 hours after infection (Peters, 1970a, after Fink and Dann, 1967).

stages of this avian malaria are developing. Gerberg *et al.* (1966) have described the process of mass rearing of *A. aegypti* for use in antimalarial drug screening. Their technique is beyond the scope of this chapter and should be read in the original by those who wish to use it. The method provides very large numbers of mosquitoes which Gerberg (1971) used in primary drug screening at the rate of up to 1000 compounds per week. It has been suggested that there is a parallel between sporontocidal and tissue schizontocidal activity. Practical experience in the screening of over 114,000 compounds has shown that this screen is, if anything, too sensitive, and many active compounds are detected, the action of which cannot later be confirmed in *in vivo* models of the same parasite.

Mosquitoes reared as described by Gerberg *et al.* (1966) and in World Health Organization (1973) are allowed to hatch from the pupae and, 3 days later, are fed on a suspension of the test compound in 10% sucrose for 2 days. They are then starved for 48 hours to increase their avidity for blood before being offered a blood meal on *P. gallinaceum*-infected chicks. Following the blood meal the mosquitoes are held in an insectary at 27°C and 80% R.H. where they again receive the sucrose–drug suspension. Nine days later gut and gland dissections are performed on samples from each cage to detect the presence of oocysts and/or sporozoites.

TABLE XI

Comparison of Three Antimalarial Screening Systems: Lowest Confirmed Sporontocidal Concentration[a,b]

Compound	WRAIR no.	Avian (%)	Simian (%)	Human (%)
Quinine	2976	–	–	–
Chloroquine phosphate	1544	–	0.1 ±	0.1
Sontoquine	7429	–	nt	–
Hydroxychloroquine	1545	–	–	–
Mepacrine	1543	–	0.1 ±	nt
Primaquine	2975	0.1	0.1	0.1 ±
Pentaquine	6021	0.01 ±	0.1 ±	0.1 ±
Pamaquine	4234	–	–	–
Isopentaquine	6020	–	–	0.01
Metachloridine	6010	0.1	0.1	0.01
Sulfadiazine	7557	0.1	0.1	0.1
Dapsone	0448	–	–	–
Proguanil	3091	0.01	0.01	0.01
Pyrimethamine	2978	0.0001	0.0001	0.0001
Lapinone	26041	–	0.1	–
Cycloguanil	5473	0.00001	0.00001	0.001

[a] Gerberg (1971).

[b] –, no sporontocidal activity; ±, variable or inconsistent sporontocidal activity; nt, not tested.

As Gerberg (1971) has pointed out, a similar system can be adopted to test for action against *P. cynomolgi* in *A. stephensi* as a model for *P. vivax*. He has also used the technique to a limited extent to examine the sporontocidal action of compounds against *P. falciparum* in this mosquito (Table XI).

4. Screening for Tissue Schizontocidal Action against Plasmodium fallax in Tissue Culture (Beaudoin et al., 1969)

The exoerythrocytic stages of avian malarias, unlike those of mammalian species, grow in cells of the reticuloendothelial system and can readily be adapted to suitable tissue culture systems. Beaudoin *et al.* (1969) described a procedure for studying the mode of action of antimalarials that could readily be adapted to drug screening of potential tissue schizontocides. Since no method has yet become available for the *in vitro* cultivation of the tissue stages of mammalian species, an avian model may still find a place in drug screening, and it is therefore outlined here.

The original procedure for tissue culture of *P. fallax* was described by Davis *et al.* (1966), whose paper should be consulted. Turkey embryonic brain monolayer cultures are grown in Leighton tubes which are sown with approximately 200,000 viable cells of which about 50% are infected with exoerythrocy-

TABLE XII

Comparison of the Level of Activity of Antimalarial Drugs against the Tissue Stages of *Plasmodium fallax* in Vitro[a]

WR no.	Drug	Number of replicate trials	Type of lesion	ED_{50} (mg/liter)
2975	Primaquine	14	I	5.30
6021	Pentaquine	3	I	3.15
6020	Isopentaquine	2	I	6.70
49577	Metabolite[b]	3	I	2.30
49808	Naphthoquinone[c]	2	I	<0.50
27653	RC12[d]	2	I	4.40
2978	Pyrimethamine	3	II	0.54
69320	Experimental drug[e]	2	II	<0.10

[a] Beaudoin *et al.* (1969).

[b] WR49577—8[(5-/isopropylamino/pentyl) amino]-5,6-quinolinediol trihydrobromide.

[c] WR49808—3-18-cyclohexyloctyl/-4-hydroxy-1,4-naphthoquinone.

[d] WR27653—4-(2-bromo-4,5-dimethoxyphenyl)-1,1,7,7,-tetraethylenetriamine.

[e] WR69320—commercially discrete compound.

tic stages of *P. fallax*. The cells are suspended in 1 ml of a complex medium described by Beaudoin *et al.* (1969). The tubes are cultured for 24 hours at 37°C in a 5% carbon dioxide–air mixture to allow the cells to flatten and attach to 11 × 22 mm coverslips in the tubes. Drugs are added to the medium in appropriate dilutions and allowed to remain in contact for 48 hours. At the end of this time the coverslips are removed, wet-fixed with 90% Zenker's solution in 10% neutral Formalin, washed in water and Lugol's iodine to remove the mercury, and then stained with Giemsa stain. Drug activity is assessed with reference to modifications of parasite morphology as compared to untreated control cultures. Minimal effective drug levels can be determined by using successive dilutions in a series of culture tubes (Table XII).

There have been no reports on the use of this model for drug screening on any significant scale.

C. Simian Malaria

1. *Plasmodium knowlesi in the Rhesus Monkey for Blood Schizontocidal Screening*

Simian models in general have the advantage over other experimental infections i.e., in birds or rodents, that the metabolic processes of the host resemble more closely those of man. Nevertheless the physiology of the parasites themselves may differ markedly from that of the parasites infecting man.

In the rhesus monkey infected with blood stages *P. knowlesi* produces a fulminating and lethal infection that has been used as the basis of a simple test for the evaluation of blood schizontocides.

Consequently it has been thought by many workers to be a good model for the study of drugs that may be effective against virulent *P. falciparum* in humans. Experience shows that this is true only to a limited degree.

The following technique was described by Richardson and his co-workers (1946), and data obtained with it were reviewed in Wiselogle (1946). An intravenous inoculum of 5×10^6 parasitized donor erythrocytes per kilogram body weight is given to young rhesus monkeys of 2–3 kg. From D0 drugs are administered twice daily for 4 days, and blood films are examined daily. Until the level of parasitemia approaches 0.01% (i.e., 1 parasite per 100 oil immersion fields), thick blood smears are examined to assess the presence of low parasite numbers. The efficiency of the treatment is judged by its ability to suppress the peak level of parasitemia, protect the animal from death, or delay death in comparison with untreated controls. As an alternative regimen the drugs may be administered once daily for 7 days commencing when the parasitemia reaches approximately 0.1%. Schmidt *et al.* (1977b) on the basis of long experience with this model have pointed out that, instead of *Macaca mulatta*, the cynomolgus monkey, *M. irus* of West Malaysian origin may be used, but not those originating in the Philip-

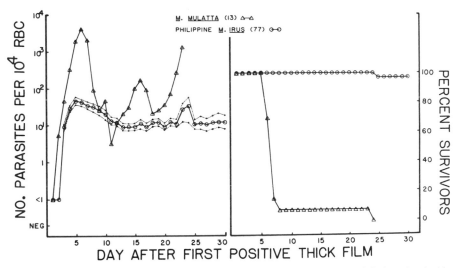

FIG. 14. Parasitemias and fates of *M. mulatta* and *M. irus* of Philippine origin inoculated with the S-M strain of *P. knowlesi*. Left-hand side, solid lines represent means, broken lines indicate ± SE values. Figures in parentheses are numbers of monkeys in groups (Schmidt *et al.*, 1977b).

pines in which *P. knowlesi* runs a relatively benign course (Fig. 14). This makes them, however, valuable for strain maintenance.

The parasitemia of *P. knowlesi,* once established in the rhesus, runs a very rapid course, so that treatment should always be commenced before the 2% level is reached (Fig. 15). From this point untreated animals usually succumb within 2 or 3 days, often in a condition characterized by peripheral vascular collapse. Several strains of this parasite are commonly used, including the Sinton–Mulligan (S-M) strain isolated from an *M. irus* of Singaporean origin in 1932, the Nuri strain (Table XIII) from West Malaysia (much used by Indian workers), and the H strain isolated from a malaria research worker naturally infected in the same country. *Plasmodium knowlesi* is little used for studies on causal prophylaxis, since the prepatent period is somewhat inconstant. No secondary tissue stages have been detected in this species.

Indian workers developed a number of lines of *P. knowlesi* resistant to drugs of the dihydrofolate reductase type (e.g., proguanil and pyrimethamine), to dapsone, and to primaquine that could be used for secondary screening. It is unlikely, however, that these lines are still available, and new ones would have to be developed if required. Since drug-resistant lines of *P. berghei* are readily available today and are probably of equal value in predicting the drug-resistance features of human malarias, it seems hardly worthwhile to utilize monkey malaria for this purpose. Moreover, we have at our disposal also drug-resistant lines of human parasites that can be studied in simian hosts (see below).

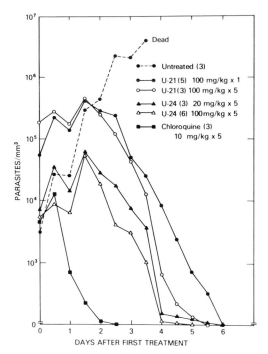

FIG. 15. Median asexual parasitemia curves in rhesus monkeys infected with *P. knowlesi*. Monkeys were treated twice a day for 5 days with either clindamycin (U-21) or *N*-demethyl-4'-pentylclindamycin (U-24) or once daily with chloroquine. Three monkeys received a single dose of clindamycin. Number in parentheses indicates number of monkeys in each group (Powers *et al.*, 1976).

TABLE XIII

Blood Schizontocidal Action against Nuri Strain of *Plasmodium knowlesi* in Rhesus Monkeys[a]

Compound	MED as base (mg/kg/day $\times$ 7)	References
Quinine	30	
Chloroquine	2.1	
Mepacrine	6	
BW 377 C 54	5.5	Sen Gupta *et al.*, 1958b
Proguanil	0.2	
Pyrimethamine	0.05[b]	Jaswant Singh *et al.*, 1954a
Sulfadiazine	0.8	
Dapsone	0.25	
Primaquine	1.1	Ramakrishnan and Satya Prakash, 1961

[a] Partly from Ramakrishnan *et al.* (1962); Peters (1970a).

[b] 0.005 for old laboratory strain.

2. *Plasmodium knowlesi in Vitro Test for Blood Schizontocidal Evaluation (Canfield et al., 1970)*

An *in vitro* procedure in which drug activity is assessed both on morphological and biochemical grounds has been described by Canfield *et al.* (1970). It is based on a technique developed by Polet (1966). Polypropylene culture tubes 17 × 100 mm in size are seeded with 0.2 ml of washed and resuspended *P. knowlesi*-infected erythrocytes drawn from a rhesus monkey with approximately a 10% parasitemia. The suspension is prepared by spinning down the donor blood when the parasites show a synchronous ring-stage infection and suspending 1.5 ml of the packed cells in 10 ml of buffered medium.

The culture medium is enriched Eagle's minimal medium with added 10% human AB group serum, antibiotics, and 20–30 μCi of methyl[^{14}C]methionine (specific activity 15 mCi/mmole) per liter, buffered to pH 7.4. Drugs to be tested are dissolved at a concentration of 0.14 mg/ml in water and adjusted to a final concentration of 10 mg/liter by adding 1 ml of drug solution to 13 ml of medium in each plastic culture tube.

The tubes are cultured at 37°C in a roller drum at 12 rpm for 18–22 hours after which they are centrifuged. The supernatant is retained for measurement of lactic acid production. Methionine incorporation is assessed with the aid of a scintillation counter. Serial drug dilutions permit drug dose–activity relationships to be plotted. Giemsa-stained smears of the infected red cells permit a count to be made of parasites that have developed toward the schizont stage.

This technique has proved valuable and relatively simple to use for evaluation of the antimalarial action of a variety of compounds including chloroquine, dihydrofolate antagonists (Canfield *et al.*, 1970) (Table XIV), and nucleic acid precursor analogs (McCormick *et al.*, 1974).

3. *Schmidt Technique for Testing Blood and Tissue Schizontocidal Action against Plasmodium cynomolgi in the Rhesus Monkey*

Sporozoite-induced *P. cynomolgi* in the rhesus monkey runs a course very similar to that of certain forms of *P. vivax* in man. Parasitemia becomes patent in 8 days and reaches a peak 8–10 days later, the primary attack lasting about 3 months or longer. Relapses occur at intervals varying from 2 to 5 weeks in untreated animals, and the total infection probably lasts for about 1 year. A similar picture is seen in the Kenyan variety of the African green monkey, *Cercopithecus aethiops*. (Schmidt *et al.*, 1977a) (Fig. 16). The infection is readily transmitted through a number of anopheline species including *A. freeborni* and *A. stephensi*. (The infection in other macaque species is very variable, and they are therefore not considered as valuable for chemotherapy studies on *P. cynomolgi* as the rhesus or African green monkey). These two

TABLE XIV

Results of *in Vitro* Antimalarial Drug Testing of Selected Compounds[a]

Class of compound and code	Name	Schizont development	Lactic acid production	Methionine incorporation
		Percent of control		
Quinoline				
WR 4809	1-Methyl-4-[4-(7-chloro-4-quinolyl-amino)benzoyl] piperazine	0	9	5
WR 30090[b]	6,8-Dichloro-2-(3',4'-dichlorophenyl)-α-(di-*n*-butylaminomethyl)-4-quinolinemethanol hydrochloride	0	83	24
WR 1544	Chloroquin	0	18	3
Phenanthrenemethanol				
WR 33063[b]	6-Bromo-α-(diheptylamino-methyl)-9-phenan-threnemethanol hy-drochloride	0	44	19
Guanyl hydrazone				
WR 5677	Dypnone guanyl hydra-zone hydrochloride	0	9	0
WR 9792	4-Trifluoromethylphenyl-4-fluorophenyl guanyl hydrazone hydro-chloride	0	2	1
Pyridine				
WR 61112	Metichloropindol	5	46	39
Pyrimidine				
WR 5949	Trimethoprim	67	86	78
WR 2978	Pyrimethamine	66	106	114
Sulfonamide or sulfone				
WR 4629	2-Sulfanilamido-3-methy-oxypyrazine	94	88	113
WR 6798[b]	4,4'-Diformamidodiphenyl sulfone	100	87	92

[a] Canfield *et al.* (1970).

[b] Not completely dissolved; the final concentration of the drug was <10 mg/liter. All other drugs were tested at 10 mg/liter.

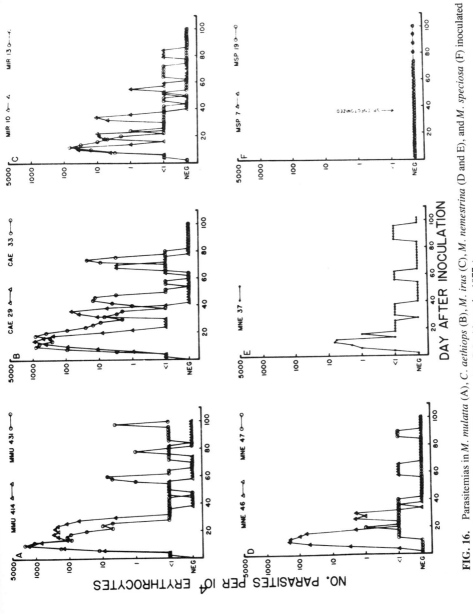

FIG. 16. Parasitemias in *M. mulatta* (A), *C. aethiops* (B), *M. irus* (C), *M. nemestrina* (D and E), and *M. speciosa* (F) inoculated with trophozoites of the B strain of *P. cynomolgi* (Schmidt et al., 1977a).

species also respond to trophozoite-induced *P. cynomolgi* infection in a similar manner. Lower infection levels are produced in other macaques.

Schmidt *et al.* (1966) inoculated *M. mulatta* intravenously with 5×10^5 sporozoites of *P. cynomolgi* derived from *A. freeborni*. Test compounds are administered from D0 through D+8, following which blood films are examined daily either until parasitemia is observed or for a period of 4–6 weeks. If they remain negative, they are rechallenged with the same infection dose. If they show parasitemia, they are included in the treatment regimen which is initiated when they reach a parasite level of 0.1–0.5%. One group of monkeys then receives treatment daily for seven consecutive days in order to observe whether the test compound acts as a blood schizontocide. If parasitemia persists or recrudesces after a short absence, chloroquine is administered for 7 days. After this the animals are observed for a further 8 weeks. If still negative after this interval, they are splenectomized to ensure that they are parasite-free (Table XV). This indicates that the test drug is active against the secondary exoerythrocytic schizonts, i.e., that the compound has produced a radical cure. Figure 17 is a ''flow diagram'' of this procedure.

TABLE XV

Causal Prophylaxis in *Plasmodium cynomolgi* (M Strain)[a]

Compound	Daily dose as base, po from D0 to D+8 (mg/kg)	Prepatent period (days)[d]
Pyrimethamine[b]	0	9, 9, 9, 10, 10, 13
	0.075	19, 24
	0.3	10, 17, 24, 27, 31, 55[e]
	1.25	23, 25, 27, 28, 34, 34
	5.0	28, 34, 43, 60[e], 68, D[e]
	20.0	23, 59[e], D, D, D, D
	Dosed from D−1 to D+7	
Primaquine[c]	1.0	None of 5 patent
Chloroquine[c]	5.0	8, 9, 9, 9, 14
RC12[c]	0	13 on 8; 1 on 9
	0.39	8, 8, 8, 8, 8
	1.56	8, 8, 9, 9, 13
	6.25	10; 9 not patent
	25.0	None of 15 patent
	100.0	None of 5 patent

[a] Peters (1970a).
[b] Schmidt and Genther (1953).
[c] Schmidt *et al.* (1966).
[d] D, died.
[e] Postsplenectomy.

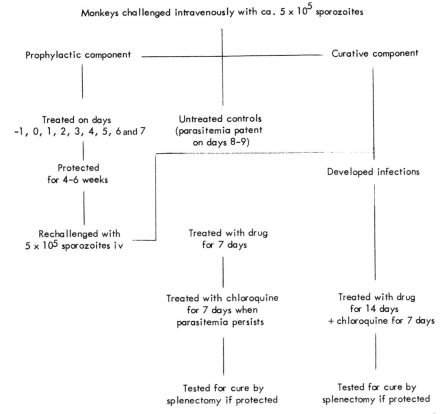

Monkeys challenged intravenously with ca. 5×10^5 sporozoites

Prophylactic component — Curative component

Treated on days
-1, 0, 1, 2, 3, 4, 5, 6 and 7

Untreated controls
(parasitemia patent
on days 8-9)

Protected
for 4-6 weeks

Developed infections

Rechallenged with
5×10^5 sporozoites iv

Treated with drug
for 7 days

Treated with chloroquine
for 7 days when
parasitemia persists

Treated with drug
for 14 days
+ chloroquine for 7 days

Tested for cure by
splenectomy if protected

Tested for cure by
splenectomy if protected

FIG. 17.   Procedure for evaluating the activity of drugs against infections with *P. cynomolgi* (L. H. Schmidt, in World Health Organization, 1973).

4. Blood Schizontocidal Test against Plasmodium cynomolgi in the Rhesus

In this simplified derivative of Schmidt's technique as described by Davidson *et al.* (1976) young rhesus monkeys first receive graded oral doses of drug suspension orally (via a nasogastric tube), starting with an empirically selected dose, e.g., 1 mg/kg. The animals receive this dose daily for two successive days. If no side effects are observed, increased doses are administered, using half-log increments until the maximum fully tolerated dose is reached (Tables XVI and XVII). At this point treatment is continued for a further 7 days if possible at one dose level lower.

Thus after determining the MTD by observation fractions of this dose are given to other monkeys that have received an intravenous inoculum of 5×10^8 parasitized donor erythrocytes. The doses are repeated at a fixed level for each

TABLE XVI

Antimalarial Activity of Quinoline Drugs in Rhesus Monkeys Infected with *Plasmodium cynomolgi*[a]

Name and compound number	Drug dose producing antimalarial effect (mg/kg/day)								Minimum curative dose (mg/kg/day)	Maximum tolerated dose (mg/kg/day)
	316	100	31.6	10.0	3.16	1.0	0.316	0.1		
Chloroquine (WR 1544)				C	MS	SS	I	I	10.0	31.6
				C	MS	I	I	I		
				C						
Amodiaquin (WR 2977)			C	MS	MS	I		I	10.0	10.0
			C	C	SS	I		I		
				MS						
Primaquine (WR 2975)			MS	MS	MS	MS	MS	I	Not curative	
			MS	MS	MS	MS	MS			
Plasmochin (WR 4234)			C	MS	MS	MS	MS	NT[b]	31.6	
			C	MS				I		
			C							
Quinine			C	MS		MS	SS	I	31.6	100
				NT[c]						
WR 30090	C	C	I	I					100	>316
	C	MS	I	I						
Endochin (WR 7295)		I	I	I					Ineffective	100
		I	I	I						

[a] Davidson *et al.* (1976).

[b] Monkey died as a result of intercurrent disease (bronchopneumonia).

[c] Monkey failed to develop adequate parasitemia prior to drug administration.

TABLE XVII

Antimalarial Activity of Sulfone and Sulfonamide Drugs in Rhesus Monkeys Infected with *Plasmodium cynomolgi*[a]

Name and compound number	Drug dose producing antimalarial effect (mg/kg/day)								Minimum curative dose (mg/kg/day)	Maximum tolerated dose (mg/kg/day)
	316	100	31.6	10.0	3.16	1.0	0.316	0.1		
Dapsone (WR 448)			C	C					10	
			MS	CS	MS	MS	MS			
			CS	MS	MS	MS	MS			
			MS	MS						
Diformyl dapsone (WR 6798)	C	C	C						31.6	>316
	CS	MS	MS	MS	MS	MS				
			MS	MS	MS	MS				
			MS							
Sulfadiazine (WR 7557)		C	MS	MS	MS	MS	MS	SS	100	
		MS	MS	MS	MS	MS	MS	I		
							C			
Sulfalene (WR 4629)		C	MS	MS	MS	MS	MS	MS	100[b]	
		C	MS	MS	MS	MS	MS	I		
							SS			
Sulfadimethoxine (WR 4873)		MS	MS	MS	I	SS			>100	
		MS	SS	SS	I	I				

[a] Davidson *et al.* (1976).
[b] The cure at 0.316 mg/kg a day has been disregarded in determining the minimum curative dose.

191

pair of monkeys for 7 consecutive days, starting 4 days after infection (i.e., D+3 through D+9). Blood films are examined daily to D+14, and then every second day. Red cell counts are also made, so that a total count of parasites per cubic millimeter of blood can be calculated. Animals that become parasite-positive are sacrificed on D+30, while negative monkeys are splenectomized. The latter are then examined every other day for 30 more days to detect subpatent parasitaemia following therapy.

The outcome of the trial is judged as shown in the tabulation:

I	Ineffective—course of parasitemia similar to that in mock-treated controls
SS	Slight suppression—parasitemia temporarily below 1000/mm^3
MS	Marked suppression—parasites absent on at least two successive days; recrudescence before D + 30
CS	Complete suppression—parsitemia became negative but reappeared after splenectomy
C	Curative—parasitemia became negative and remained so up to at least 30 days after splenectomy

Both in the previous test and in this one the parasite used was the subspecies *P. cynomolgi bastianellii* which was first isolated in 1957 from an *M. irus* originating from Pahang. It should be remembered that this subspecies readily infects humans, producing a vivaxlike infection.

5. Test for Gametocytocidal and Sporontocidal Action against Plasmodium cynomolgi in the Rhesus and Anopheles maculatus

In a series of studies Omar and his associates examined the gametocytocidal and sporontocidal action of drugs against *P. cynomolgi*. The hosts were the rhesus monkey and *Anopheles maculatus*. The technique they used was not aimed at primary drug screening but rather at secondary evaluation. Young rhesus monkeys received intravenous inocula of 2 ml of donor blood heavily infected with *P. cynomolgi bastianellii*. Batches of 2- to 3-day-old mosquitoes (75 per batch) were allowed to feed when numerous gametocytes were present. They fed just before administration of the test drugs, at various hours during the day of treatment, and then daily just before subsequent treatments. After feeding the insects were given 10% Karo syrup *ad lib* and held in an insectary at 25°C and 80% R.H. Giemsa-stained smears were made and examined from stomachs 24 and 48 hours after the blood meal to detect changes in the ookinetes. Batches were dissected at various intervals after feeding to determine the exact point in the cycle at which the drugs were exerting their effects. Dissections of midguts were made for oocysts from D+6 and D+9, and of glands for sporozoites from D+12 to D+18. Material was also fixed in Carnoy's solution, embedded, sectioned, and stained by the Giemsa technique to demonstrate morphological changes.

With this technique Omar *et al.* (1973) showed that primaquine exerted a marked sporontocidal action when given even in small doses and that this action appeared within 4 hours of initial treatment (Table XVIII). However, larger doses exerted their sporontocidal action even sooner, although gametocytes remained in the monkey's blood for a further 2 or 3 days. Omar *et al.* (1974) showed that proguanil and pyrimethamine exerted their effects on the developing oocysts (Table XIX). Omar and Collins (1974) found that the pyrocatechol RC12 was sporontocidal when mosquitoes fed on drug-treated animals but not when the insects fed on RC12 solutions after taking an infective blood meal from untreated animals.

D. Human Malaria

1. *In Vitro test of Blood Schizontocidal Action against Plasmodium falciparum (Rieckmann et al., 1968b)*

a. **Original (Macro-) Technique.** When Rieckmann and his colleagues first described this procedure for determining the blood schizontocidal action of drugs against *P. falciparum in vitro,* the source of the parasitized blood used was human volunteers. The test has since been somewhat modified and adapted as a method of monitoring the response of naturally acquired infections to chloroquine under field conditions. From the point of view of drug screening it is debatable whether the Rieckmann test should be considered part of primary screening or, as in my opinion, only a step to be adapted at the stage of secondary or tertiary screening. In any case, the availability of numerous drug-resistant as well as drug-sensitive strains of *P. falciparum* now makes this kind of test particularly valuable, since the activity of a compound *in vitro* can be checked directly against the target organism and a forecast can be made of its potential value in the treatment or prevention of infections with parasite strains resistant to the drugs in common use (Table XX). Moreover, two sources of parasitized blood other than humans are now available, first, ongoing *in vitro* cultures of *P. falciparum* (see Volume 2, Chapter 6), and second, infections maintained in *Aotus* monkeys (see next section).

The principle of this test, which is an adaptation of the old Bass and John's method (1912), is to incubate defibrinated blood containing young ring forms of *P. falciparum* in the presence of glucose and a range of concentrations of test drug in shallow layers in small tubes exposed to air for 24 hours. In control tubes the young parasites mature toward schizogony, and the proportion of schizonts can be assessed in stained thick blood films made at the end of the 24-hour

TABLE XVIII

Effect of a Single Dose of Primaquine (1.95 mg Base/kg/day Equivalent to 45 mg Base for Humans) on Gametocytes and Sporogony of *Plasmodium cynomolgi* in *Anopheles maculatus*[a]

Time after treatment (hours)	Parasites (per mm³)	Gametocytes (per 100 WBC)[b]	Ookinetes[c] Formation (+'s)	Ookinetes[c] Gut penetration (+'s)	Gut dissections Pos/Dis	Gut dissections Percent positive	Gut dissections Mean oocysts/ + gut	Gland dissections Pos/Dis	Gland dissections Percent positive	PGI[b]
X-152[d]										
0	23,450	72	3	3	25/25	100	150 (4–428)[g]	8/8	100	3.9
1			3	3	18/20	90	107[e] (7–270)	6/10	60	3.1
4			1	1	6/30	20	1.2[f] (1–2)	0/8	0	0
8			1	1	2/25	8	1.0[f]	0/8	0	0
24	58,000	12	1		2/32	6	1.5[f] (1–2)	0/6	0	0
48	6,600	16	1		3/51	6	1.3[f] (1–2)	0/22	0	0
72	370	0			1/22	5	1.0[f]	0/9	0	0
96	420	0			0/40	0	0	0/16	0	0
120	40	0			0/32	0	0	0/9	0	0
X-173										
0	18,000	15	3	3	27/30	90	88.7 (1–250)	11/12	92	4.0
1			3	3	26/30	86	77.3[e] (1–216)	12/12	100	3.8
3			3	3	25/30	83	59.0[e] (5–161)	9/15	60	3.5
4			2	2	24/30	80	12.3[e] (1–41)	5/20	25	3.2

Hour									
8			1	9/50	18	1.3[f] (1–3)	0/20	0	0
24	6,300	6	1	3/43	7	1.0[f]	0/20	0	0
48	220	0		2/43	5	1.5[f] (1–2)	0/20	0	0
72	110	0		4/48	8	1.5[f] (1–3)	0/18	0	0
96	40	0		2/40	5	1.5[f] (1–2)	0/20	0	0
120	110	0		0/57	0	0	0/20	0	0
216	2,700	0	1	9/30	30	2.0 (1–4)	6/14	43	3.7
X-182									
0	94,400	92	3	33/33	100	265 (2–630)	7/7	100	3.6
1			3	29/35	82	168[e] (2–435)	17/21	81	3.8
2			3	21/36	58	33[e] (1–149)	5/13	59	3.8
4			1	3/34	9	1.3[f] (1–2)	0/14	0	0
8			1	5/30	17	2.8[f] (1–7)	0/15	0	0
24	280,000	52		1/39	3	1.0[f]	0/12	0	0
48	31,000	20		3/44	7	1.3[f] (1–2)	0/16	0	0
72	8,000	0	1	13/30	43	3.7[e] (1–9)	14/21	67	3.2
96	1,000	2	1	14/30	47	2.5[e] (1–6)	10/25	40	3.2
120	18,500	2	2	13/30	43	4.2 (1–11)	7/23	34	3.0

[a] Omar et al. (1973).
[b] WBC, white blood cell; PGI, positive gland index.
[c] Number of plus signs indicates relative intensity of parasites observed in six mosquitoes (1–9: 1+; 10–99: 2+; more than 99: 3+).
[d] This monkey was treated after previously being used as a control. See Fig. 1.
[e] Some retarded or degenerate oocysts present in addition to normal oocysts.
[f] Retarded or degenerate oocysts.
[g] Figures in parentheses denote ranges.

TABLE XIX

Effect of Proguanil (5.6 and 11.3 mg Base/kg/day Equivalent to 150 and 300 mg in Humans) on Gametocytes and Sporogony of Plasmodium cynomolgi in Macaca mulatta and Anopheles maculatus, Respectively[a,b]

Time after treatment (hours)	Parasites (per mm³)	Gametocytes (per 100 WBC)	Ookinetes Formation (+'s)	Ookinetes Gut penetration (+'s)	Gut dissections Pos/Dis	Gut dissections Percent positive	Gut dissections Mean oocysts/+ gut	Gland dissections Pos/Dis	Gland dissections Percent positive	Gland dissections PGI
X-109 [5.6 mg base/kg/day(×5)]										
0	34,000	2	3	3	25/25	100	115 (1–275)	13/18	72	3.3
1			3	3	2/20	10	1.5*(1–2)	0/9	0	0
3			3	3	5/27	18	1.0*	0/8	0	0
24	660	0	2	1	5/30	17	1.6*(1–3)	0/10	0	0
48	0	0	0	0	2/20	10	1.0*	0/6	0	0
72	0	0	0	0	0/20	0	0	0/10	0	0
96	0	0	0	0	2/20	10	3.0*(1–5)	0/7	0	0
120	0	0	0	0	2/20	10	1.0*	0/10	0	0
X-108 [11.3 mg base/kg/day (×5)]										
0	120,000	75	3	3	25/25	100	438 (60–970)	20/20	100	3.8
1			3	3	12/30	40	1.5#(1–4)	1/19	5	3.0
2			3	3	12/32	38	2.4*(1–5)	0/42	0	0
3			3	3	13/30	43	1.7*(1–5)	0/40	0	0
5			3	3	11/30	37	1.6*(1–4)	0/20	0	0
8½			3	3	12/34	35	1.2*(1–2)	0/30	0	0
9			3	3	7/34	20	1.5*(1–3)	0/16	0	0
24	46,000	48	3	1	1/60	2	1.0*	0/17	0	0
48	750	4	1	0	2/50	4	1.5*(1–2)	0/12	0	0
72	0	0	0	0	3/51	6	1.0*	0/10	0	0
96	0	0	0	0	1/47	2	2.0	0/13	0	0
120	0	0	0	0	3/43	7	1.0	0/18	0	0

[a] Omar et al. (1974).

[b] #, Some normal oocysts in addition to retarded and degenerate oocysts; *, retarded or degenerate oocysts; figures in parentheses indicate ranges; +, number of plus signs indicates relative intensity of parasites observed in six mosquitoes (1–9: 1+; 10–99: 2+; more than 99: 3+); PGI, positive gland index.

TABLE XX

The *in Vitro* Activity of Experimental Antimalarial Compounds against Strains of *Plasmodium falciparum* with Varying Degrees of Sensitivity to Pyrimethamine and Chloroquine[a]

Class	Drug	Strain of *P. falciparum*[b]	Concentration (μg of salt per liter of blood)[c]												
			2500	1000	500	250	100	50	25	10	5	2.5	1.0	0.5	0.25
Inhibitory drugs	Chloroquine diphosphate	Viet Nam (Marks)	+++	+	0										
		Malaya (Camp.)		+++	++	+	0								
		Uganda I				+++	+	0							
	WR 30090	Viet Nam (Marks)	++	+	0										
		Uganda I	+++	+	+	0									
	WR 142490	Viet Nam (Marks)				+++	+	0							
		Uganda I				+++	+	0							
	WR 122455	Viet Nam (Marks)				+++	+	0							
		Uganda I				+++	+	0							
Dihydrofolate reductase inhibitors	Pyrimethamine isethionate	Viet Nam (Marks)	0												
		Malaya (Camp.)		+++		++	+								
		Uganda I				+++	+	0							
	Cycloguanil hydrochloride	Viet Nam (Marks)					++	+	0						
		Malaya (Camp.)					+++	++	+	0					
		Uganda I							+++	+++	++				
	WR 38839	Viet Nam (Marks)						+++	++	+	0				
		Malaya (Camp.)							+++	++	+	0			
		Uganda I									+++	+	0		
	WR 99210	Viet Nam (Marks)										+++	+++	++	+
		Malaya (Camp.)										+++	++	0	0
		Uganda I										+++	++	+	0

[a] Unpublished data from Dr. K. H. Rieckmann, based on the technique described by Rieckmann *et al.* (1968) (World Health Organization, 1973).

[b] Viet Nam (Marks): highly resistant to chloroquine and pyrimethamine; Malaya (Camp.): resistant to pyrimethamine; Uganda I: sensitive to chloroquine and pyrimethamine.

[c] +++, >90% parasites affected by drug; ++, 50–90% parasites affected by drug; +, <50% parasites affected by drug; 0, no drug effect (as control).

incubation (Fig. 18). By comparing the proportions of schizonts in drug-containing tubes with those in the controls, a dose–activity curve can be calculated and plotted. For simple screening it suffices to take arbitrary screening concentrations and a standard drug for comparison. The technique works best with compounds such as chloroquine that act rapidly and have a steep dose–activity regression line. With antimetabolites such as cycloguanil the interpretation can be more difficult. The technique as described by the authors requires 10–15 ml of parasitized blood, and this is an obvious drawback in relation to its use for field studies in man, or for screening. The stages in the test are as follows (Rieckmann *et al.*, 1968b; Rieckmann, 1971):

1. A series of screw-cap, flat-bottomed glass vials 6 cm tall and 1.5 cm in internal diameter are prepared. Each contains 5 mg glucose and a range of quantities of the drug to be tested. In the case of chloroquine, the quantities used could range from 0.5 to 5.0 nmoles/ml blood. Glucose and drug are added to the vials in aqueous solution, and the water is then allowed to evaporate at a temperature not exceeding 40°C.

2. Parasitized blood is defibrinated in sterile Erlenmeyer flasks containing glass beads by rotating gently for about 5 minutes.

3. Aliquots of 1 ml parasitized blood are transferred to each vial, the contents of which are then swirled gently to dissolve and mix the glucose and drug.

4. The vials are then held in an incubator or water bath at 38°–40°C for 24 hours. They are *not* agitated during incubation.

5. After 24 hours the contents of the vial are further agitated to resuspend the parasitized red cells. Thick films are prepared and stained by the Giemsa technique.

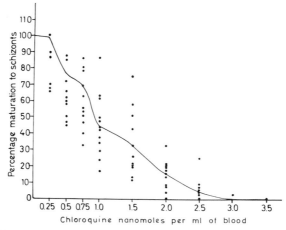

FIG. 18. Effects of chloroquine added *in vitro* upon maturation of asexual erythrocytic forms of strains of *P. falciparum* in Thailand using the Rieckmann macrotechnique (Sucharit *et al.*, 1977).

6. Schizonts (trophozoites containing more than two chromatin masses) and total asexual parasites up to at least 100 in each specimen thick film are counted, and the proportion of schizonts calculated. It is advisable to use duplicate vials for each drug concentration and the drug-free controls.

7. The values for test samples are divided by the values for the control samples, and the results are expressed as percentages.

b. Modified (Micro-) Technique. The large quantity of blood required in the original Rieckmann test is obviously a disadvantage. He and his co-workers have recently described a modification whereby only 50 μl of blood is required, a quantity that can readily be collected with the aid of a simple calibrated hematology pipet from a finger prick sample. The details are as follows (Rieckmann *et al.*, 1978).

Dilutions of the test compound are placed in the flat-bottomed wells of disposable, plastic, microtiter plates and then dried and stored dry ready for use. A culture medium is prepared by adding to RPMI 1640 medium sodium bicarbonate (2 mg/ml), HEPES buffer (6 mg/ml), and gentamicin sulfate (4 μg/ml). To 50 μl of this mixture is added in each well 5 μl of parasitized blood. After the plastic lid has been placed on the plate, the latter is shaken to dissolve the test compound and mix the blood and medium. It is then placed in a desiccator in which a candle is burned (as in Trager and Jensen's blood culture technique, Volume 2, Chapter 6) until the fumes escape and the flame begins to die. The stopcock is then closed, and the desiccator is placed in an incubator at 38°–39°C for 24–30 hours. A the end of this period the microtiter plate is removed, and thick smears made from the contents of each plate are stained with Giemsa. The proportion of schizonts is assessed in each smear and compared with those in control wells containing no drug, as in Rieckmann's original technique, the schizonts being counted against 500 white cells. Rieckmann *et al.* (1978) use Microtest II plates made by Falcon Plastics, Oxnard, California; RPMI 1640 powdered TC medium made by Gibco, Grand Island, New York; and an Eppendorf pipet to measure 5-μl samples of blood, supplied by Brinkmann Instruments, Westbury, New York. In their first published experiments they used chloroquine diphosphate (0.1–25 ng) dissolved in 25 μl distilled water in wells having a diameter of 6.5 mm. The samples examined were blood from *Aotus* monkeys infected with either the chloroquine-sensitive Uganda Palo Alto strain or the chloroquine-resistant Viet Nam Oak Knoll strain of *P. falciparum* (Table XXI). The former proved in repeat experiments to be at least 10 times more sensitive to chloroquine than the latter. While the heaviness of the infection did not seem to influence the results significantly, subsequent experience has indicated that parasite density will have to be allowed for.

If this test on further evaluation in the field upholds the promise of the first report, it will be an invaluable tool not only for monitoring the chloroquine

TABLE XXI

Effects of Chloroquine on Two Strains of *Plasmodium falciparum* in Vitro[a]

Strain of *P. falciparum*[b]	Hematocrit (vol %)	Parasites (per mm³)	Schizonts (per 500 leukocytes in control samples)[c]	Percentage maturing to schizonts and nanograms of chloroquine diphosphate per well[d]											
				0.1	0.3	0.5	1.0	1.5	2.0	2.5	5.0	10.0	15.0	20.0	25.0
Uganda Palo Alto (FUP)	58	58,000	52	86	93	19	4	0	0	0					
	49	106,000	260	73	73	78	49	1	0	0					
	41	4,920	98	93	73	14	0	0	0	0					
	38	2,340	150			69	40	0	0	0					
Viet Nam Oak Knoll (FVO)	33	19,800	184								92	66			0
	30	24,000	98								98	51			0
	40	32,000	1258							94	93	82			0
	34	1,020	31							102	75	63	21	5	0
	17	940	35								80	60	26	0	0

[a] Rieckmann *et al.* (1978).

[b] Parasites were obtained during the course of infection of two *Aotus* monkeys infected with the FUP strain of *P. falciparum* and three *Aotus* monkeys infected with the FVO strain of *P. falciparum*.

[c] Mean of two replicates.

[d] Percentage of asexual parasites, relative to the mean of two control replicates (100%), that matured to schizonts.

response of naturally acquired infections of *P. falciparum* in man, but also for monitoring other drugs and for secondary, if not primary, *in vitro* drug screening.

Powell and Berglund (1974) tried unsuccessfully to adapt Rieckmann's original technique to *P. vivax*. They were hindered by the inconsistent morphological changes induced in the parasites following the period of incubation (24 hours), probably related to the lack of synchronicity inherent in this parasite in many human infections. They found it impossible to select a practical end point upon which to base their drug–dose activity data. Nevertheless, as anticipated, they observed that chloroquine inhibited maturation of the asexual parasites to some degree over the range of concentrations studied. However, this inhibition was by no means complete even at a chloroquine concentration of 2 nmoles/ml.

2. In Vitro Tests of Blood Schozontocidal Action against Plasmodium falciparum

a. Method of Richards and Williams (1975).   These authors adapted the method by which schizontocidal action against *P. berghei in vitro* is judged by the effect of a compound on the incorporation of [^{3}H]leucine by the parasites (see description in Section III,A,7 p. 172). Their experiments were somewhat complicated in that they examined both the *in vivo* action of drugs and then removed blood at various intervals after treatment of the hosts and cultivated it for a further 24 hours in the presence of [^{3}H]leucine to measure the viability of the parasites. The hosts in their experiments were *Aotus trivirgatus* monkeys infected with a chloroquine-sensitive West African strain of *P. falciparum*.

Animals were treated either with oral chloroquine sulfate (40, 20, or 10 mg base/kg on three successive days) or the test compound (an amidino urea) at the corresponding dose levels. Blood was collected from each monkey and from untreated controls (0.5 ml per animal) 18 hours after the first dose. It was diluted 1:6 in the culture medium without first passing the sample through a cellulose column to remove leukocytes (because of the small quantity of blood taken). The rest of the procedure was as described in Section III,A,7.

As employed by the authors this test was valuable in demonstrating the viability of the apparently normal parasites observed in the peripheral blood *in vivo* for several hours following initial treatment with the amidino urea. It could readily be adapted for the screening of blood schizontocides *in vitro* against various strains of *P. falciparum*, using either parasitized blood from *Aotus* or from *in vitro* cultures. So far there are no reports of its having been used for this purpose.

b. Method of Richards and Maples (1979).   The technique for the continuous culture of *P. falciparum in vitro* introduced by Trager and Jensen (1976) has been utilized in the development of an elegant procedure for evaluating the activity of antimalarials *in vitro* which is simpler than that described in Section III,A,7.

The basic culture technique is that described by Trager and Jensen (see Volume 2, Chapter 6). Human blood of group A^+ collected into acid citrate dextrose or citrate phosphate dextrose is washed twice in culture medium RPMI 1640 and centrifuged at 800 *g* for 10 minutes, or is passed through a cellulose column to remove the leukocytes (Williams and Richards, 1973), and then washed twice. After resuspending in an equal volume of RPMI 1640 medium the cells are then added at a concentration of 10% to the cultures.

Drugs to be tested are dissolved in RPMI 1640, sterilized by filtration through an 0.2-μm cellulose acetate filter, and then diluted to produce the appropriate concentrations in RPMI medium. In their report the authors state that pyrimethamine base had to be dissolved in 0.5% lactic acid to give a final concentration of 10^{-2} *M* from which further dilutions could be made in RPMI 1640. The lactic acid was found to have no action on the parasites in culture.

To 0.1 ml of a 1% concentration of stock *P. falciparum* culture was added 1.4 ml of drug-containing RPMI 1640 medium. The mixtures were incubated at 37°C in desiccators in which the oxygen tension was reduced by burning wax candles to extinction. Every 24 hours the medium was changed; the first time the medium was replaced with further drug-containing medium, and the second and third times with medium containing no drug. On each occasion the cultures were monitored on Giemsa-stained blood films.

As shown in Fig. 19, this procedure permits an accurate determination to be made not only of a drug's absolute activity on parasite viability but also lends

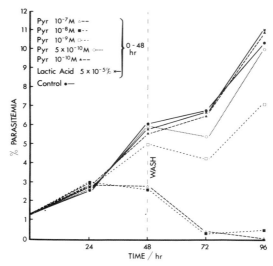

FIG. 19.   Effect of pyrimethamine on *P. falciparum in vitro* (Richards and Maples, 1979).

itself to a simple determination of the dose–activity relationship. Since high concentrations of drugs can be used, the technique is valuable for the detection of even a low level of activity, which may be invaluable in the early stages of drug screening and drug design. Very small quantities of drug are required, so that the method is economical and allows a new compound to be tested against the target organism itself, thus sparing the use of primates for this purpose. The technique could, of course, also be adapted as a bioassay for the level of a drug or its active metabolites in the blood of a treated animal or person.

3. The Use of Aotus trivirgatus for Screening of Blood Schizontocides against Plasmodium falciparum or Plasmodium vivax (Schmidt, 1973)

The adaptation of human malaria parasites to monkeys has provided an invaluable series of models in which drugs can be evaluated directly against the target organisms *in vivo*. Of all the animals in which *P. falciparum* and other human parasites can develop, the most valuable for research is the owl or night monkey, *A. trivirgatus*. Other species of Old and New World monkeys that will support the development of human malarias are reviewed by Young *et al.* (1975). Of the several subspecies of this animal, the Colombian *A. trivirgatus griseimembra* appears to be the most susceptible, at least to *P. falciparum* (see Fig. 20).

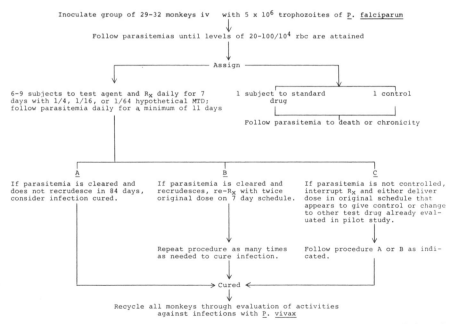

FIG. 20.   Schema for pilot studies of the activities of various chemical compounds in owl monkeys infected with trophozoites of *P. falciparum* and *P. vivax* (Schmidt, 1973).

Schmidt (1973) has pioneered the use of *A. trivirgatus* in drug screening and established the following models for infections with *P. falciparum* and *P. vivax*. An important prerequisite for using these small animals (they grow up to 1200 g) is their careful management in the laboratory and conditioning by good feeding, housing, and careful handling. They are highly susceptible to many infections including various species of *herpesvirus* and should be kept away from other species of monkeys. Schmidt (in World Health Organization, 1973) has contributed the following notes on their care and handling:

> Owl monkeys appear to thrive poorly when caged alone. They should therefore be caged in groups of 5–6 if cages of 1 m³ or slightly greater volume are available. Individual aggressive animals may need to be isolated temporarily to avoid fighting. The animal quarters should be kept darkened and quiet at a constant temperature of 22–27°C and at least 50% relative humidity. After being allowed to settle down for about a week the monkeys can be individually tattooed across the abdomen so that they can be recognized easily without unnecessary handling.
>
> On arrival in the laboratory, instead of their natural diet of fruits owl monkeys are fed initially on a mixture of fruits and vegetables, supplemented with brewers' yeast and monkey chow. The latter is given after being soaked in reconstituted dried milk (10% in water) and drained in a sieve. A little vanilla flavouring makes the chow more appetizing until the animals become accustomed to the taste. Then the diet is gradually changed until it consists only of the monkey chow-milk mix, which must contain adequate vitamin D_3. On this regimen a 700 g male will gain about 15 g weekly up to about 1 kg. During the next year it will gain another 100 or 200 g and reach a maximum weight of approximately 1200 g.
>
> After about a month the haemoglobin is measured and any anaemia treated by the administration of vitamin B_{12} and multivitamin preparations. Blood films are examined for the presence of anaemia, microfilaria (at least 4 species of *Dipetalonema* occur in *Aotus*), trypanosomes (about 1 film in 50 is positive, probably with *T. rangeli*), and *Haemobartonella*. Natural malaria infections have not been seen in *Aotus trivirgatus*.
>
> Gloves are used to catch individual animals and are disinfected before being reused for animals of another cage. Blood for making blood films, etc., may be collected from the marginal ear veins, which become distended in malaria-infected monkeys. For intravenous inoculation or venesection the mid-saphenous vein on the back of the leg is used. Between 4 and 5 ml can readily be withdrawn into a heparinised syringe. The animals should be handled gently.
>
> To prepare blood inocula 1 ml is withdrawn from a monkey with approximately 20% parasitaemia and appropriately diluted with iced saline.
>
> Drugs are administered orally through a urethral catheter to animals in 10 ml of physiological saline and the contents of the tube are washed down with a further 5 ml of saline.

Infections of either *P. falciparum* or *P. vivax* can be induced in the *Aotus* by syringe passage, but it may be necessary for primary isolations to use immunosuppressed or splenectomized animals. Once the parasites have become adapted to the simian host, infections can readily be induced by syringe transfer of infected blood to intact animals. Numerous drug-sensitive as well as drug-resistant strains of these parasites are available (Schmidt, 1973; Young *et al.*, 1975). Schmidt gives a detailed account of the course of such infections in untreated monkeys. *Aotus* is in short supply and will remain so until good husbandry methods are developed to enable us to breed adequate numbers in captivity. In the meantime the fullest use should be made of any available animals. Survivors of experiments with *P. falciparum* can, for example, after an adequate interval be reused for studies on *P. vivax*.

Animals in which the parasites are used for strain passage receive an inoculum of 5×10^4 parasitized red cells intravenously. When the parasitemia reaches between 10 and 20%, blood is collected for passage, animals succumbing at a parasite level between 15 and 30%. For drug experiments recipient monkeys are given an intravenous inoculum of 5×10^5 infected red cells on D0. By D+3 *P. falciparum* will usually become patent, reaching 0.2–1.0% by D+5 in early morning blood films. Therapy commences at this stage, drugs being given orally to unanesthetized animals (as illustrated by Schmidt, 1973) about midday and repeated daily for a total of 7 days. If the parasitemia continues to increase after the animals have received treatment for 3 days, the dose or the drug is changed. Blood films are made daily and, in monkeys that become parasite-free with treatment, are continued for 3 days longer, then twice weekly for 2 more weeks and once weekly up to 3 months from the last treatment or retreatment. When animals remain positive on D+6, daily films are examined until 3 days after they become negative, and then twice weekly and weekly up to 3 months (Tables XXIII and XXIII).

The MTD is interpolated from data obtained in models used for primary screening (e.g., the Rane test) in other models, usually the mouse. Usually three dose levels are used, equivalent to $\frac{1}{4}$, $\frac{1}{16}$, $\frac{1}{64}$ of the MTD, if sufficient animals are available, with two animals in each group and two mock-treated controls. If the top dose is ineffective (by the third treatment day), the dose for these animals

TABLE XXII

The Capacity of WR 142490 to Cure Established Infections with Various Strains of *Plasmodium falciparum* and *Plasmodium vivax*[a]

Strain	Susceptibility to			CD_{90} for WR 142490, daily dose [mg/kg body weight ($\times 7$)]
	Chloroquine	Pyrimethamine	Quinine	
Plasmodium falciparum				
Malayan Camp-CH/Q	R I	R III	R I	3.125
Viet Nam Oak Knoll	R III	S	R III	3.125
Viet Nam Smith	R III	R III	R III	5.0
Plasmodium vivax				
New Guinea Chesson	S	S	S	2.5
Viet Nam Palo Alto	S	R III	S	2.5

[a] Schmidt (1973).

TABLE XXIII

The Capacity of WR 158122 to Cure Established Infections with Various Strains of *Plasmodium falciparum* and *Plasmodium vivax*[a]

	Susceptibility to			
Strain	Chloroquine	Pyrimethamine	Quinine	CD$_{90}$ for WR 158122, daily dose [mg/kg body weight (×7)]
Plasmodium falciparum				
Malayan Camp-CH/Q	R I	R III	R I	0.39
Viet Nam Oak Knoll	R III	S	R III	0.098
Viet Nam Smith	R III	R III	R III	>6.25
Plasmodium vivax				
New Guinea Chesson	S	S	S	0.39
Viet Nam Palo Alto	S	R III	S	6.25

[a] Schmidt (1973).

is doubled, and those on the lower doses receive a different drug. If a lower dose is effective, the dose can be titrated further downward in other animals. When sufficient monkeys are available, different drug-resistant strains of *P. falciparum* can be used. Animals on the lowest doses of an active drug can be used to inoculate clean animals which then receive a larger dose to look for changes in drug response indicating the buildup of resistance to the test drug. The schedule of treatment of the various groups is summarized in Fig. 21.

A similar procedure can be followed for the study of drug action against *P. vivax*.

Schmidt has found that the MTD as obtained in the Rane test, or the effective dose when this is much lower, provides a useful indicator of the MTD in *Aotus*. If, for example, the MTD of a drug in the Rane test is approximately 700 mg/kg, this is taken as the total dose for the *Aotus* to be given over 7 days, i.e., 100 mg/kg daily, and fractions of this, e.g., 25, 6.25 mg/kg then give the ¼, $\frac{1}{16}$ etc., levels, respectively.

Hayes and Ward (1977) have reported that *P. falciparum* can be transmitted by mosquito bite to *A. trivirgatus* if the animals are first splenectomized and given a supplement of DL-methionine in the diet (0.2 g 5 days a week for 6 weeks). This might open the way for use of this experimental host for studies on potential causal prophylactic agents were *Aotus* monkeys not in such short supply. Rossan and Baerg (1975) have demonstrated that an *Aotus*-adapted strain of *P. falciparum* can infect the howler monkey (*Alouatta villosa*), but studies on this model are still at an early stage.

Rossan *et al.* (1975) have shown that *P. vivax* in the squirrel monkey, *Saimiri*

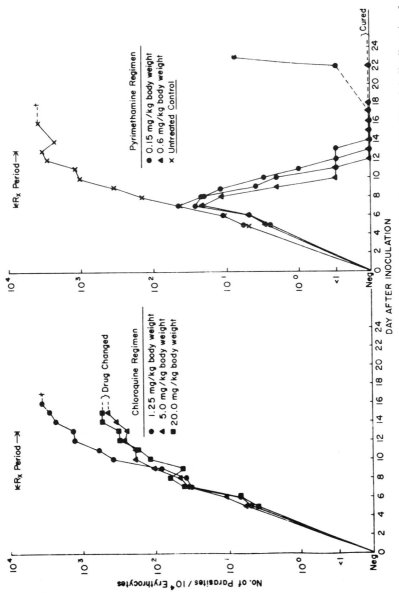

FIG. 21. Representative responses of infections of *A. trivirgatus* with trophozoites of the Viet Nam Oak Knoll strain of *P. falciparum* to treatment with chloroquine and pyrimethamine (Schmidt, 1973).

TABLE XXIV

Chemotherapy of Trophozoite-Induced Infections of *Plasmodium vivax* (Achiote Strain) in Unaltered *Saimiri sciureus*[a]

Experiment no.	Monkey no.	Treatment initiated		Response	
		Patent day	Parasitemia (per mm^3)	Days to clear	Negative days examined[b]
Chloroquine (10, 10, 5 mg base/kg in 3 days)					
1	5885	3	1,100	3	52
	6409	5	1,040	4	175
	5881	7	1,160	2	15
	5890	7	1,760	2	21
	5882	8	940	2	67
	5900	8	3,850	3	73
Chloroquine (10 mg base/kg in 1 day)					
2	5895	5	1,120	2	126
	5896	6	1,160	3	38
	5886	7	1,070	3	194
	6386	8	1,590	1	161
Pyrimethamine (1 mg/kg in 1 day)					
3	5203	6	1,190	6	176
	5879	6	2,610	6	24
	5986	6	3,060	5	17
	5988	7	4,210	5	72
	5982	13	5,150	4	11

Experiment no.	Monkey no.	Untreated controls, primary attack		Relapse(s)	
		Patent period (days)	Maximum parasitemia (per mm^3)	Subpatent period(s) (days)	Negative days examined after final patent period
1	5892	24	87,130	40	103
	5876	39[c]	69,420		
2	5897	24	40,280	12, 33	23
	5898	55	76,530		22
3	5921	33[c]	37,540		
	5889	45	93,210	17, 31	105

[a] Rossan *et al.* (1975).

[b] No relapses occurred in treated monkeys.

[c] Died during patency after maximum parasitemia.

sciureus, provides a potentially valuable model for chemotherapy (Table XXIV). In this host (as well as in *Aotus*) sporozoite-induced infections relapsed after treatment with chloroquine alone and were radically cured by chloroquine followed by primaquine, as in man. Since this New World monkey can be colonized in captivity, it could be of considerable interest in the future for antimalarial drug screening, especially for antirelapse drugs.

E. Clinical Trials in Man

Clinical trials of antimalarials in man have evolved in parallel both with advances in other medical fields (e.g., the decrease in neurosyphilis following the introduction of penicillin) and changes in medical ethics regarding the use of volunteers for drug experiments. Increasingly since the thalidomide disaster in the 1950s governmental regulatory agencies have tightened up on the requirements both for clinical trials and new drug registration, while at the same time increasingly rigid ethical requirements have made it ever more difficult to initiate any testing of new compounds, particularly where the tests also involve deliberate infection of volunteers with pathogenic organisms.

As pointed out by the World Health Organization (1973), the objective of clinical trials (stage IV screening) is to determine first the safety and then the efficacy of selected antimalarial agents. Screening in man follows the six phases set out at the start of this section. Rigid protocols must be established and approved by an independent ethical committee for each phase of the study from phase 1, clinical pharmacology, through preliminary trials in infected volunteers, pilot studies in naturally infected, partially immune subjects in the field (Fig. 22), and hospital patients, and then extended field trials. Finally it is necessary to establish an efficient monitoring system for reporting any untoward side effects of the new drug once it is used en masse, and to take remedial action if indicated (e.g., withdrawal of the compound where serious adverse reactions become apparent).

Up to 1939 the majority of phase-2 studies of antimalarials were carried out not simply in volunteers but also in patients with neurosyphilis who were receiving therapeutic malaria to kill their spirochetes with the aid of an induced fever (see Peters, 1970a). Although the most important clinical studies on antimalarials from 1939 onward were carried out in volunteers [e.g., the Australian antimalarial program in Cairns headed by Fairley (1945)], occasional reports continued to appear of trials in neurosyphilitics. This held no particular danger as long as the malaria infections with which these patients were being treated still responded to an alternative drug, e.g., chloroquine or quinine. However, it became quite a different matter when tests were made on patients infected with strains of *P. falciparum* that were highly resistant to chloroquine, and in some cases, partially resistant to quinine, since failure of the new compound under test could also put

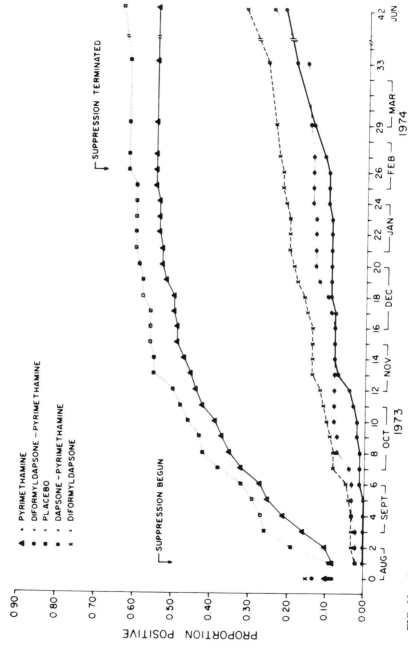

FIG. 22. Cumulative proportion of subjects infected with *P. falciparum* by study group. Example of a phase-3 pilot field trial in semi-immune subjects (Pearlman *et al.*, 1975).

the subject's health if not life seriously at risk. Nevertheless, such trials are necessary, but they should only be carried out in otherwise healthy, informed volunteers under strictly monitored conditions and by an experienced research team (Table XXV).

For many years from 1939 onward prisoners in certain jails, notably in the United States, were permitted under certain conditions to volunteer for inclusion in trials of new antimalarial drugs. Thus it was relatively easy to carry out phase-1 and -2 studies in a relatively short period of time. A great debt is owed to these volunteers and to the prison authorities who permitted this system to operate. Unfortunately, these facilities are no longer available in the United States, which provided a leading example of this type of volunteer program. Military personnel too have formed an invaluable source of volunteers, particularly during World War II when important new compounds such as mepacrine, chloroquine, and proguanil were being tested. Soldiers were also included in certain trials of primaquine when its value as a radical curative agent was being evaluated, especially against the Korean strains of *P. vivax* (Vivona *et al.*, 1961). More recently the value of drug combinations in the prevention of chloroquine-resistant *P. falciparum* (Black, 1973) and of new drugs in the prevention and treatment of such infections (Canfield and Rozman, 1974), have been carried out in military units in Southeast Asia.

1. Causal Prophylactic Action

Healthy human subjects are exposed to the bites of infected colony-reared *Anopheles* mosquitoes infected with *P. falciparum* or *P. vivax*. Test drugs are administered usually from the day before infection (D−1) daily up to 6 days after infection (D+6). In order to avoid exerting drug action on the sporozoites the first treatment dose may be delayed until a few hours after the infection is given. Usually each volunteer receives bites from 10 or more heavily infected mosquitoes. The "interrupted bite" technique, first described by Coatney *et al.*

TABLE XXV

Falciparum Malaria in Thailand—Comparison of Cure Rates[a]

Drugs	Average initial parasite count (per mm^3)	R III	R II	R I	S	Cure rate[b] (%)
Pyrimethamine + sulfadoxine	60,300[c]	4	0	2	33	85
Pyrimethamine + diformyldapsone	16,900[c]	2	2	9	10	43

[a] Doberstyn *et al.* (1976). Patients who did not complete follow-up examinations were not included in this table.

[b] The difference in cure rates was statistically significant ($\chi^2 = 9.67$, $p < 0.01$).

[c] The average initial parasite counts were significantly different ($t = 8.4$, $p < 0.001$).

(1947) and Alving *et al.* (1948), is useful in ensuring an equitable distribution of infective sporozoites among subjects.

Each mosquito kept in a separate container is permitted to probe through the skin of two, three, or four subjects in turn but only allowed to engorge fully after feeding on the last one. Bites are arranged so that each subject in the group receives if possible an equal number of first, second, third, etc., bites. If a mosquito refuses to probe, a substitute insect is brought in. After feeding the insects are dissected, and sporozoite densities in the salivary glands are determined using the following gradings: 1–9 sporozoites +; 10–99 ++; 100–199 +++; 1000 or more ++++. The "infectivity" of the group of mosquitoes used is the total of the + signs for all 10 infective insects. Blood films (thick and thin) are made and examined daily from D+7 until patency, or up to a predetermined time limit.

Using this procedure Rieckmann *et al.* (1974) demonstrated that a single 1-g dose of mefloquine hydrochloride produced a suppressive cure against a chal-

TABLE XXVI

Prophylactic Activity of a Single Dose of 1 g of Mefloquine Hydrochloride against the Viet Nam (Marks) Strain of *Plasmodium falciparum*[a]

Group	Volunteer	Weight (kg)	Interval between drug administration and sporozoite inoculation (days)	Day of patency after sporozoite inoculation
I	1	75	2	None
	Control	56		12
II	2	62	14	None
	3	78	14	None
	Control	66		11
	Control	74		11
III	4	79	14, 16	None
	5	69	14, 16	None
	Control	86		12
	Control	92		14
IV	6	73	21	34 (55)[b]
	7	86	21	17 (38)[b]
	Control	65		9
	Control	59		12
V	8	73	21	37 (58)[b]
	Control	63		10
	Control	74		9

[a] Rieckmann *et al.* (1974).

[b] Numbers in parentheses represent days between drug administration and the onset of patent parasitemia.

lenge by sporozoite-induced *P. falciparum* made up to 16 days after medication (Table XXVI). A challenge 21 days after medication resulted only in a suppression of the parasitemia. (In another series of volunteers these workers confirmed *in vitro* the long duration of activity of mefloquine in the serum—up to 35 days after a single dose.)

2. Blood Schizontocidal Action

It is preferable to infect test subjects through mosquito bite as described above, but blood-induced infections can be used if mosquito infections cannot be used. In the latter case a few milliliters of donor blood containing approximately 5×10^5 asexual parasites are injected intravenously. It is essential that the donors be Australia antigen-negative and free of other infectious diseases as far as can be determined. Rieckmann (quoted in World Health Organization, 1973) gives each recipient γ-globulin as a precaution.

Once a patent parasitemia has developed, the volunteer recipient commences oral therapy with the test drug which he receives at a dose previously determined on the basis of preliminary animal screening and phase-1 clinical trials. The drug is given over a period of 3–7 days during which the recipient's parasitemia and general condition are carefully monitored according to a precisely laid down protocol. Quinine is usually kept in readiness in case the subject becomes hyperpyrexial or fails to respond to the new compound, so that dangerously high parasite levels cannot be reached. It is often considered advisable to use partially immune volunteers for the initial phase-2 tests of a new compound. Thick and thin blood films are examined several times daily as long as the parasitemia persists, and then daily for at least 60 days after in order to exclude any recrudescence of parasitemia. (Blood schizontocidal studies against *P. vivax* require a different timing, since relapses are liable to result in certain strains from the presence of secondary tissue schizonts, as well as recrudescences from surviving asexual parasites in the blood.)

3. Antirelapse (Tissue Schizontocidal) Action

For such studies it is advisable to use a strain of *P. vivax* with a short-term relapse pattern such as the New Guinea Chesson strain, in order to avoid the necessity of long periods of observation (e.g., over 1 year in the case of North Korean infections). Following infection by sporozoite bite parasitemia is allowed to develop. The subjects then receive the test drug, usually over a period of 14 days. (Presumably this timing has been adopted for comparison with the "standard" 14-day therapeutic regimen of primaquine.) Blood films and general physical parameters are monitored as above. Test compounds believed not to possess a significant blood schizontocidal action may have to be given after the parasitemia has been cleared with chloroquine, or together with chloroquine (e.g., the study by Clyde *et al.*, 1974, on the pyrocatechol RC12).

Miller *et al.* (1974) and Contacos *et al.* (1974) have employed this procedure to compare the drug response of different strains of *P. vivax* to various regimens combining chloroquine and primaquine. The first workers found that the standard 14 days of primaquine (15 mg base daily) together with chloroquine was followed by a relapse in 2 out of 57 prison volunteers infected with various Central American strains of *P. vivax.* Contacos's group showed that eight weekly doses of 300 mg chloroquine base with 45 mg primaquine base radically cured all 10 volunteers infected with a South Viet Nam strain of this parasite, but only 1 out of 3 infected with the Chesson strain.

Clyde and McCarthy (1977) demonstrated that it was not necessary to give primaquine for 14 days, but that a 7-day course of 60 mg base following chloroquine (1.5 g base over 3 days) was equally effective in producing a radical cure of Chesson strain infection. (However, not all subjects can tolerate such a large daily dose.) On the other hand, Contacos *et al.* (1973) showed that a 5-day course of primaquine (14 mg base/day) with chloroquine had no tissue schizontocidal effect on a Pakistani strain of *P. vivax* in nonimmune volunteers.

Trenholme *et al.* (1975) has observed that a single dose of 1 g of mefloquine hydrochloride, which produces a suppressive cure of some strains of sporozoite-induced *P. falciparum* (Table XXVII), will not give a radical cure of sporozoite-induced Chesson strain *P. vivax* infection even in partially immune subjects. This compound possesses good blood schizontocidal action against this parasite but clearly no action against the secondary exoerythrocytic stages.

Clyde *et al.* (1976) found that weekly doses of 250 mg mefloquine hydrochloride suppressed vivax malaria only as long as the prophylactic dose was continued. Less frequent drug dosage was not even suppressive. On the other hand, the same dosage produced a suppressive cure of *P. falciparum* infection (Table XXVIII).

4. Gametocytocidal and Sporontocidal Action

The value of antimalarials as gametocytocides or sporontocides is in their use in limiting transmission of the parasites in an endemic area. Every new antimalarial should be evaluated for its activity against gametocytes, especially those of chloroquine-resistant *P. falciparum* against which only primaquine is of general value. The test drug is administered only after the gametocytes have reached a density of about $100/mm^3$, an alternative blood schizontocide such as quinine being given if necessary to damp down asexual parasitemia in the meantime. Both the direct influence of the test compound on the morphology and number of gametocytes and any effect on the development of gametocytes in mosquitoes fed on the volunteers after drug administration should be observed. Mosquito feeds should be made at various intervals both before and after the drug is given, and the subsequent effects noted on the development both of oocysts and sporozoites (Fig. 23). If possible, an attempt should be made also to see whether any

TABLE XXVII

Response of 35 Nonimmune Volunteers Infected with *Plasmodium falciparum* to Treatment with Mefloquine[a]

Strain of *P. falciparum*	Dose of mefloquine hydrochloride		No. treated	Asexual parasites (per mm³)[b,c]	Maximum rectal temperature (°C)[b]	Clearance time (days)		No. cured
	mg	mg/kg[b]				Fever[b,d]	Asexual parasites[b]	
Ethiopian (Tamenie)	400	5.4 (4.6–6.2)	2	1,610 (1,520–1,700)	41.5 (41.5–41.5)	5.5 (5–6)	4.0 (3–5)	1
Vietnam (Marks)	400	5.5 (3.9–7.5)	8	2,195 (240–8,880)	40.4 (39.8–40.6)	4.1 (2–6)	5.1 (2–7)	1
Cambodian (Buchanan)	400	5.6 (5.2–5.9)	2	2,835 (2,550–3,120)	40.3 (40.1–40.6)	5.0 (4–6)	5.0 (4–6)	0
Ethiopian (Tamenie)	1,000	10.4 (7.7–12.5)	3	810 (520–1,130)	40.1 (39.4–40.9)	5.0 (4–6)	3.0 (2–4)	3
Vietnam (Marks)	1,000	14.6 (13.6–15.4)	8	3,437 (760–8,480)	41.0 (40.6–41.6)	5.25 (4–7)	3.1 (3–4)	8
Cambodian (Buchanan)	1,000	13.9 (10.7–17.2)	4	10,090 (740–28,200)	41.2 (40.9–41.3)	4.5 (4–6)	4.75 (4–7)	2[e]
Cambodian (Buchanan)	1,500	21.2 (16.8–26.2)	8	8,437 (830–18,750)	40.1 (39.1–41.3)	3.2 (2–6)	4.0 (3–5)	8

[a] Trenholme *et al.* (1975).
[b] Mean, with range in parentheses.
[c] Maximum parasite count during the first 48 hours of treatment.
[d] Interval between treatment and the first day of a 48-hour period during which the rectal temperature remained below 38°C.
[e] The individuals who were not cured received 10.7 and 13.2 mg of mefloquine per kilogram and those who were cured received 14.5 and 17.2 mg of the drug per kilogram.

TABLE XXVIII

Prophylactic Effect on *Plasmodium falciparum* of Mefloquine Given Weekly[a]

Dose (mg)	Volunteer[b]	Days of first and last weekly dose	Days of mosquito challenge	Results
250	1. 31, C, 109	0 and 49	0	Suppressive cure
	2. 43, C, 95	0 and 49	0	Suppressive cure
	3. 35, C, 75	0 and 49	0	Suppressive cure
	4. 40, C, 76	0 and 49	0	Suppressive cure
	5. 29, N, 98	0 and 49	0	Suppressive cure
	6. 27, C, 70	0 and 49	0	Suppressive cure
	7. 29, C, 73	0 and 49	0	Suppressive cure
	8. 35, C, 84	0 and 49	0	Suppressive cure
	9. 27, C, 84	0 and 49	0	Suppressive cure
	10. 44, C, 86	0 and 35	0, 3, 6	Suppressive cure
None	11. 28, C, 85		0	Parasitemia on day 9
	12. 40, C, 67		0	Parasitemia on day 10
	13. 36, C, 77		0	Parasitemia on day 10
500	15. 32, C, 120	0 and 49	0 and 4	Suppressive cure
	16. 27, N, 85	0 and 49	0 and 4	Suppressive cure
	17. 34, C, 68	0 and 49	0 and 4	Suppressive cure
	18. 42, C, 73	0 and 49	0 and 4	Suppressive cure
None	19. 33, C, 75		0	Parasitemia on day 10

[a] Clyde *et al.* (1976).

[b] The number assigned the volunteer is followed by his age (in years), his race (C, Caucasian; N, Negro), and his weight (in kilograms). Volunteers 1 to 13 were exposed to one batch of mosquitoes, and volunteers 15 to 19 were exposed to another.

sporozoites that do mature are actually infective by allowing such mosquitoes to bite other, previously uninfected volunteers.

5. *In Vivo* Tests for Chloroquine Susceptibility of *Plasmodium falciparum* in Man

The serious nature of chloroquine resistance in *P. falciparum* has necessitated the design of an empirical procedure for the monitoring of response to this compound in man. The following test has been designed for this purpose and is known as the WHO standard field test (1973).

In the simplest form, the "7-day test," patients receive an oral dose of chloroquine totaling 25 mg/kg over a 3-day period (i.e., 10, 10, and 5 mg/kg or 600, 600, and 300 mg base for a 60-kg adult, and correspondingly less for children). Blood films, thick and thin, are taken daily, starting just before the first test dose and continuing for 7 days. A simple urine test is carried out to ensure that the drug has been taken and absorbed. The response to this treatment

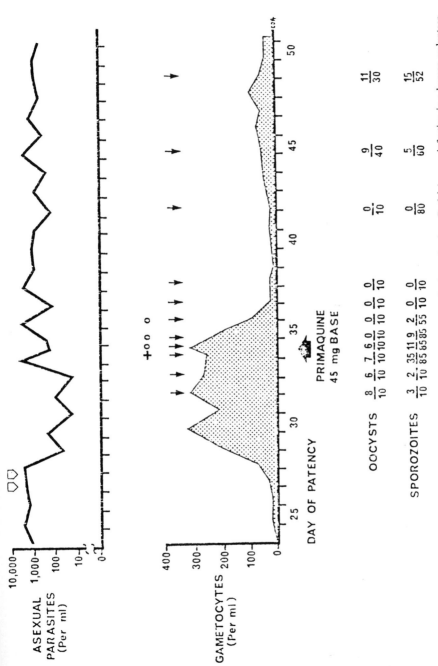

FIG. 23. Gametocytocidal and sporontocidal action of a single 45-mg dose of primaquine in a *P. falciparum* infection in a human volunteer. Open arrows indicate a dose of 540 mg quinine base. Solid arrows indicate mosquito feeds resulting in feeds later infective to humans (+) or noninfective (○). Lower figures show proportions of mosquitoes with oocysts or sporozoites seen on dissection (Rieckmann *et al.*, 1968a).

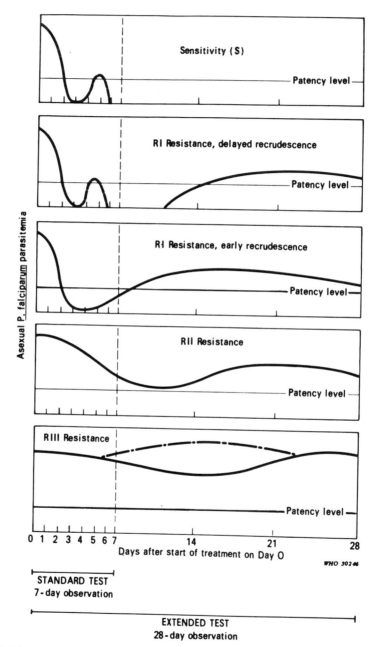

FIG. 24. Response to WHO field test for sensitivity of *P. falciparum* to chloroquine *in vivo* in man (World Health Organization, 1973).

is recorded as indicated in Fig. 24. In the 7-day test it is not possible to distinguish between a sensitive parasite giving an S response (i.e., clearance of asexual
parasitemia within 7 days of initiation of treatment without subsequent recrudescence) from an R I response (i.e., clearance of asexual parasitemia as in sensitivity, followed by a recrudescence after 7 days). It will distinguish an R II response
(i.e., a marked reduction in asexual parasitemia but no clearance within 7 days)
and an R III (no marked reduction or a rise in asexual parasitemia within 7 days).
Naturally the clinical condition of the patient must take preference over the test,
and appropriate measures must be taken in the presence of an R II or R III
response if necessary (see Section VI, C, 2).

Whenever possible the "extended test" should be carried out. This entails
extension of the observation period to 28 days and permits differentiation between an S, an R I with delayed recrudescence, and an R I with an early
recrudescence response. Further details of the World Health Organization field
test are to be found in the original report (1973). Data obtained with this test
correlate well, although not precisely, with data obtained by the Rieckmann *in
vitro* macro test, as can be seen in Fig. 25.

A simple test for the detection of chloroquine in the urine was designed by Dill
and Glazko (Lelijveld and Kortmann, 1970). The Dill–Glazko reagent consists of
50 mg eosin (yellowish) added to 100 ml chloroform (reagent quality) to which 1
ml 1 N hydrochloric acid is added. The mixture is shaken until the chloroform
becomes a light-yellow color, after which the chloroform solution is separated in
a separating funnel from the acid and stored in a glass-stoppered brown bottle.

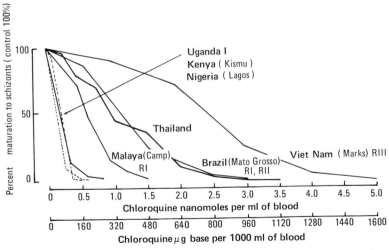

FIG. 25. Responses obtained in three sensitive African strains of *P. falciparum,* strains of West
Malaysia, Brazil and Viet Nam, as compared with strains of Thailand, using the Rieckmann
macrotechnique *in vitro* and the WHO field test *in vivo* (Sucharit *et al.,* 1977).

About 10 drops of the reagent are added to 2 ml of urine in a testtube. The contents are shaken vigorously for a few moments. The presence of chloroquine in the urine is indicated by a change in color from yellowish to violet-red in the chloroform layer which precipitates after the shaking.

IV. PHARMACOLOGY AND MODE OF ANTIMALARIAL ACTION

The various aspects of the mode of action of antimalarial drugs may be studied as provided in the following outline:

1. General pharmacology
   Pharmacodynamics
      Absorption by host
      Absorption by parasites
   Tissue distribution
   Drug metabolism
2. Molecular pharmacology
   Structural changes
   Reaction with nucleic acids
   Interaction with enzymes
   Complexing with metabolic intermediates or substrates
3. Secondary actions on host physiology
   Interaction with host enzymes
   Antitoxic effects
   Interaction with host immunity
   Relation to host erythrocyte metabolism
4. Drug potentiation and antagonism
5. Structure–activity relationships

The investigation of the mode of action of any given antimalarial compound may be seen therefore to include all the classic techniques of pharmacology, pharmacodynamics, and toxicology, in addition to more specialized procedures for observing the action of the drug on the host–parasite complex. Only the latter will be considered in detail here, since exploration of the molecular pharmacology of antimalarials makes particular demands on our imagination and ingenuity. First, however, a few points need to be made about the less specific characteristics of the drugs in common use.

A. General Pharmacology

The general pharmacology of the main compounds in humans has been reviewed in such texts as that of Goodman and Gilman (1970) and in more specialized reviews by Findlay (1951) and Peters (1970a). It has also been

reviewed in the work of Black *et al.* (1979). The structural formu
pounds referred to in the text are shown in Fig. 26.

1. Quinine

When administered by mouth, quinine salts pass unchanged through the
stomach but are quickly and almost completely absorbed through the upper
intestinal tract and circulate as a base. Up to 5% of the drug rapidly appears in the
urine in the parent form, while quinine circulating in the tissues is rapidly
metabolized by the liver so that little remains in the body 48 hours after a single

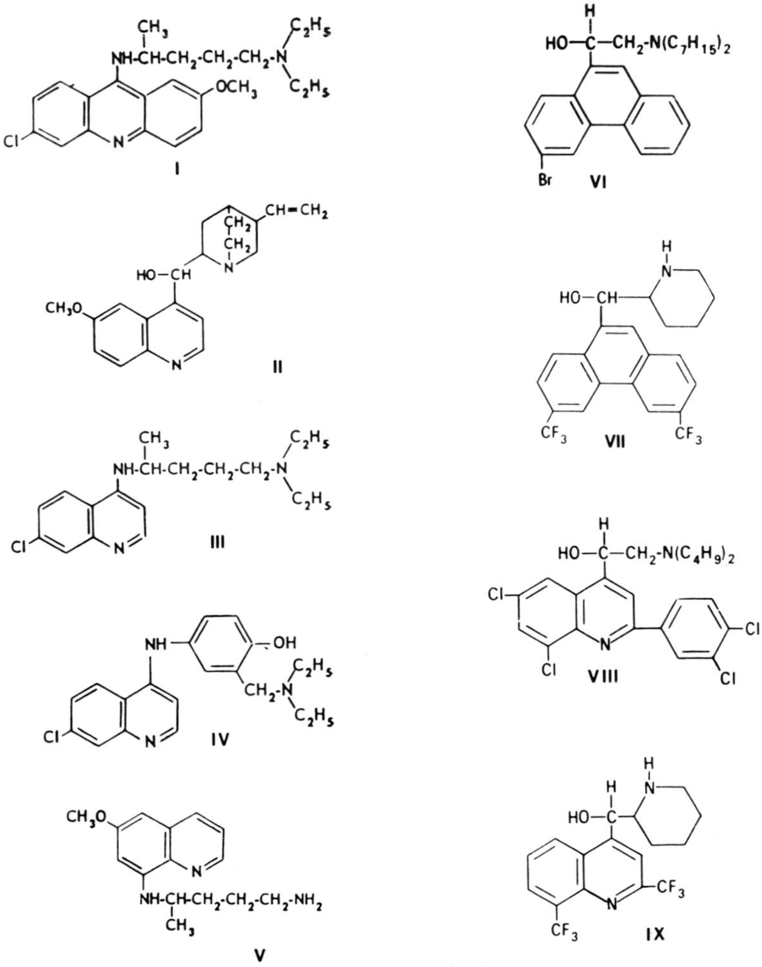

FIG. 26a. I, Mepacrine; II, quinine; III, chloroquine; IV, amodiaquin; V, primaquine; VI, WR 33063; VII, WR 122455; VIII, WR 30090; IX, mefloquine (WR 142490).

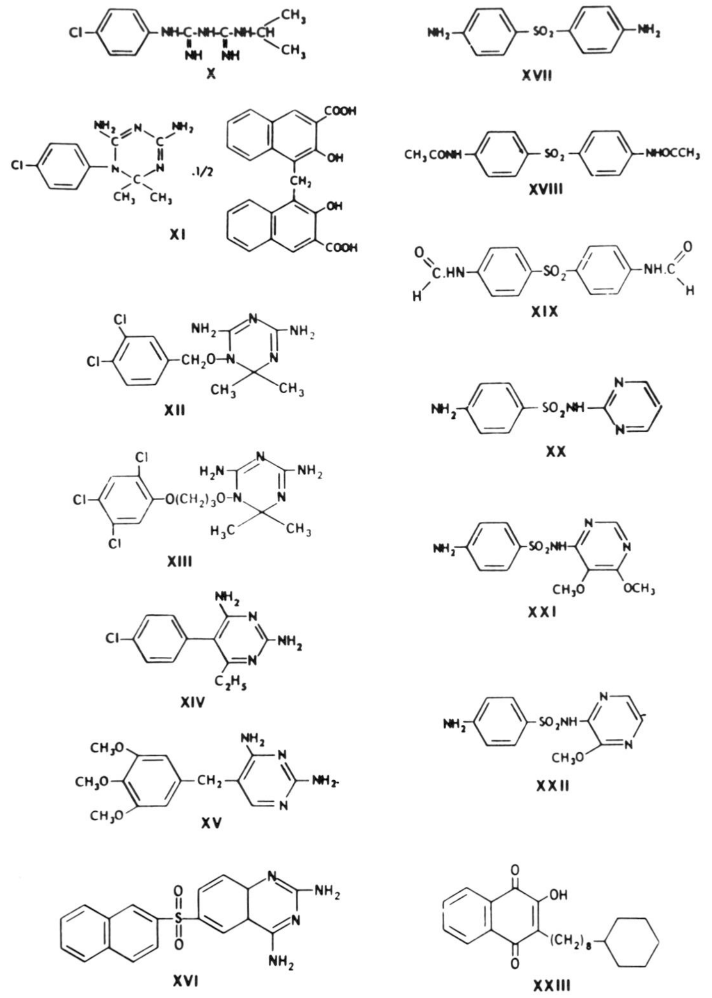

FIG. 26b.   X, Proguanil; XI, cycloguanil embonate; XII, clociguanil; XIII, WR 99210; XIV, pyrimethamine; XV, trimethoprim; XVI, WR 158122; XVII, dapsone; XVIII, acedapsone; XIX, diformyl dapsone; XX, sulfadiazine; XXI, sulfadoxine; XXII, sulfalene; XXIII, menoctone.

dose. In man a peak plasma concentration is reached within 1–3 hours after an oral dose, the half-life being on the order of 10 hours (Table XXIX). In the plasma the quinine is bound to plasma proteins.

A mean plasma level between 3 and 5 mg/liter is required to control parasitemia, but higher levels may be required in infections with some strains of *P. falciparum*. In man higher plasma levels are associated with toxic side effects that include giddiness, blurred vision, deafness, and ringing in the ears (cin-

TABLE XXIX

Approximate Biological Half-Lives of Some Antimalarials in Different Hosts[a]

Compound	Mouse, sc	Human, po
Chloroquine phosphate	~18 hours	120 hours
Mepacrine methanesulfonate		~100 hours
Quinine sulfate		5.7–10 hours
Primaquine phosphate		~4 hours
Mefloquine hydrochloride		2–3 weeks
Pyrimethamine		80 hours (35–175)
Trimethoprim	12–17 hours	9 hours
Cycloguanil pamoate	4–8 weeks	~18 weeks (im)
Sulfadiazine	11 hours	16.7 hours
Sulfalene		65 hours
Sulfadoxine	38 hours	120–200 hours
Dapsone		25 hours
Diformyl dapsone		30 hours
Diacetyl dapsone		~10 weeks (im)
Tetracycline		9 hours

[a] Data from various sources.

chonism). Intravenous injection may cause a sudden fall in blood pressure as a result of acute vasodilatation, and fatal collapse. Excessive oral dosage may cause temporary blindness or deafness which may occasionally leave a residual impairment of vision or hearing. An idiosyncrasy in man in regard to quinine which is rare is manifested by urticarial or erythematous rashes, pruritus, fever, gastric distress, and dyspnoea.

Quinine has a complex action on skeletal muscle, acting directly by increasing the tension response to single maximal stimuli but also increasing the refractory period by a curarelike action at the motor end plate. This is said by Guerra (1977b) to contribute to its rapid relief of the severe shivering that accompanies the cold stage of a malarial paroxysm.

2. Chloroquine

Chloroquine and similar 4-aminoquinolines are rapidly and almost completely absorbed from the gastrointestinal tract, following which they are localized in tissues where they become concentrated in cell lyososomes. Chloroquine shows a special affinity for melanin-containing tissues in which it is selectively concentrated. It is only slowly released from the binding sites to be metabolized and excreted. Chloroquine is also highly concentrated in malaria-infected erythrocytes and in leukocytes. Degradation of the side chain occurs to form secondary and primary amines. In man following daily administration of chloroquine about 10% is excreted in the feces and 60% in the urine where 60–70% of the material is probably parent compound, about 3% primary amine, and the rest secondary amine degradation products. An effective blood concentration is reached in man within 2–3 hours if a loading dose of 600 mg base is employed, followed 6 hours later by half that dose and another 300 mg base after another 6 hours. The therapeutically effective plasma concentration in man is on the order of 15–30 μg base/liter but is higher against infections with chloroquine-resistant species. Active and toxic dose levels of chloroquine and other antimalarials against rodent malaria are provided in Table XXX.

Like quinine, chloroquine has a complex pharmacological action, the most important from a clinical point of view being its antiinflammatory properties which are perhaps related to its ability to stabilize lysosomal membranes. Its influence on the function of prostaglandins has not been clarified. The second important action is a decrease in the conduction velocity of cardiac muscle, although this is less than that seen with quinidine. Intravenous administration or rapid absorption of a large intramuscular injection may be followed by acute hypotension and collapse, so that great caution should always be exercised in its use other than by the oral route, especially in infants and young children.

Secondary effects associated with the chronic administration of chloroquine are mainly associated with the skin. Pruritus, headache, nausea, and blurring of the vision may occur following therapeutic dosage, but malarial prophylactic dosage is usually well tolerated. Chronic administration of the high doses formerly used for the treatment of collagen diseases such as rheumatoid arthritis may lead to an accumulation of drug in various tissues of the eye, and severe retinitis, often irreversible, may occur even some time after chloroquine intake has ceased. Because of its fixation in the tissues, especially those containing melanin, chloroquine tends to accumulate, and it has been suggested that the cumulative dosage in man should not be allowed to exceed 100 g in any indication.

3. Primaquine

Primaquine in man is rapidly absorbed and rapidly excreted, peak plasma levels being achieved about 30–60 minutes following a single oral dose. The drug is probably rapidly metabolized, but its metabolites have not yet been identified and it is uncertain whether the drug functions directly or through one or more metabolites. It has a short half-life of about 4 hours, and very little drug is fixed in the tissues.

Two types of toxic side effects are exerted by primaquine. The first is related to the gastrointestinal tract, high doses causing anorexia, nausea, epigastric pain, and sometimes severe abdominal cramps. The second type of side effect is related to the genetic background of the individual. A congenital deficiency of the enzyme NADH-methemoglobin reductase leads to marked cyanosis following a dose of primaquine, or of other oxidant drugs such as sulfonamides and sulfones. Individuals with a hereditary glucose-6-phosphate dehydrogenase defi-

TABLE XXX

Blood Schizontocidal Levels of Antimalarials against *Plasmodium berghei* in the 4-Day Test in Mice, Compared with Their Toxicity[a,b]

Compound	Route	Activity [mg/kg/day ($\times$4)]			LD$_{50}$ ($\times$1)	Reference[c]
		ED$_{50}$	ED$_{90}$	MFTD ($\times$4)		
Chloroquine	sc	2.1	3.7	~100	150	
phosphate	po		2.8–4.6		250	(1)
Amodiaquin	sc	1.6	2.2	>100		
hydrochloride	po		3.1–3.4			(1) (2)
Mepacrine methane-	sc	4.2	5.5	>60	300	
sulfonate	po		4.3		500–800	(1)
Mepacrine						
hydrochloride						
Cycloquine	sc	0.4	0.5	>30		
phosphate						
Primaquine	sc	2.1	3.4	>60		
phosphate	po		1.5		130–169	(2)
WR 33063	sc	8.2	2.5	>600		
WR 122455	sc	4.6	9.4	>100		
	po	2.8	4.3	100		
WR 30090	sc	6.0	9.5	>300		
	po	2.1	2.7	>30		
Mefloquine	sc	4.6	9.4	>100		
hydrochloride	po	2.8	4.3	>100		
Pyrimethamine base	po	1.2–3.5			150–200	(1)
	ip	0.3	0.6	>60		
Proguanil	sc	>MFTD	>MFTD	~10	20 (im)	
hydrochloride	po		10–25		60–80	(3)
Cycloguanil	sc	3.5	8.5	~30		
hydrochloride	po		30–32			(2)
Sulfadiazine	sc	0.03	0.2	>100		
	po		2.6–9.6		>10,000	(1)
Sulfaphenazole	sc	1.2	2.8	>1000		
Sulfadoxine	sc	0.05	0.1	>>30	2,900	
Dapsone	sc	0.1	0.4	>10	430 (ip)	
	po		1.3			(2)
Diformyl dapsone	sc	0.2	0.7	~100		
Menoctone	sc	1.0	1.5	~100		

[a] Unpublished data of the writer except where otherwise stated.

[b] MFTD, maximum fully tolerated dose.

[c] Key to references: (1) Personal communication Dr. M. Heiffer, WRAIR. Dose b.d. $\times$ 3 days; (2) Thompson, various papers. Dose b.d. $\times$ 3 days; (3) Hill (1963) in Schnitzer and Hawking (1963).

ciency may develop an acute hemolytic episode following the administration of primaquine, and as many as 20% of the older circulating red cells may be destroyed, to be replaced following compensatory hematopoiesis.

4. Proguanil

Proguanil (also called chlorguanide in the United States) has relatively few nonspecific or adverse pharmacological effects, and its antimalarial action is accounted for by its rapid conversion to a dihydrotriazine derivative known as cycloguanil. Proguanil in humans is rapidly absorbed through the upper gastrointestinal tract and is eliminated relatively slowly, mainly in the urine and feces in which about 40% is lost as parent substance. The half-life of the dihydrotriazine metabolite, which is a powerful inhibitor of dihydrofolate reductase, is much shorter than that of proguanil itself. Its toxicity is very low, high doses sometimes causing anorexia, vomiting, or diarrhea. Rarely acute overdosage may cause hematuria. Unlike man, mice appear not to metabolize proguanil readily, so that the drug is comparatively ineffective as an antimalarial in rodents.

5. Pyrimethamine

Pyrimethamine is also a potent inhibitor of the enzyme dihydrofolate reductase, but it is an extremely efficient antimalarial since it displays a far greater affinity for the parasite enzyme than that of its mammalian host. Pyrimethamine is rather slowly absorbed from the intestinal tract and is then highly bound to proteins in the tissue fluids. This has the effect of greatly prolonging its biological activity, so that a single oral dose of as little as 25 or 50 mg in man may exert its antimalarial action for 1 week or more. After a single oral dose of 100 mg only 20–30% of the drug is excreted in the urine over the next 40 days. While clinical observations suggest that a mean plasma level of between 250 and 750 μg/liter is an effective blood level, *in vitro* studies show that as little as 10 μg/liter may be enough to stop development of the trophozoites of a drug-sensitive line of *P. falciparum* (see Table XX).

Excess dosage of pyrimethamine can in time lead to a deficiency of folic acid in the host which, in turn, results in a failure of hematopoiesis and megaloblastic anemia. This effect is readily countered by the administration of folinic acid. Gross overdose of pyrimethamine sometimes occurs in young children who inadvertently consume the almost tasteless white tablets. Acute poisoning is manifested by central nervous system toxicity including convulsions.

Pyrimethamine displays a marked potentiating effect (Fig. 27) when given with an appropriate sulfonamide or sulfone, because the two compounds act by blocking sequential steps in the pathways leading to the *de novo* synthesis of purines and pyrimidines by the plasmodia.

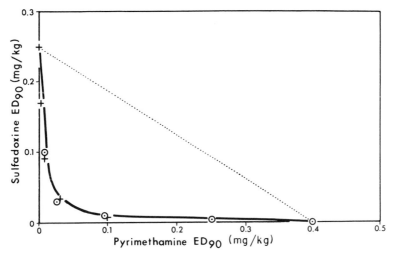

FIG. 27. Potentiation of suppressive action against *P. berghei* erythrocytic infection in mice. Ordinates and abcissae show the daily doses given for 4 days (D0 to D+3). The figures are plotted from data in Table XXXII to show the ED_{50} or ED_{90} of the sulfonamide when given alone or with different doses of pyrimethamine (+) or of the latter when given with different doses of the sulfonamide (⊙). A simple additive effect would be present if the points fell on the dotted lines joining the respective ED values for the individual compounds. Points below this line indicate potentiation of activity, and points above indicate drug antagonism (Peters, 1968b).

B. Molecular Pharmacology

1. Structural Changes

As noted in Section I, the discoverer of the malaria parasite, Laveran (1893), was himself the first to observe under the light microscope the morphological changes induced in the intraerythrocytic plasmodia by quinine. Since that time many such observations have been made, not only with quinine but with each successive new antimalarial as it appeared. Among others, Black (1946) was prominent in drawing attention to the morphological changes brought about by the contact of various antimalarials with *P. falciparum in vitro,* and Thurston (1951, 1953) described their action on blood stages of *P. berghei* in mice. Other references are listed by Ladda (1966). Antimalarials may be roughly grouped according to these simple observations:

Group 1   Clumping of malaria pigment (hemozoin) rapid and very marked at normal treatment doses *in vivo* or therapeutic concentrations *in vitro*. All asexual stages affected. Mepacrine, chloroquine, and other 4-aminoquinolines.

Group 2   Clumping less coarse, developing more slowly, and associated
              with generalized evidence of cell death (pycnosis and fragmen-
              tation of nuclei, vacuolization of cytoplasm, etc.). All stages
              affected except mature *P. falciparum* gametocytes. Quinine,
              mefloquine, WR 122455, primaquine (and other 8-amino-
              quinolines).

Group 3   Blockage of asexual cycle during schizogony leading to the
              production of uniformly large asexual parasites within 24–72
              hours (depending on the duration of the cycle in the particular
              species). Subsequent disintegration of parasites. Proguanil,
              pyrimethamine, sulfones, and sulfonamides.

Beaudoin *et al.* (1969) described two classes of drug-induced morphological
effects on exoerythrocytic schizonts of *P. fallax* growing in tissue culture. These
were (1) vacuolization of parasite cytoplasm (8-aminoquinolines, menoctone,
RC12); and (2) initial staining changes in the nucleus and pycnosis, followed by
the degeneration of cytoplasm; younger parasites were not seen (possibly because
of blockage of schizogony) (pyrimethamine).

With the advent of electron microscopy the effects of drugs on the ultrastructure of parasites could be investigated. One of the first reports was that of Ladda
(1966), but some of his observations were possibly misleading because of the
unphysiological conditions employed. Subsequently Macomber *et al.* (1967) and
Warhurst and Hockley (1967) demonstrated that the primary lesion induced by
chloroquine in *P. berghei* and *P. cynomolgi* was the aggregation of hemozoin
into a cytolysosome, which corresponded with the coarse pigment clumping
observed at the light microscope level (Fig. 28). Similar changes follow exposure
of the parasites to other 4-aminoquinolines and to mepacrine.

The action of quinine on *P. berghei* was described by Davies *et al.* (1975).
They observed swelling and vesiculation of the outer parasite membranes, a
decrease in electron density of the granules of hemozoin, and a swelling of the
vesicles within which they were situated. Blebbing of the nuclear membrane was
also observed. Similar changes followed exposure of the parasites *in vivo* to the
phenanthrenemethanol compound WR 122455 (Davies *et al.*, 1975) and to mefloquine (Fig. 29) (Peters *et al.*, 1977a). Porter and Peters (1976) also remarked
on the coarsening of the hemozoin induced by WR 122455 as seen with the light
microscope. This is associated with the forming of hemozoin granules into
groups of two or three in each vesicle, but not with the type of cytolysosome
formation brought about by chloroquine.

Primaquine and menoctone primarily affect the mitochondria-like organelles
of *P. berghei* trophozoites (Howells *et al.*, 1970). Numerous membranous
whorls appear in the cytoplasm, and it is suggested that they may play a role in
overcoming the damage to the mitochondrial enzyme system. Similar endoplas-

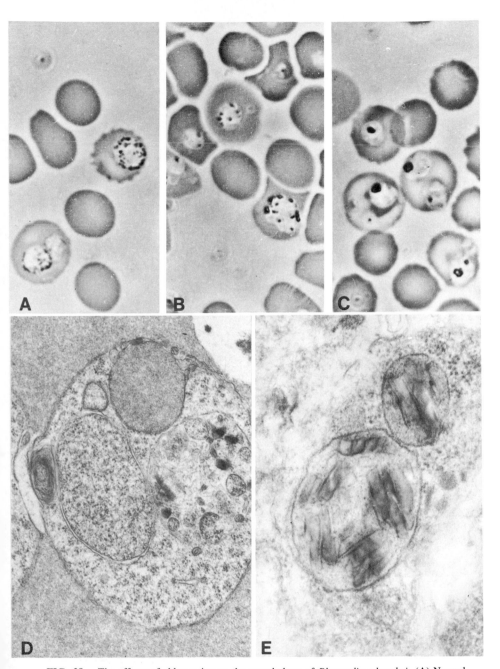

FIG. 28. The effects of chloroquine on the morphology of *Plasmodium berghei*. (A) Normal trophozoites with scattered pigment grains. ×2000. (B) Trophozoites showing fine clumping of pigment 20 minutes after exposure to chloroquine. ×2000. (C) Trophozoites showing coarse clumping of pigment 80 minutes after exposure to chloroquine. ×2000. (D) Chloroquine-induced autophagosome (coarse pigment clumps) in a trophozite of *P. berghei*. ×38,000. (E) Pigment clumps in the residual body of a schizont of normal, untreated *P. berghei*. ×60,000.

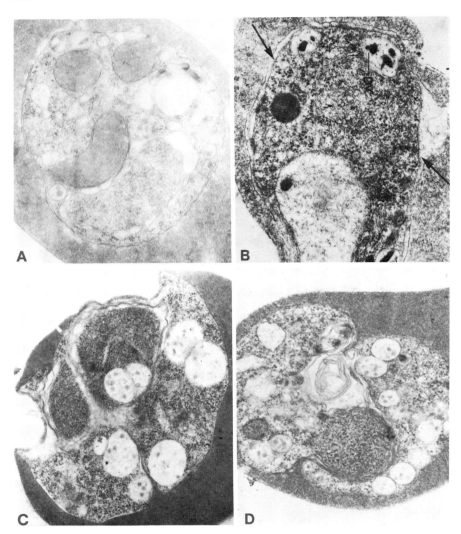

FIG. 29. *Plasmodium berghei* trophozoites following exposure to mefloquine, quinine, and WR 122455. (A) Trophozoite following exposure to mefloquine for 9 hours. ×25,000. (B) Trophozoite following exposure to quinine for 24 hours. ×45,000. (C and D) Trophozoite following exposure to WR 122455 for 24 hours. ×25,000.

mic reticular changes were reported earlier by Ladda (1966). Beaudoin and Aikawa (1968) also recorded damage to mitochondria in the exoerythrocytic stages of *P. fallax* in tissue culture under the influence of primaquine (Fig. 30).

Aikawa and Beaudoin (1968) demonstrated that pyrimethamine interrupted nuclear division of *P. gallinaceum* at metaphase. A similar effect on the

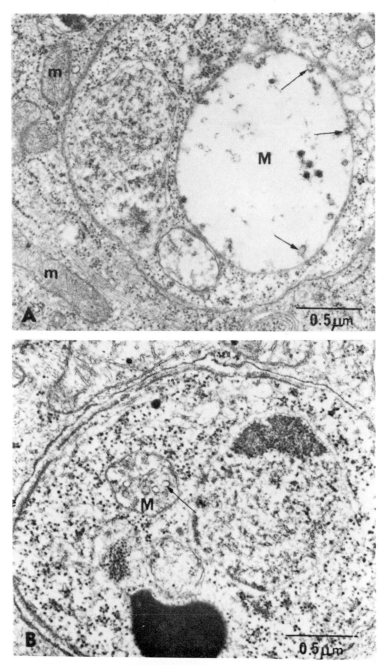

FIG. 30. (A) Action of primaquine on *P. fallax* exoerythrocytic parasites in tissue culture. A trophozoite 48 hours after exposure to primaquine. A swollen mitochondrion (M) with its cristae (arrows) is noticeable; the mitochondria (m) of the host cell appear to be unaffected. (B) An exoerythrocytic trophozoite from a control culture; note a mitochondrion (M) with the microrubular type of crista (arrow) (Beaudoin and Aikawa, 1968, Copyright American Association for the Advancement of Science).

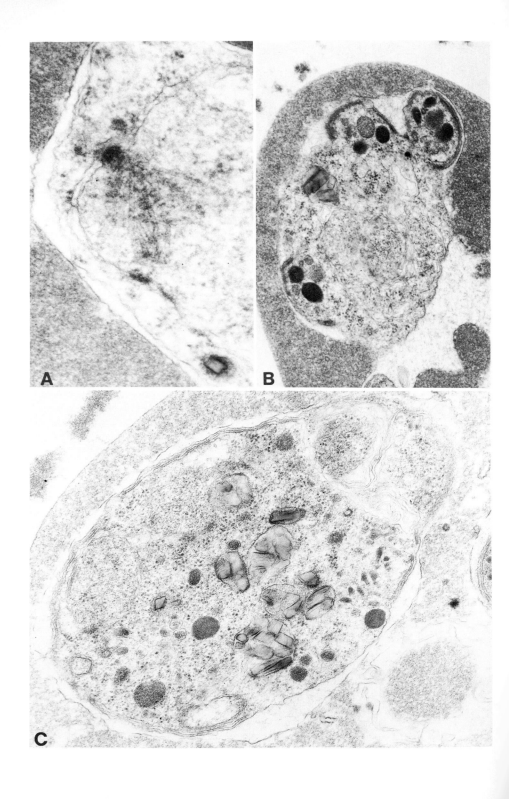

schizogony of *P. berghei* has been found by Peters (1974a) (Fig. 31) in oocysts of *P. yoelii nigeriensis*.

2. Biochemical Effects

a. Chloroquine-Induced Pigment Clumping. The observation of structural changes induced by drugs gives only an indication of the possible manner in which they act at the molecular level. Biochemical techniques must be employed to follow up these indications. One of the first logical experiments to identify the significance of the pigment clump formed under the influence of chloroquine was described by Warhurst and Williamson (1970) who were able to demonstrate that the phenomenon was associated with a breakdown of parasite RNA into smaller fragments. However, the most valuable offshoot from the observations on chloroquine-induced hemozoin clumping was the evolution by Warhurst and his colleagues of a technique whereby this phenomenon could be exploited to probe the nature of the biochemical reactions of the malaria parasite within its host erythrocyte, and the influence of various biochemical and chemotherapeutic factors on these reactions either *in vivo* or *in vitro*. Warhurst (1973) quite correctly described chloroquine-induced pigment clumping (CIPC) as a valuable experimental tool. The procedure for examining the influence of other compounds on CIPC *in vitro* is as follows (Warhurst *et al.*, 1974).

i. Culture Medium and Incubation. To 10 ml of culture medium 199 diluted to 100 ml with distilled water are added 0.2 glucose, 0.148 g sodium bicarbonate, 1 ml 200 m*M* glutamine, and 11 ml fetal bovine serum (membrane filter-sterilized). The mixture, after equilibration at 37 °C for 30 minutes with a 95% air–5% carbon dioxide mixture (the pH should be 7.4), is distributed in quantities of 3.9 ml into 10 × 1 cm acid-washed neutral glass test tubes fitted with silicone rubber stoppers. These are further gassed and equilibriated at 37 °C for 15 minutes.

Blood is removed in a heparinized syringe from an infected mouse anesthetized with ether, by axillary puncture, and 0.04 ml is added to each culture tube. The tubes are then mechanically rotated at 12 rph at 37°C. The maintenance of this temperature is essential, pigment clumping being inhibited at higher temperatures. It is not essential to maintain absolute sterility, since the cultures are incubated for no more than 1–2 hours.

ii. Chloroquine-Induced Clumping. The blood–culture medium mixtures are equilibrated for a further 10 minutes. Chloroquine phosphate is then added in

---

FIG. 31. *Plasmodium yoelii nigeriensis* erythrocytic forms 24 hours after treatment with pyrimethamine (5 mg/kg intraperitoneally). (A) Arrested nuclear divisions in preschizont showing spindle figure. ×80,000. (B) Arrested schizont showing some degree of merozoite differentiation. ×40,000. (C) Arrested preschizont. ×50,000 (from Peters and Howells, 1978).

0.1 ml of 0.85% sodium chloride (w/v) at a concentration 40 times that of the desired final concentration. Saline is added to the control tubes, and then all the tubes are mixed by inversion and replaced on the roller apparatus. Duplicate or triplicate series are run for each test. The drug is allowed to act for 80 minutes. When the influence of other compounds or conditions on CIPC is to be examined, a final concentration of 10^{-6} M chloroquine is normally used. The agents are made up in the desired concentrations in saline and, like the chloroquine itself, added to the cultures in 0.1 ml at 40 times the required final concentration. An additional 0.1 ml saline is added to the controls. The other compounds can be added at a standard 15 minutes before the chloroquine if a dose–response curve is being worked out or, in time course studies, from 30 minutes before to 70 minutes after adding the chloroquine. After the chloroquine is added the mixtures in all the tubes, including the controls and those without chloroquine, are incubated for a further 80 minutes.

   iii. Preparation of Blood Films and Interpretation.   When incubation has been completed, the contents of the tubes are centrifuged at 700 g for 5 minutes. The supernatant is poured off, and the tubes are briefly inverted over filter paper to drain off any remaining supernatant. A drop of fetal bovine serum is then added to resuspend the pellet, and thin blood smears are prepared in the usual manner from the suspension. The unfixed, unstained blood smears are examined under an oil immersion lens using a green filter. Pigmented parasites in the red cells are counted and classified into those containing fine, granular, or coarse pigment as shown in Fig. 32. "Fine" pigment is usually seen as 20–50 grains per parasite, "granular" as about 6–24, and "clumped" as 1–4. A minimum of 50 pigmented parasites are counted on each blood film, and the percentage of the three different types of pigment is recorded.

   The percentage of clumping in cultures treated with chloroquine is calculated by subtracting the percentage in the saline controls from that in the chloroquine-treated tubes. This value is compared with the percentage in tubes treated with both chloroquine and other compounds to obtain the percentage inhibition caused by the other drugs, using the following formula:

$$\text{Percent inhibition} = 100 - \frac{\text{Percent clumped with drug plus chloroquine}}{\text{Percent clumped with chloroquine alone}} \times 100$$

   Some drugs themselves cause pigment clumping. Values less than 10% above control values are not considered significant.

   The time course of CIPC with chloroquine alone is illustrated in Fig. 33 which shows that clumping of the malaria pigment was complete within 60–80 minutes at a chloroquine concentration of 10^{-6} M.

   Using this technique Warhurst (1973) and co-workers have shown that a

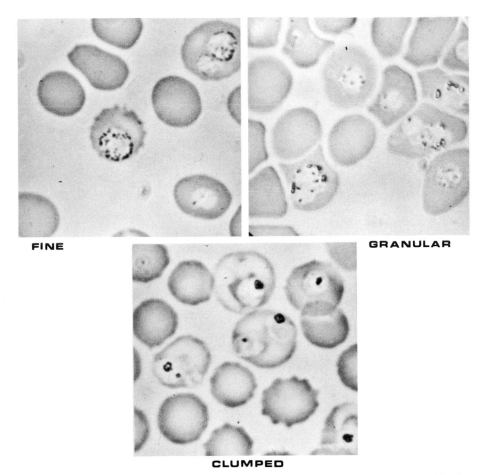

FINE   **GRANULAR**

CLUMPED

FIG. 32. Drawings of infected erythrocytes from unfixed, unstained thin films of mouse blood after incubation in 199 medium. The distinction between fine, granular, and clumped pigment is illustrated (Warhurst *et al.*, 1974).

variety of cytotoxic agents inhibit CIPC and have concluded that the autophagic vacuole formed during this process requires active cellular synthesis and a functional glycolytic cycle. They have also postulated from their observations that chloroquine binds to the parasite–host cell complex at three different sites. One of these appears similar to the "high-affinity binding site" described by Fitch (1969), 50% clumping being produced by a concentration of 4.5×10^{-8} M. CIPC is inhibited by a concentration of 10^{-5} M chloroquine or above, which Warhurst *et al.* (1972) believe may relate to the second binding site described by Fitch. A third type of site appears to be associated with the red cell itself and only comes into operation at a concentration of 10^{-3} M or above. Chloroquine-

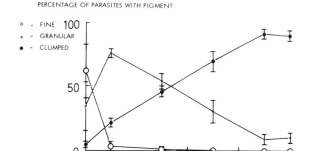

PERCENTAGE OF PARASITES WITH PIGMENT

o - FINE
. - GRANULAR
• - CLUMPED

TIME (MINUTES) FROM EXPOSURE TO CHLOROQUINE

FIG. 33. Ordinate: Percentage of infected erythrocytes showing fine, granular, or clumped pigment after incubation for varying periods in 10^{-6} M chloroquine. Abscissa: Time in minutes during which chloroquine was allowed to act. Two experiments; $n = 4$. Standard deviation of mean indicated (Warhurst *et al.*, 1974).

resistant *Plasmodium* is now known to be associated with a fall in the binding capacity of the high-affinity binding sites. The precise location of the various chloroquine-binding sites is still a moot question.

A variety of antimalarial drugs which, like chloroquine, can be doubly protonated at physiological pH also induce hemozoin clumping (e.g., amodiaquine and mepacrine), but quinine and quininelike compounds such as mefloquine and WR 122455 do not have this property. Warhurst and Thomas (1957b), however, have demonstrated that they are competitive inhibitors with chloroquine in the CIPC test. Mefloquine was the most active of the series studied, being about 100 times more effective than quinine (Fig. 34).

Homewood *et al.* (1972b) utilized the CIPC technique to explore the various factors concerned with electron transport in *P. berghei* (see Section III, B, 2) while Peters *et al.* (1975a) classified a wide variety of potential blood schizontocides as being "chloroquinelike" or "quininelike" in their mode of action, depending upon whether they caused clumping themselves or inhibited CIPC. Those that were clearly chloroquinelike generally exhibited cross-resistance against chloroquine-resistant strains of *P. berghei*. Those that were quininelike were usually active against such strains, as are, for example, quinine and mefloquine.

Einheber *et al.* (1976), who confirmed Warhurst's observations on the inhibition of CIPC by quinine, mefloquine, and antimalarials of this general type *in vivo*, went a stage further and showed that CIPC that had already taken place *could be reversed* by such compounds. The clumped pigment appeared to disaggregate and break up again into individual granules of hemozoin in individual vesicles. The reversal commenced within 30–80 minutes of administering the

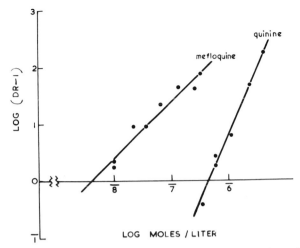

FIG. 34. Graph showing relationship between concentration of mefloquine and quinine and log of expression (DR−1). DR represents the dose ratio, i.e., the factor by which the concentration of chloroquine must be raised when mefloquine or quinine is used as a competitive antagonist in the *in vitro P. berghei* clumping test (based on data from Warhurst and Thomas, 1975a). Note the straight-line relationships in this figure (Peters *et al.*, 1977a).

inhibitor which was given, in each case, 80 minutes after the chloroquine (i.e., at a time when the CIPC was complete). Electron microscopy suggested that the individual hemozoin-containing vesicles were formed by a pinching off from the main aggregation. The effectiveness of the compounds in reversing CIPC was, strangely, unrelated to their inherent efficacy as antimalarial agents. These workers have suggested that this property could be of practical value in demonstrating that such compounds, administered orally, have been absorbed, i.e., as an indicator of the bioavailability of a preparation.

b. DNA Binding. The interaction of a compound with DNA is readily demonstrated by examining the ultraviolet spectrum of the compound alone and after allowing it to interact with DNA extracted from an appropriate organism. The techniques employed are quite standard and do not need to be detailed here. A number of workers have demonstrated that 4-aminoquinolines such as chloroquine, mepacrine, and quinine intercalate with DNA and have argued that this is the way such compounds exert their antimalarial action (see, e.g., Hahn *et al.*, 1966). There is no question that many compounds with this type of structure do bind with DNA extracted from a variety of sources including species of *Plasmodium*. However, morphological and biochemical observations, some of which have been referred to above and which are reviewed at length by Peters (1970a), make it unlikely that the interaction of such drugs with parasite DNA is

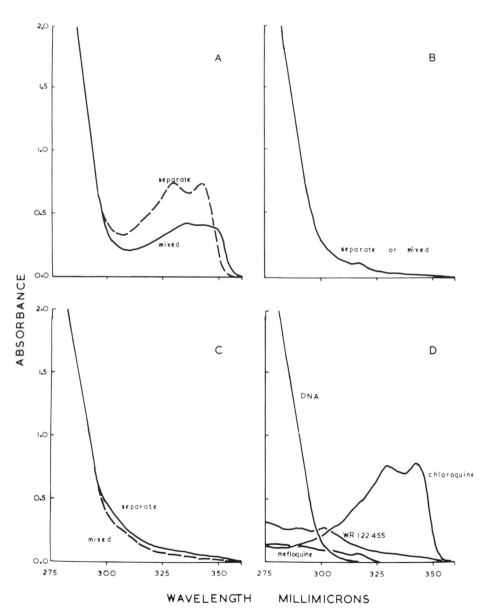

FIG. 35. The ultraviolet spectra of DNA alone and in the presence of antimalarial drugs. The DNA is sigma *Escherichia coli* DNA. Baseline adjusted between readings. Reactions carried out in $0.01\ M$ phosphate buffer at pH 7.4. (A) Interaction of $1.7 \times 10^{-5}\ M$ chloroquine phosphate with $2.2\ M$ DNA phosphate. "Separate" indicates spectrum produced by 2.4 ml of $3.3 \times g\ 10^{-4}\ M$ DNA phosphate in a 3-cm cell plus 1.2 ml of $5 \times 10^{-5}\ M$ chloroquine in a 1-cm cell. "Mixed" indicates spectrum produced after mixing the DNA and the chloroquine in the same cells. (B) Lack

anything but a terminal event in the life of the intracellular organism. One of the most potent 4-quinolinemethanols, mefloquine, has been shown by Davidson *et al.* (1975) and Peters *et al.* (1977a), unlike quinine, chloroquine, and the phenanthrenemethanol WR 122455, not to intercalate with DNA (Fig. 35).

c. Interaction with Other Parasite or Host Structures. From their recent investigations of the influence of various metabolic inhibitors on CIPC, Warhurst and Thomas (1978) have concluded that chloroquine, after being concentrated in the cytoplasm of malaria parasites at the high-affinity binding site, is transferred to or interacts with a mitochondrial site, and that this initiates the pigment-clumping process. They also have confirmed an earlier suggestion by Homewood *et al.* (1972a) that a pH gradient is involved in the entry of chloroquine into the parasite–red cell complex. This suggestion is complementary to other recent observations by the same authors on mepacrine which otherwise appears to function in much the same way as chloroquine. Warhurst and Thomas (1975a) have found that the fluorescence of mepacrine appears initially in the region of the paired organelles (rhoptries) of the merozoites of *P. berghei* and *P. falciparum* when parasitized blood is exposed to the drug *in vitro* and examined under ultraviolet light. Later fluorescence appears at the host–parasite interface but never in association with the host membranes [this contrasts with the suggestion of Fitch *et al.* (1974) that the red cell membrane is an important antimalarial binding site]. The interest of the mepacrine observations lies in their possible significance in the light of recent reports that the rhoptries contain a specialized histidine-rich protein (Kilejian and Jensen, 1977) and that they may be involved in the process by which merozoites invade new host erythrocytes (Miller, 1977). Both chloroquine and mepacrine have a complex mode of action. While both are capable of acting against developing trophozoites and young gametocytes [e.g., gametocytes up to the sixth day of development in *P. falciparum* (Smalley and Sinden, 1977)], they have been thought to have no effect on mature schizonts or mature gametocytes. From these new observations it appears quite possible that these compounds have yet a further point of action, namely, in interfering with the invasion of new host cells by the merozoites. This speculation, however, remains to be confirmed.

---

of interaction between $1.7 \times 10^{-5} M$ mefloquine with $1.5 \times 10^{-4} M$ DNA phosphate. Spectrum produced by a mixture of the drug and DNA in the same cells and spectrum produced by 2.4 ml of $2.3 \times 10^{-4} M$ DNA phosphate in a 2-cm cell plus 1.2 ml of $5 \times 10^{-5} M$ mefloquine in a 1-cm cell. Note that the two curves superimpose, indicating that there is no interaction. (C) Interaction of $1.7 \times 10^{-5} M$ WR 122455 with $1.5 \times 10^{-4} M$ DNA. "Separate" indicates spectrum produced by 2.4 ml $2.3 \times 10^{-4} M$ DNA phosphate in a 1-cm cell. "Mixed" indicates spectrum produced after mixing the DNA and WR 122455 in the same cells. WR 122455 was dissolved first in ethyl alcohol; the final concentration of alcohol was 1%. (D) Ultraviolet spectra of chloroquine, mefloquine, WR 122455, and DNA alone. Drugs were $5 \times 10^{-5} M$ in a 1-cm cell, DNA phosphate $2.3 \times 10^{-4} M$ in a 2-cm cell (Peters *et al.*, 1977a).

The mature schizont is released from its host cell when the latter undergoes lysis, a process that is apparently facilitated (or even precipitated) by the accumulation within the parasitized erythrocytes of octadecanoic fatty acids. Laser (1946) showed that certain antimalarial drugs could delay the hemolysis caused by such lipids in red cells *in vitro*. It is now evident, however, that the hemolytic action of oleic acid is normally inhibited by the buffering action of various proteins including the red cell's hemoglobin. Laser *et al.* (1975) have recently suggested that certain antimalarials including quinine exert their antimalarial action by preventing the buffering action of proteins in the red cells, thus permitting an accumulation of haemolytic fatty acids which causes premature lysis of the parasitized cells and release of immature schizonts, hence interruption of their growth. It must be noted, however, that the drug concentrations used in their experiments were significantly higher than those encountered in practice, and it is questionable whether a quinine–fatty acid complex formation forms an important component of this drug's antimalarial activity.

d. Inhibition of Metabolic Pathways.   The *in vitro* techniques for demonstrating the influence of drugs on various metabolic pathways are those of classic enzymology and do not need to be given here in detail. To some degree such actions can be shown also *in vivo* by employing judicious mixtures of potential antimetabolic agents and the metabolites with which they are believed to interfere. This was best demonstrated in the case of *P. berghei* and the influence of a milk diet deficient in *p*-aminobenzoic acid (PABA), an essential metabolite for *Plasmodium* (Maegraith *et al.*, 1952). The influence of different supplements of PABA on *P. berghei* developing in mice maintained on a milk diet was clearly demonstrated by Kretschmar (1965) among others.

The specific inhibitors of PABA utilization in bacteria and *Plasmodium* are sulfonamides. These can readily be shown to compete directly with PABA in mice infected with *P. berghei,* and indeed the level of response of such an infection to a given sulfonamide can be taken as a "bioassay" of the level of PABA in the animal's diet.

Inhibitors of plasmodial dihydrofolate reductase such as pyrimethamine also can be, in turn, antagonized by the administration of dihydrofolate to the infected animals. Ferone (1970) has shown that, *in vitro,* this reaction is basically competitive provided that the drug, enzyme, and substrate are incubated together (Table XXXI). If the drug and enzyme are incubated alone and dihydrofolate then added, a noncompetitive double reciprocal plot is obtained. It is common practice in fact to carry out this latter procedure when testing for drug and metabolite antagonism, and the conclusions may thus be misleading.

One of the more interesting reports on metabolic inhibitors to appear in recent years was that of Wan *et al.* (1974) who described a series of 5,8-quinolinequinones designed specifically as antagonists of coenzyme Q_8.

TABLE XXXI

Inhibition of Dihydrofolate Reductases by Pyrimethamine and Trimethoprim[a]

Drug	Concentration for 50% inhibition of different enzymes $(\times 10^{-8}\ M)$[b]			
	Rat liver	Mouse erythrocyte	E. coli	P. berghei
Pyrimethamine	70	100	250	0.05
Cycloguanil	nd	160	nd	0.36
Trimethoprim	26,000	100,000	0.5	7

[a] After Ferone et al. (1969).
[b] nd, Not done.

Ubiquinone-8 has been found in *P. lophurae, P. knowlesi, P. cynomolgi,* and *P. berghei,* and it seems likely that it is common to all *Plasmodium* species. It does not occur in mammals which, instead, utilize ubiquinone-10. Thus synthetic analogs of ubiquinone-8 might be expected to be selectively toxic to the parasites, and this hypothesis seems to be borne out by the data of Wan *et al.* (1974). They have not, however, reported whether the antimalarial action of the potent 5,8-quinolinequinones they describe can be antagonized (competitively or otherwise) by ubiquinone-8. Surprisingly, no reports have appeared on the further development of this very interesting series of antimalarial agents.

When two enzyme inhibitors function sequentially at different points on the

TABLE XXXII

Activity of Sulfadoxine and Pyrimethamine, Alone and in Combination, with Erythrocyte Infection Rate as Percentage of Controls on D+4.[a]

Sulfadoxine, as base (mg/kg)	Pyrimethamine, as base (mg/kg)						
	0	0.003	0.01	0.03	0.10	ED_{50}	ED_{90}
0	100	87.5	63.7	58.8	28.2	0.03	0.40
0.003	90.0	62.7	59.7	65.8	22.6	0.02	0.25
0.01	91.8	70.0	74.0	45.7	6.0	0.025	0.095
0.03	62.6	24.4	41.0	29.8	0.19	0.008	0.025
0.10	30.8	16.5	6.1	0.9	0	0.0015	0.007
ED_{50}	0.04	0.015	0.019	0.008	0.0014		
ED_{90}	0.25	0.17	0.09	0.035	0.006		

[a] Mean control infection 11.8 ± 1.1%. Peters (1968b).

same metabolic pathway, a potentiating effect can usually be demonstrated. Such an effect is readily seen when a sulfonamide is administered *in vivo* in association with a dihydrofolate reductase inhibitor such as pyrimethamine. Peters (1968b) has shown *in vivo* that pyrimethamine and sulfadoxine (sulformethoxine) potentiate each other's effect against *P. berghei* in mice very markedly, while Ramkaran and Peters (1969b) have observed the same effect against *P. berghei* developing in *A. stephensi*. Using their *in vitro* technique in which the uptake of [^{14}C]orotic acid into DNA was measured in *P. knowlesi* exposed to the drugs, McCormick and Canfield (1972) observed a similar strong potentiation in trimethoprim and sulfalene. In all these experiments the data obtained for the various drug combinations were plotted as bolograms which indicate whether two drugs in combination display a synergistic action, an additive effect, or antagonize each other. The examples in Table XXXII and Fig. 27 show how the data are analyzed and graphed.

V. EXPERIMENTAL DRUG RESISTANCE

A. Techniques for the Experimental Induction of Drug Resistance

A wide variety of procedures have been used to develop lines of *Plasmodium* with resistance to antimalarial drugs. Both animal and *in vitro* models have been employed, and in the former diverse methods have been used to reduce host immunity, hence improve the chances of survival of very low numbers of parasites. Peters, 1970a classified the diverse procedures as given in Table XXXIII.

In practice two of these approaches are most commonly used, namely, the application of slowly increasing drug selection pressure on parasites in successive animal passages, and single applications of large drug doses, with passage of relapsing infections. The outcome of the two procedures using a single drug against a given parasite may differ considerably, presumably because a variety of different mechanisms may be called into play to enable the organisms to survive the drug's action. In the following pages some examples will be given of these two basic procedures in different *Plasmodium* species.

1. Progressively Increased Drug Dosage

This technique is widely used to produce lines of rodent malaria parasites resistant to different antimalarial drugs. In the form described by Peters (1965a), who used it to produce lines of *P. berghei* resistant to chloroquine, to cycloguanil, and to primaquine, the steps are as follows.

Mice are infected with the appropriate parasite, e.g., *P. berghei,* on D0, using intraperitoneal inocula of approximately 10^7 infected donor erythrocytes. The

TABLE XXXIII

Classification of Techniques for Inducing Drug Resistance[a]

1. *In vitro* (not yet applicable)
2. Semi-*in vitro* (not yet reported; could be used with or without the aid of a mutagenic agent)
3. Tissue culture (not yet reported in *Plasmodium* but used successfully to produce pyrimethamine resistance in *Toxoplasma gondii* by Cook, 1958)
4. *In vivo*
    4.1. Serial passage
        4.1.1. Single treatment (or course of treatment) per passage
            i. Constant dose
                a. Intermittent exposure (in alternate passages)
                b. Constant exposure (e.g., drug–diet method)
            ii. Low dosage increased progressively (favors adaptation)
            iii. High dosage
                a. Rapid passage (favors selection of mutants)
                b. Passage in relapse (favors selection of mutants)
        4.1.2. Multiple treatment (or course) in each passage
            i. High infection rate
                a. Low dosage increased progressively at each relapse
                b. High doses, passage in relapse (favors selection of mutants)
            ii. Low infection rate (latent infections)
                a. Low dosage increased progressively (unfavorable to production of resistance)
                b. Constant dose (unfavorable to production of resistance)
    4.2. Single treatment
    4.3. Hybridization
        4.3.1. In vertebrate host (Yoeli *et al.,* 1969)
        4.3.2. In invertebrate host (Greenberg and Trembley, 1954; Greenberg, 1956)
5. Indirect methods
    5.1. Withhold essential metabolites (Ramakrishnan *et al.,* 1956)
    5.2. Produce resistance to other compounds working on same metabolic pathways or by similar mechanisms of action.

[a] Peters (1970a).

animals receive four consecutive daily doses of drug on D0, D+1, D+2, and D+3, starting with a dose level shown by trial and error to permit parasitemia to build up in treated animals to approximately 1% by D+6 (i.e., 1 week later). Three parallel groups of five animals per group are used for each weekly passage. One group receives this dose, one a higher dose, and one no drug at all. With successive passages it will usually be found that the parasites can tolerate an increasingly high dose, so that the dose can be increased progressively, usually maintaining one group on the highest tolerated dose and exposing the second treated group to the tentatively increased level. At each passage the three groups of mice (including those that are to remain untreated in the passage) are infected with parasites that have survived the highest dose level. The untreated group is

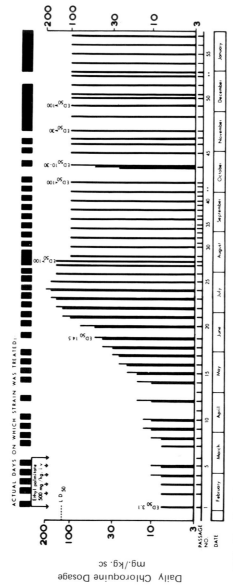

FIG. 36. Evolution of chloroquine-resistant (RC) strain of *P. berghei* in the albino mouse. Note the logarithmic dosage scale; **indicates two passages from the same donor (i.e., passages 42 and 53 each were duplicated) (Peters, 1965a).

kept as a reserve in case no parasites survive in either treated group, as sometimes happens if the doses are increased too rapidly. In the latter case it may be necessarily actually to reduce the dosage for a passage or two, or at least to hold it constant. Figure 36 shows the rate at which the chloroquine-resistant RC strain of *P. berghei* was built up in this manner. It should be noted that the drug-resistant lines of *Plasmodium* established may be less virulent than the parent organisms, and allowance may have to be made for this. The resultant drug resistance may prove to be more or less stable if the parasites are subsequently passaged in the absence of drug selection pressure. However, this may be also a function of time, the line stabilizing with continual drug pressure in later passages.

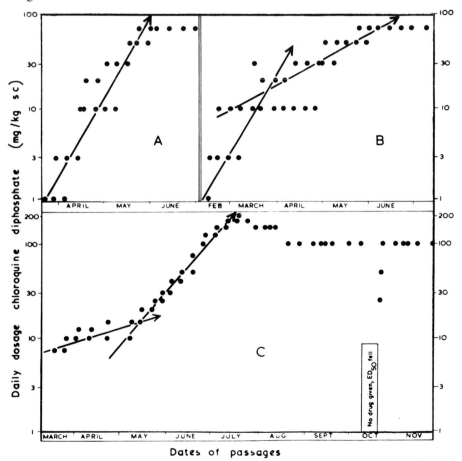

FIG. 37. The acquisition of chloroquine resistance in *P. berghei* as reflected by the dosage given in succeeding passages. (A) NK65 strain, line 41A. (B) NK65 strain, line 41. (C) Old laboratory strain N, RC line (Peters, 1968a).

The rate at which a drug-resistant line develops may be monitored either by plotting the maximum dose levels the parasites can tolerate in succeeding passages (as in Fig. 37) or by carrying out a standard 4-day test on material from the drug-treated line and comparing the ED_{50} and ED_{90} with those of the original parent material.

This technique may also be used to compare the rates at which resistance develops to single drugs used alone with the rates at which it develops to the compounds in a fixed or variable combination. Thus it was shown that the simultaneous administration of chloroquine and pyrimethamine had no influence on the rate at which resistance developed to the pyrimethamine component, whereas a mixture of chloroquine and sulfaphenazole considerably slowed down the rate at which resistance developed to the sulfonamide (Fig. 38). It should be noted that in these experiments the chloroquine dosage could not be raised very much without endangering the survival of the resistant lines. Resistance to chloroquine alone developed rapidly in a parallel group of animals infected with the same parent *P. berghei* line.

In contrast to these experiments, studies with a fixed combination of sulfadoxine and pyrimethamine in a 3:1 ratio showed that the use of this potentiating combination slowed down the emergence of resistance to the individual components very considerably (Peters, 1957b).

2. Relapse Technique

The second widely used method for selecting drug-resistant plasmodia is to treat the infected host with a single large dose of the drug, to wait for parasitemia to recrudesce, and then to passage into clean hosts. The parasites are then allowed to build up to a reasonably high level, and the hosts are again treated with the same high dose of drug, the procedure being repeated in subsequent passages. This technique can readily be combined with a bioassay for monitoring the changing response to the drug. Such an approach was described by Peters who combined a simple relapse technique using chloroquine in mice infected with various lines of *P. berghei* and *P. yoelii* with a modification of the bioassay technique of Warhurst and Folwell (1968). In the latter the time from the day of infection required for parasitemia to reach the 2% level is compared in groups of *Plasmodium*-infected mice in treated and untreated groups. The delay in this period caused by administration of a single large drug dose at the time of infection is recorded as the 2% delay time, and changes in this period are plotted against succeeding passages. An example of this technique as originally applied is shown in Fig. 39.

It was subsequently discovered in fact that this technique had selected out a second parasite that had remained mixed in a cryptic state with several lines of *P. berghei* from Katanga and that is now recognized as being an undescribed subspecies of *P. yoelii* (Peters et al., 1978).

A

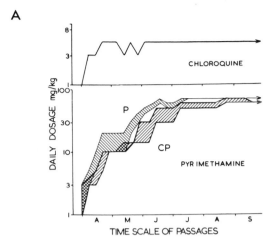

B

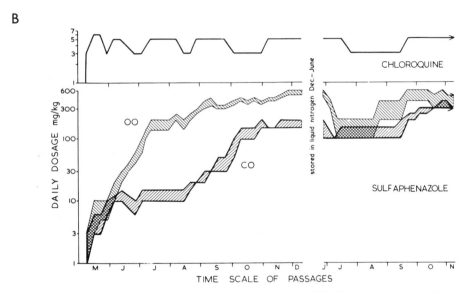

FIG. 38. Levels of resistance developed by *P. berghei* NK 65 strain to various drug combinations. (A) Pyrimethamine administered alone (P) or combined with a suboptimal dose of chloroquine (CP). (B) Sulfaphenazole alone (OO) or combined with a suboptimal dose of chloroquine (CO). Shaded areas in bottom part of each figure indicate the range of doses used in each passage. The solid line at the top of the figures indicates the chloroquine dosage applied to the CP and CO lines, respectively (Peters *et al.*, 1973).

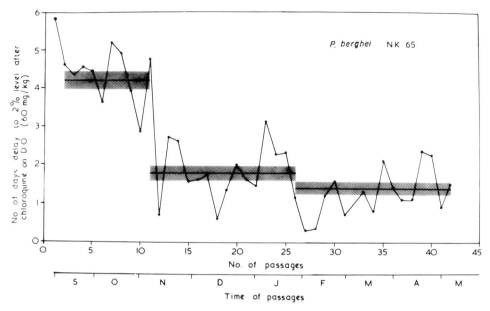

FIG. 39. The rate of acquisition of chloroquine resistance in *P. berghei berghei* NK65 strain, 185 line, as reflected by changes in the delay from infection to a 2% parasitemia after administration of a single dose of 60 mg/kg chloroquine phosphate, subcutaneously on D0. In the shaded areas, the central line indicates the mean delay times over the corresponding group of passages, and the shaded areas the range of these values (Peters, 1968a).

Many authors have employed a relapse technique in a variety of models, ranging from avian to human parasites. The frequency of potentially drug-resistant mutants in a parasite population controls the rate at which resistant lines develop under these conditions. Single exposures to pyrimethamine, for example, have led to the development of resistant lines of *P. berghei* in mice (Diggens, *et al.*, 1970), *P. cynomolgi* in rhesus monkeys (Schmidt and Genther, 1953), and *P. malariae, P. vivax,* and *P. falciparum* in man (Young, 1957; Young and Burgess, 1959; Burgess and Young, 1959). The relapse technique may in fact be applied to any *Plasmodium*–drug–host system. Recently Glew *et al.* (1978), for example, applied a similar procedure to produce a quinine-resistant line of *P. falciparum* in *Aotus* monkeys. They started with a quinine-sensitive isolate from Panama, which was cured by a 14-day course of 125 mg/kg daily for 14 days. After seven serial passages under drug pressure during a period of 6 months a line developed that produced an R I response in 3, an R II in 5, and an R III in 4 animals out of 12 treated with 125 mg/kg for 14 days. The resistant parasites were as virulent as the drug-sensitive parent line.

Since there is a marked similarity in the mode of action of the new antimalarial, mefloquine, and quinine, this experience should be taken as a warning of the

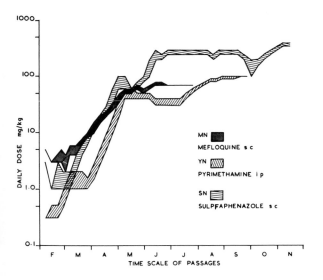

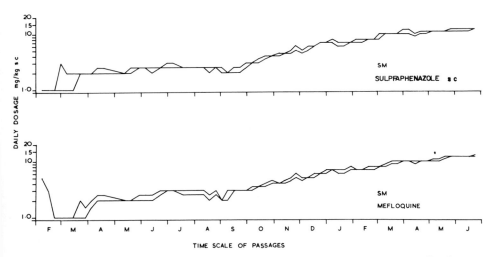

FIG. 40. (Top) Rate of acquisition by *P. berghei* N strain of resistance to mefloquine, pyrimethamine, and sulfaphenazole when the drugs are used alone. Consecutive passages were exposed to increasing drug doses given daily for 6 days of each week, the passage being made on the seventh day. (Bottom) Influence of combining mefloquine with sulfaphenazole on the rate of acquisition of resistance to each drug by *P. berghei* N strain in consecutive passages. Top lines indicate maximum levels of sulfaphenazole and bottom lines those of mefloquine on the mixtures at each passage (Peters *et al.*, 1977b).

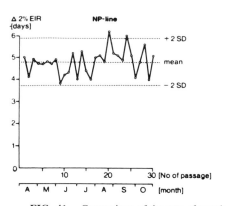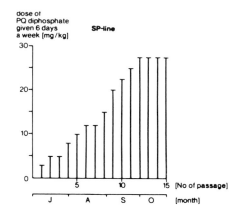

FIG. 41. Comparison of the rate of acquisition of primaquine resistance by *P. berghei* using (left) relapse technique and (right) increasing dosage. Note the rapid increase in resistance in the right-hand figure compared with the failure to change the level of drug sensitivity in the left-hand figure (Merkli and Peters, 1976).

danger that resistance to mefloquine might also develop quite rapidly under favorable circumstances if this drug comes into general use alone for the treatment of *P. falciparum*. Development of resistance to mefloquine can, however, be slowed down if the drug is given in combination with various other antimalarials, for example, sulfonamide (Fig. 40).

A marked difference was found when *P. berghei* was exposed to primaquine using in parallel the first method described above of applying a gradually increasing drug selection pressure and the second relapse technique. Merkli and Peters (1976) failed to produce resistance in 30 passages by the latter technique but readily produced a resistant line by the first procedure (Fig. 41).

B. Genetic Analysis of Drug Resistance

All early attempts to determine the genetic basis of drug resistance in avian malaria were based on a somewhat empirical analysis of the rate at which resistance could be induced in blood-passaged parasites, mainly of *P. gallinaceum* in chicks. In more recent years a critical analysis of the genetics of malaria parasites has been made, mainly by research workers in Edinburgh using lines of rodent malaria with genetic markers consisting not only of drug response characters but also biochemically characterized isoenzymes. Drug resistance markers have in fact been used as tools for studying the genetics of malaria parasites rather than the converse.

Bryson and Szybalski (1955) produced a classification of the possible modes of origin of drug resistance as given in Table XXXIV.

TABLE XXXIV

Classification of Possible Modes of Drug Resistance[a]

A. Resistance primarily dependent upon change in genotype
    i. Mutation
        Spontaneous (the expression of the mutant may be delayed by "phenomic lag";
            i.e., several generations may elapse between the genetic event and its pheno-
            typic expression)
        Induced (usually by nonspecific mutagenic agents rather than the drug itself,
            but the latter is possible if subinhibitory drug concentrations are used)
    ii. Genetic exchange (chromosomal or extrachromosomal)
        By gametes (sexual recombination)
        By "unpackaged" DNA
        Transduction
        Transformation
B. Resistance dependent upon nongenetic change in phenotype (i.e., inducible organisms)
    i. Induction of a new physiological function
        Production of inducer-inactivating enzymes
        Single enzyme
        Chain of enzymes
    ii. Elimination of a cytoplasmic particle
    iii. Accumulation of a drug-inactivating factor
    iv. Selection of an alternative physiological function, e.g., selective change in the rela-
        tive emphasis upon two or more preexistent enzymatic pathways, leading to the for-
        mation of an essential metabolite
    v. "Reorganization of the cytoplasm" (a general term quoted from Beale to cover a
        variety of phenotypic adaptations leading to resistance, e.g., altered membrane
        structure and permeability)
C. Resistance involving no adaptive change
D. Borderline cases
E. Resistance dependent upon composite changes (the most likely process in most cases of
    drug resistance)

---

[a] Peters (1970a), after Bryson and Szybalski (1955).

A number of these possibilities have now been explored in malaria parasites, and simple Mendelian inheritance of certain characters has been confirmed. Nongenetic factors also appear to be responsible for certain types of experimentally determined drug resistance, but transfer of drug resistance through a mechanism resembling episomal transfer in bacteria appears so far to have been excluded.

1. Older Studies in Avian Malaria

Bishop (1958, 1959) utilized clones of *P. gallinaceum* in an attempt to define the genetic basis of resistance to metachloridine. These parasites were passaged by blood inoculation into series of chicks in which they were exposed to drug selection pressure. No attempt was made to cross sensitive and resistant parasites through genetic exchange in vector mosquitoes, although Bishop did employ cyclic transmission to determine the stability of her drug-resistant lines. Bishop concluded that the size of inoculum but not the level of drug pressure was the factor that determined the rate at which resistance emerged. From her comparative experiments she determined that mutants resistant to metachloridine were present in her original line of *P. gallinaceum* at a frequency of less than 1 in 5 × 10^7 parasites, and probably in less than 1 in 10^9.

A further step in the analysis of drug resistance was taken by Greenberg and Trembley (1954) who attempted to hybridize two lines of *P. gallinaceum* in *A. aegypti*. In addition to pyrimethamine and metachloridine resistance they used as a genetic marker the character of virulence in one of the two lines. From a series of complicated experiments in which they made sequential cyclic passages of several infections of *P. gallinaceum,* not attempting to clone their material, Greenberg (1956) concluded that pyrimethamine resistance and the other strain characters (notably those for virulence) were transmitted by four independent genes carrying resistance to metachloridine, transferability, and virulence on the one hand, and pyrimethamine resistance on the other. He suggested that the first three characters might be grouped on one chromosome and the last on another. Alternatively all four genes might lie on the same chromosome but at opposite poles. Unfortunately this work is no longer considered conclusive, especially since it was not based on cloned material.

2. Genetics of Resistance in Rodent Malaria

a. Extranuclear Transmission of Resistance. Of the various possible modes of extranuclear production of drug resistance listed by Bryson and Szybalski (1955) (see Table XXXIV), there is some evidence suggesting that, under certain circumstances, an adaptive process can be induced under drug pressure. The type of chloroquine resistance associated with the application of gradually increasing chloroquine dosage, i.e., in the RC type of *P. berghei* line, is highly unstable in the absence of drug pressure and, in the early stages of the development of this type of resistance the parasites rapidly revert to a normal level of sensitivity. However, as noted by Peters (1970a), this type of resistance became stable after several hundred passages under drug pressure, suggesting that the initial mechanism of inheritance of RC resistance had been replaced by or reinforced by a mutational change. It is noteworthy too that there are a number of physiological differences between the RC parasites and the parent strain, both in the metabolism of the parasite itself and in its relationship with its host cell (Peters, 1965b; Howells *et al.,* 1972).

The rapidity with which chloroquine resistance appeared to spread in *P. falciparum* suggested to various observers that an unusual type of mechanism might be responsible for its inheritance, and the possibility that an episomal type of factor was concerned clearly called for an investigation. One direct method of searching for such factors is to isolate the DNA from the parasites by classic separation techniques and to search for extranuclear, "satellite" DNA in density gradients prepared by ultracentrifugation. This procedure was carried out by Chance *et al.* (1972) with a line of *P. yoelii,* and a small satellite particle was apparently found. However, this observation could not be repeated in subsequent experiments, and in a recent paper Chance *et al.* (1978) reported they had found no further evidence of a satellite DNA in a variety of naturally or experimentally derived chloroquine-resistant lines of *P. berghei* and *P. yoelii.*

Using quite a different approach Yoeli *et al.* (1969) set up a complex experiment to determine whether pyrimethamine resistance could be transmitted through an extranuclear mechanism. They passaged a pyrimethamine-resistant *P. vinckei* through mice which were simultaneously infected, also by syringe passage, with a pyrimethamine-sensitive line of *P. berghei.* In subsequent passages they passed the parasites through a series of "filters" designed to eliminate drug-sensitive *P. berghei,* and at the end of their experiments they concluded that the resistance factor had been passed from the *P. vinckei* to the *P. berghei.* Since this could only have taken place at a time when both a pyrimethamine-resistant *P. vinckei* and a drug-sensitive *P. berghei* trophozoite were, by chance, invading the same host erythrocyte, they termed the phenomenon "synpholia." However, one of their filters consisted of a single exposure to a high dose of pyrimethamine aimed at eliminating any drug-sensitive *P. berghei* that may have been passaged. As could be anticipated and as Diggens *et al.* (1970) subsequently proved, this process alone is enough to select preexisting pyrimethamine-resistant mutants. Thus this piece of evidence suggesting the transmission of pyrimethamine resistance by an extranuclear process cannot be held valid. There is in fact no evidence so far to indicate that episomal resistance transfer exists in the genus *Plasmodium.*

b. Mendelian Inheritance of Drug Resistance. The foundations for study of the genetic nature of drug resistance in rodent malaria were laid by the pioneering work of Carter who characterized a number of isoenzymes by which different species, subspecies, and strains of these parasites could be identified. Carter's observations are summarized in Table XXXV (Beale *et al.,* 1978).

The first essential in using these parasites for genetic studies is to clone the parasites. Diggens (1970), using a micromanipulation technique, showed that mice infected intravenously with a single trophozoite of *P. berghei* could develop an infection, and this has been amply confirmed subsequently by the work of Beale's group. They in fact use the following dilution technique to produce clones.

TABLE XXXV

Isolates of Rodent Malaria Species and Subspecies Available in the Laboratory[a]

Plasmodium species and subspecies	Isolate	Host species[b]	Origin			Enzyme composition			
			Host specimen	Region of capture	Date of capture	GPI	6PGD	LDH[c]	GDH[c]
P. berghei	K173	*G. surdaster*	K173	Katanga	1948	3	1	1	3
	SP11	*A. d. millecampsi*		Katanga	1961	3	1	1	3
	Anka	*A. d. millecampsi*		Katanga	1966	3	1	1	3
	Luka	*A. d. millecampsi*		Katanga	1966	3	1	1	3
	NK65	*A. d. millecampsi*		Katanga	1964	3	1	1	3
P. y. yoelii	17X	*T. rutilans*	17X	Central African Republic	1965	1	4	1	4
	32X	*T. rutilans*	32X	Central African Republic	1965	1	4	1	4
	33X	*T. rutilans*	33X	Central African Republic	1965	2	4	1	4
	55X	*T. rutilans*	55X	Central African Republic	1965	1	4	1	4
	86X	*T. rutilans*	86X	Central African Republic	1965	1	4	1	4
	146X	*T. rutilans*	146X	Central African Republic	1965	1	4	1	4
	5AD	*T. rutilans*	AD	Central African Republic	1969	1,2	4	1	4
	3AE	*T. rutilans*	AE	Central African Republic	1969	1	4	1	4
	3AF	*T. rutilans*	AF	Central African Republic	1969	1	4	1	4
	1AK	*T. rutilans*	AK	Central African Republic	1969	1	4	1	4
	1AR	*T. rutilans*	AR	Central African Republic	1969	2	4	1	4
	2AZ	*T. rutilans*	AZ	Central African Republic	1969	1	4	1	4
	14BE	*T. rutilans*	BE	Central African Republic	1969	1	4	1	4
	1BF	*T. rutilans*	BF	Central African Republic	1969	2	4	1	4
	1BG	*T. rutilans*	BG	Central African Republic	1969	1	4	1	4
	2BR	*T. rutilans*	BR	Central African Republic	1970	2	4	1	4

	Clone	Species	Code	Location	Year				
	2CF	*T. rutilans*	CF	Central African Republic	1970	2	4	1	4
	2CL	*T. rutilans*	CL	Central African Republic	1970	1	4	1	4
	2CN	*T. rutilans*	CN	Central African Republic	1970	1,10	4	1	4
	5CP	*T. rutilans*	CP	Central African Republic	1970	1	4	1	4
	2CU	*T. rutilans*	CU	Central African Republic	1970	1	4	1	4
	2CX	*T. rutilans*	CX	Central African Republic	1970	1	4	1	4
P. y. killicki	193L	*T. rutilans*	193L	Brazzaville	1966	1	4	1	1
	194ZZ	*T. rutilans*	194ZZ	Brazzaville	1968	1	4	1	1
P. y. nigeriensis	N67	*T. rutilans*	N67	Nigeria	1967	2	4	1	2
P. c. chabaudi	54X	*T. rutilans*	54X	Central African Republic	1965	4	3	3	5
	864VD	*T. rutilans*	864VD	Central African Republic	1970	4	3	4	5
	3AC	*T. rutilans*	AC	Central African Republic	1969	4	2,3	2,4	5
	2AD	*T. rutilans*	AD	Central African Republic	1969	4	2	3,5	5
	16AF	*T. rutilans*	AF	Central African Republic	1969	4	2	5	5
	AJ	*T. rutilans*	AJ	Central African Republic	1969	4	3	2	5
	1AL	*T. rutilans*	AL	Central African Republic	1969	4	2	2	5
	1AM	*T. rutilans*	AM	Central African Republic	1969	4	2	3	5
	1AQ	*T. rutilans*	AQ	Central African Republic	1969	4	3	2	5
	1AS	*T. rutilans*	AS	Central African Republic	1969	4	2	3	5
	4AT	*T. rutilans*	AT	Central African Republic	1969	4	3	2,3	5
	1BC	*T. rutilans*	BC	Central African Republic	1969	4	3	4	nt
	40BE	*T. rutilans*	BE	Central African Republic	1969	4	3	2	5
	BJ	*T. rutilans*	BJ	Central African Republic	1969	4	2	4	5
	1BK	*T. rutilans*	BK	Central African Republic	1969	4	7	2	5
	1BS	*T. rutilans*	BS	Central African Republic	1970	4	2	5	5
	2CB	*T. rutilans*	CB	Central African Republic	1970	4	3	4	5
	2CE	*T. rutilans*	CE	Central African Republic	1970	4	3	3,4	5
	2CP	*T. rutilans*	CP	Central African Republic	1970	4	2	4,5	5

(continued)

TABLE XXXV—*Continued*

Plasmodium species and subspecies	Isolate	Host species[b]	Host specimen	Region of capture	Date of capture	Enzyme composition			
						GPI	6PGD	LDH[c]	GDH[c]
P. c. adami	2CQ	T. rutilans	CQ	Central African Republic	1970	4	3	5	5
	4CR	T. rutilans	CR	Central African Republic	1970	4	2	3	5
	2CW	T. rutilans	CW	Central African Republic	1970	4	3	4	5
	556KA	T. rutilans	556KA	Brazzaville	1970	8	2	8	5
	408XZ	T. rutilans	408XZ	Brazzaville	1972	8	2	10	5
P. v. vinckei	v-52	A. d. millecampsi		Katanga	1952	7	6	6	6
	v-67	A. d. millecampsi		Katanga	1967	7	6	6	6
P. v. petteri	1BS	T. rutilans	BS	Central African Republic	1970	9	5	7	6
	2BZ	T. rutilans	BZ	Central African Republic	1970	9	5	7	6
	2CR	T. rutilans	CR	Central African Republic	1970	5,9	5	7	6
	2CE	T. rutilans	CE	Central African Republic	1970	5	5	7	nt
P. v. lentum	170L	T. rutilans	170L	Brazzaville	1966	6	5	7	6
	483L	T. rutilans	483L	Brazzaville	1966	6	5	7	6
	194ZZ	T. rutilans	194ZZ	Brazzaville	1968	6	5	7	6
	408XZ	T. rutilans	408XZ	Brazzaville	1972	11	5	9	6
P. v. brucechwatti	1-69	T. rutilans	1-69	Nigeria	1969	6	6	9	6
	N48	T. rutilans	N48	Nigeria	1967	6	6	9	6

[a] The isozyme composition and details of origin of each isolate are given. Beale *et al.* (1978).
[b] *G. surdaster, Grammomys surdaster; T. rutilans, Thamnomys rutilans; A. d. millecampsi, Anopheles dureni millecampsi.*
[c] nt, not tested.

i. Cloning. Blood is collected from a donor animal with a rising parasitemia and diluted with cold Ringer's solution and fetal calf serum in a 1:1 proportion to yield a concentration of one or fewer parasitized red cells in each 0.1 ml of the diluent. Mice are then given an intravenous inoculum of 0.1 ml of the diluted blood. Blood films are made and examined for parasitemia after 7 days in infections with *P. yoelii* and after 10 days with *P. chabaudi*. Application of the Poisson distribution tables reveals whether the mice on the average have been infected with one, two, or three parasites. For example, if the aliquots contain only one parasite, approximately 63% of the recipients will become infected, and 58% of these will be clonal infections; if each inoculum contains on an average only 0.1 parasite, only 10% of the mice will become infected, but of these 96% will be clones.

ii. Hybridization. Lines to be hybridized are passed simultaneously through *A. stephensi* by allowing them to feed on mice that have been doubly infected with both the parasites under study. The assumption (now adequately proved) is that male and female gametes of either line will meet at random and fuse to form homozygotes or heterozygotes which will subsequently mature and produce a mixed population of infective sporozoites. The mosquitoes containing mature sporozoites are used to infect clean mice. When the parasitemia becomes patent in these animals, the parasites are cloned and passaged into a further series of mice. The infections that develop subsequently in these mice are characterized in two ways, first by determining the nature of certain key isoenzymes, and second by observing their response to a standard discriminating dose level of the drug in question. The procedure is illustrated in Fig. 42 which also shows how controls are produced for comparison with possible hybrids.

Since blood-induced infections of the two lines may not produce similar gametocyte numbers at the same time in a single animal, the infections can be raised in separate mice, and gametocyte-containing blood can be mixed and fed to mosquitoes by means of a standard pattern of artificial membrane feeder. In either case, if genetic recombination takes place in the gut of the insects, approximately 50% of the zygotes will be hybrids, while the remainder should contain equal proportions of the two parental lines.

iii. Enzyme Variants. The four enzymes that have proved most useful in hybridization studies have been glucose phosphate isomerase, 6-phosphogluconate dehydrogenase, lactate dehydrogenase, and NADP-dependent glutamate dehydrogenase. The various forms of these enzymes are determined by electrophoresis on starch or acrylamide gels using such techniques as those described by Carter (1973) who has assigned number to the enzyme variants as shown in Fig. 43.

Starting from cloned material Morgan (1974) has shown that pyrimethamine

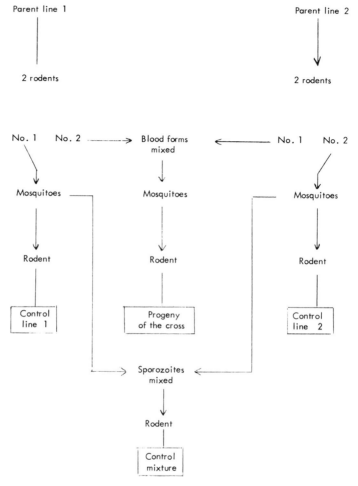

FIG. 42. Procedure used in making cross-preparing and control samples (Beale *et al.*, 1978).

resistance occurs as a mutant character which is transmitted in Mendelian fashion in *P. yoelii*. The mutation is stable and has been shown by other workers (in *P. berghei*) to be associated with a modified parasite dihydrofolate reductase (Ferone *et al.*, 1969). An increased level of the enzyme was also found in resistant parasites. Morgan's (1974) data suggest, as did those of Bishop (1962) for *P. gallinaceum*, that the mutant occurs with a frequency of less than 1 in 10^9 parasites. Another worker in Beale's group hybridized two lines of *P. chabaudi*, distinguishable on isoenzymes, one of which was sensitive to pyrimethamine and sulfadiazine and the other of which was resistant to both drugs, in an attempt to

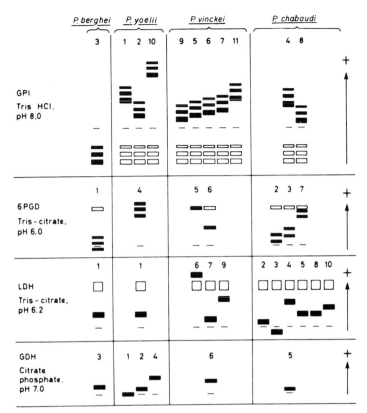

FIG. 43. Electrophoretic forms of glucose phosphate isomerase (GPI), 6-phosphogluconate dehydrogenase (6PGD), lactate dehydrogenase (LDH), and NADP-dependent glutamate dehydrogenase (GDH), using selected systems of electrophoresis (modified from Carter, 1973, and unpublished). Parasite bands are solid; those of the rodent host (mouse) are open. Not all enzyme variants can be distinguished by the electrophoresis systems illustrated here (Beale *et al.*, 1978).

resolve the question of why some lines resistant to one drug are cross-resistant to both, and some not. MacLeod (in Beale *et al.*, 1978) showed that resistance for the two drugs recombined separately. His data suggested that mutants could appear at three separate loci, two of which were associated with resistance to both drugs but at different levels, and the third of which was associated with resistance to sulfonamide alone.

Recently Rosario (1976), working with the same Edinburgh group, has shown that a low level of chloroquine resistance in *P. chabaudi* is a stable character, also inherited in Mendelian fashion. In a subsequent study Rosario *et al.* (1978) demonstrated that, while pyrimethamine-resistant *P. chabaudi* had possibly a slight biological disadvantage when mixed with sensitive parasites in the same mice, chloroquine-resistant parasites showed a distinct biological advantage. The potential implications of this finding in relation to chloroquine-resistant *P. falciparum* in man (if the same principles apply) are obvious. There are two sets of experimental evidence suggesting that chloroquine may also enhance the infectivity of chloroquine-resistant gametocytes in the vector. Ramkaran and Peters (1969a) observed this phenomenon with *P. yoelii* in *A. stephensi,* while Wilkinson *et al.* (1976) reported similar findings with *P. falciparum* in *A. balabacensis.* When all these factors are taken together, it seems hardly necessary to seek further mechanisms such as episomal chloroquine resistance transfer in *P. falciparum* to explain the rapid spread of this problem throughout large parts of the tropics.

VI. GUIDE TO PROPHYLAXIS AND TREATMENT IN MAN

The survival of an attack or multiple attacks of malaria endows the victim with a measure of protection from both humoral and cellular elements of the host's immune processes. It is not intended to pursue this topic further in this chapter, since it is dealt with at length elsewhere in Volume 3, Chapter 3. It should be pointed out, however, that drugs alone will *not* necessarily free the host organism of malaria parasites, no matter how efficient they may be, and that chemotherapy is only an adjunct to the host's inherent immune response. This said, it must also be stressed that antimalarial drugs are relatively more effective in helping to clear parasitemia in an individual who possesses some degree of immunity. This of course can readily be demonstrated experimentally in immunologically deprived animals or, conversely, by treating reinfections in partially immune ones. The recommendations for chemoprophylaxis or chemotherapy are therefore rather different depending upon the immune status of the individuals or communities concerned.

A word of caution is needed also. In an area where the level of endemicity has been radically reduced by energetic malaria control measures, the level of communal immunity to infection will decrease with time. A marked fall in antibody titers is likely after about 3 years, and after that time the population will become decreasingly immune, hence increasingly susceptible to new infection. They will also require the doses of antimalarials normally recommended for nonimmunes. This is the situation currently seen in India where, over the last few years, there has been an enormous resurgence of malaria, mainly *P. vivax.* Indian physicians are finding that the traditional "presumptive" single dose of chloroquine is no longer sufficient to abort an acute attack of vivax malaria, and full courses of this compound must often be given. This phenomenon is not to be confused with drug resistance. Drug resistance, incidentally, is usually first detected in nonimmune visitors to endemic areas, the local people responding well to even small doses of drugs by virtue of their acquired immunity, at least until such time as the level of drug resistance becomes excessively high. Such a situation exists today, for example, in Thailand.

A. Malaria Prophylaxis in Nonimmunes

1. In the Absence of Drug Resistance

The recommended dosages of commonly used antimalarials in this situation are summarized in Table XXXVI. Further details of drug formulations and synonyms will be found in the monograph on malaria chemotherapy by Black *et al.* (1980), as well as recommendations for dosages in infants and children.

2. In the Presence of Chloroquine-Resistant Falciparum Malaria

It is unusual for chloroquine-resistant falciparum malaria to be the only species of malaria transmitted in a particular locality and, as a rule, *P. vivax* is also present. In some cases *P. malariae* may also occur. *Plasmodium ovale* is rare anywhere except in West Africa. The first essential is for the traveler or his or her physician to become familiar with the recorded situation of drug response or resistance in the area involved. This information is readily obtainable from WHO (1976b), from the Center for Disease Control (1978), or (in most cases) from the health authorities of the country concerned. The general distribution of chloroquine-resistant falciparum malaria is shown in Fig. 44.

TABLE XXXVI

Dosage of Various Drugs for General Protection[a]

Drug	Interval	Dosage (mg) and age (years)					
		Over 16	11–16	7–10	4–6	1–3	Under 1
Proguanil salt[b]	Daily	100	100	75	50	50	25
or							
Chloroquine base	Weekly	300	225	150	100	75	37
or							
Amodiaquin base	Weekly	400	300	200	133	100	
or							
Mepacrine[c]	Daily	100	75	50	25		
or							
Pyrimethamine[b]	Weekly	25	25	18	12	6	

[a] Peters (1970a), after Covell *et al.* (1955).

[b] Contraindicated in areas where the prevailing malaria is known to be resistant to either of these drugs.

[c] Beginning 10 days before exposure to infection. With the other drugs listed, it is essential to begin the course at least one day prior to exposure.

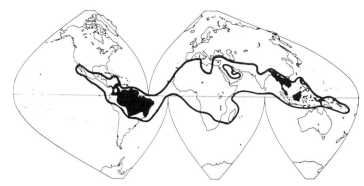

FIG. 44. Approximate distribution of malaria and chloroquine-resistant *P. falciparum* in 1978.

Most strains of *P. falciparum* that are resistant to chloroquine are also resistant to antifolates such as pyrimethamine and proguanil when these are used alone. They respond, however, to potentiating combinations of sulfonamides or sulfones with antifolates. Unfortunately, *P. vivax* is not very responsive to sulfonamides, and even such combinations may fail completely to protect against vivax infection. Nevertheless, the best protection against chloroquine-resistant malaria at present available is one of the following combinations: sulfadoxine-pyrimethamine (20:1 ratio), Fansidar (Roche); sulfalene–pyrimethamine (20:1 ratio), Kelfimeta (Pharmitalia); and dapsone–pyrimethamine (8:1 ratio), Maloprim (Wellcome) (see also the note on mefloquine, Section VI, C, 2.

The first two combinations contain 500 mg sulfonamide and 25 mg pyrimethamine in one tablet; the third preparation contains 100 mg dapsone and 12.5 mg pyrimethamine. Adults should take one tablet once weekly, children proportionally less.

It has been suggested that, in order to ensure protection also against *P. vivax*, these preparations could be taken in addition to chloroquine. My view is that it is safer to omit the chloroquine, knowing that if, by ill chance, a vivax infection is acquired, it can readily be treated with chloroquine and primaquine.

In all cases it is essential to commence prophylaxis at least 1 week before entering the endemic area, to take the medication regularly throughout exposure as prescribed, and to continue it for 4 weeks after leaving the endemic area. The purpose of this is to ensure that drug is present in the body throughout the preerythrocytic development cycle of any *P. falciparum* that may have been contracted just before leaving the endemic area, and for a week or two longer to cover the contingency of any possible, slower developing liver schizonts being present. There being no secondary tissue cycle in this species, this regimen should ensure a suppressive cure, if not causal prophylaxis. With this regimen, as indeed with any, suppression of a cryptic vivax infection may be followed several weeks or months after the arrest of medication by parasitemia resulting from the maturation of secondary exoerythrocytic schizonts. In this eventuality the individual should be treated as described in the next section.

Sulfonamide-hypersensitive individuals should not take the combinations described above. The best that can be offered for them at present is to take amodiaquin, which may have an action marginally superior to that of chloroquine against resistant strains, and to treat with quinine and tetracycline any parasitemia that may happen to break through (see below).

In the doses prescribed here pyrimethamine is not known to have any adverse effects in pregnancy. On principle, however, caution must be exercised in giving advice on prophylaxis or treatment to a woman in the early stages of pregnancy, bearing in mind the relative risks of malaria infection and drug prophylaxis to mother and fetus.

B. Malaria Prophylaxis in Semi-Immunes

In semi-immune populations chemoprophylaxis may be considered either for the protection of selected high-risk groups of the population such as infants, under fives, and pregnant and nursing mothers, or in terms of mass drug administration as part of a campaign of malaria control. The issues are complex and beyond the scope of this chapter. Reference should be made to WHO manuals on this question (World Health Organization, 1973; Black *et al.*, 1980). No really satisfactory drugs are available at the present time for mass drug administration, the resistance problem apart, since all current preparations have to be given at too frequent intervals for regular coverage to be ensured.

C. Treatment of Malaria in Nonimmunes

1. Drug-Sensitive Infections

The drug of choice for the treatment of an acute attack of malaria due to any species is chloroquine. Quinine should be reserved for those who are severely ill, such as individuals with excessively high parasitemia levels (over 100,000 parasites/mm^3), hyperpyrexia, or cerebral malaria, or for other special indications. The adult dosage of chloroquine (in terms of base) given orally is 600 mg at once followed by 300 mg after 6 hours and 300 mg daily for the next 2 days.

If quinine is indicated because of the severity of the illness, it should be given in a dextrose saline intravenous infusion of quinine dihydrochloride at the rate of 490 mg base (for practical purposes this can be taken as 500 mg) in 500 ml dextrose saline over a 4-hour period (Table XXXVII). This may be repeated two to three times in 24 hours to a total dose of 0.98–1.47 g/day.

Chloroquine too may be given in a slow intravenous infusion at a dose of 5

TABLE XXXVII

Intravenous Quinine and Fluid Infusion in Falciparum Malaria: Guidelines for Daily Dosage[a]

Weight of patient (kg)	Daily quinine dose (mg)	Daily volume of fluid (ml)[b]	No. of infusions[c]	Infusion rate (ml/hour)	Infusion rate [drops/minute (approx)]
5	100	200	1	25	10
10	200	200	1	50	20
25	500	500	2	63	25
50	1000	1000	2	125	50

[a] Hall (1976). Standard daily dose of quinine base is 20 mg/kg. Standard ampule contains about 500 mg quinine base. Recommended daily intravenous fluid intake is 20 ml/kg (40 ml/kg in small children).

[b] Normal saline is recommended.

[c] Standard infusion time is 4 hours for each infusion.

mg/kg body weight. As soon as possible, parenteral therapy should be replaced with oral therapy.

General supportive therapy may have to be given, especially in severe falciparum infections. This may include a packed red cell transfusion to compensate for the acute hemolytic amemia, peritoneal or hemodialysis in the event of renal failure, and other procedures the details of which should be sought in the papers of Clyde (1974), Hall (1976), and Black *et al.* (1980).

In order to ensure a radical cure of vivax malaria it is necessary to administer not only chloroquine as a blood schizontocide, but also primaquine—15 mg base daily for 14 days or up to 22.5 mg base for people infected in southwest Pacific areas. The primaquine can be commenced from the third day of treatment. Caution must be exercised in individuals known to have genetic deficiency of the enzymes glucose-6-phosphate dehydrogenase or NADH methemoglobin reductase. The former type of deficiency can cause severe hemolysis when primaquine (or many other drugs) is administered, and the latter produces cyanosis. Radical cure may be obtained of vivax malaria in glucose-6-phosphate dehydrogenase-deficient subjects by treating them with single weekly doses of 300 mg chloroquine base plus 45 mg primaquine base for eight consecutive weeks (Table XXXVIII), although this may not always succeed against southwest Pacific strains. This is well tolerated by such individuals, since primaquine only causes hemolysis of older erythrocytes, and compensatory hematopoiesis makes up any red cell loss between doses.

2. Chloroquine-Resistant Falciparum Infection

Sulfonamide–antifolate combinations are effective in treating uncomplicated acute infection with chloroquine-resistant strains of *P. falciparum*. The oral dose

TABLE XXXVIII

Efficacy of Chloroquine (300 mg Base)–Primaquine (45 mg Base) Given Prophylactically-
Suppressively or Therapeutically Once Weekly for Eight Consecutive Weeks to Volunteers
Exposed to Infection with a South Viet Nam Isolate of *Plasmodium vivax* by the Bites
of Mosquitoes[a]

Treatment classification	Prepatent period, median (days)	Parasite count at time of treatment (per mm^3)	Parasite clearance (hours)	Number protected or cured/total number
Suppressive-prophylactic				9/10[b]
Therapeutic	9–17 (11)	50–4250	24–72	10/10

[a] Contacos *et al.* (1974).
[b] One volunteer developed patent infection on day 455. Day 0 is day of exposure to infection.

of sulfadoxine–pyrimethamine, which is the combination with which most experience has been reported, is two or three tablets given in 24 hours, the larger dose being for heavier subjects. Some authorities recommend that treatment commence with oral quinine, 540 mg base (two tablets of quinine sulfate) being given every 8 hours for 2 or 3 days, followed by sulfadoxine–pyrimethamine.

If the severity of the condition necessitates parenteral therapy, the treatment of choice is quinine as described in Section VI, C, 1 above, followed by oral quinine and sulfadoxine–pyrimethamine as soon as practical.

If sulfonamides are precluded because of a prior history of sulfonamide hypersensitivity, treatment should be started with quinine for 2 or 3 days, followed by 7 days of therapy with tetracycline hydrochloride (1–2 g daily) *or* doxycycline (0.2 g daily) *or* minocycline (0.1–0.4 g daily) (Clyde, 1974).

Several reports indicate that a single dose of 1.5 g mefloquine hydrochloride achieves a radical cure in almost every patient infected with chloroquine-resistant falciparum malaria (Trenholme *et al.*, 1975; Hall, 1976) (see Table XXVII). Hall (1976) reported that 29 of 31 patients were cured with mefloquine alone in a clinical study in Thailand, but that the other 2 patients, both of whom had very high parasite counts, responded more slowly. He therefore recommends (Hall, 1977) that therapy be initiated in severe cases with quinine, followed by a single dose of mefloquine, which has a very long half-life in humans. Rieckmann *et al.* (1974) (see Table XXVI) noted a significant blood schizontocidal effect against *P. falciparum in vitro* in serum samples taken from subjects 35 days after they had taken a single dose of only 1 g mefloquine. While in this study mefloquine did not display true causal prophylactic properties, it did suppress sporozoite-induced infections with the highly chloroquine-resistant Viet Nam (Marks) strain of *P. falciparum* for more than a month. A monthly dose of 1 g or repeated fortnightly doses of 0.5 g also produced suppressive cure of infections with the Viet Nam (Smith) strain (Clyde *et al.*, 1976) (see Table XXVIII). Unfortunately, at the time of writing mefloquine has not yet been released for general use. *Plasmodium vivax* is somewhat less susceptible to mefloquine's suppressive action than *P. falciparum* (Clyde *et al.*, 1976).

D. Treatment of Malaria in Semi-Immunes

1. Drug-Sensitive Infections

The recommended doses for the treatment of acute malaria in a semi-immune adult are summarized in Table XXXIX.

To prevent relapses of vivax malaria in semi-immunes, various regimens of primaquine ranging from 5 to 14 days have been applied. The success of these regimens depends upon the strain of *P. vivax*, as well as upon the immune status of the patient. In India, for example, the 5-day course is probably followed by about a 10% relapse rate (Table XL).

2. Chloroquine-Resistant Falciparum Malaria

Experience shows that it is probably safest to treat semi-immune patients infected with chloroquine-resistant *P. falciparum* in the same manner as nonimmunes. In addition it is advisable to administer a single dose of 45 mg primaquine base to any who have persisting gametocytemia in order to render these parasites noninfective, hence help to reduce the pool of infection and transmission.

VII. FUTURE RESEARCH DIRECTIONS

In 1975 a group of experts was called together to form the first Task Force on the Chemotherapy of Malaria as part of the function of the new WHO Special

TABLE XXXIX

Single-Dose Therapy for Dispensary Patients[a]

	Dosage (mg) and age (years)					
Drug	Adult	Over 12	6–12	3–6	1–3	Under 1
Chloroquine *or*	600 base	450–600	450	300	225	37–75
Amodiaquine	600 base	400–600	400	300	200	100–150

[a] Peters (1970a), after Covell *et al.* (1955).

TABLE XL

Radical Curative Efficacy of Primaquine Daily for Five Consecutive Days against a West Pakistan Strain of *Plasmodium vivax*[a]

		Infection days[b]		
Volunteer	Primary attack	Chloroquine, 1500 mg base total dose	Primaquine, 15 mg base daily	Relapse
BR	10	13–15	16–20	121
DU	12	15–17	18–22	177
FO	15	17–19	20–24	181
HO	13	16–18	19–23	174
SP	11	14–16	17–21	150

[a] Contacos *et al.* (1973).
[b] Day of exposure to infection by mosquito bite was day 0.

Programme for Research and Training in Tropical Diseases, now commonly known as the TDR program (1976a). This group attempted to analyze the gaps in malaria chemotherapy and to formulate a program of research designed to fill these gaps. The main practical problems that the group identified were the following:

1. Many strains of *P. falciparum* are resistant to a wide spectrum of the currently available antimalarial drugs.

2. None of the standard antimalarials have proved successful for mass drug administration to protect large communities, irrespective of the resistance problem.

3. Primaquine, the only available drug for the radical cure of vivax malaria, is far from ideal because (a) it is rapidly excreted and must be given for several days and (b) it is toxic, particularly to certain enzyme-deficient individuals.

4. Commercial organizations have little interest in developing antiparasitic drugs today because of the exorbitantly high cost of drug development, the severe regulations governing the clinical use of new drugs, and the slender chance of recovering development costs for a product that will be largely used in the poorest countries of the developing world.

It was felt that, apart from further study of the promising compounds now emerging from the massive antimalarial drug screening and development program of the U.S. Army, and of a few isolated compounds from certain pharmaceutical companies, little new could be expected from random drug screening without exploiting radically new ideas and new approaches to the problem. The task force (now renamed the Scientific Working Group or SWG) drew up a program that included the following areas.

A. Improvement of Existing Drugs Already in Clinical Use

The emphasis here was on the development of formulations or chemical modifications by which the duration of action of existing compounds could be extended, the principle being that it would be extremely valuable for mass drug administration use to have a preparation, a single dose of which would give protection for at least 3 months. The idea behind this is that the regular distribution to whole communities of a single dose at intervals of three or more months might be logistically and economically feasible as one means of reducing the quantum of malaria in a community, whereas long and bitter experience has shown that more frequent doses have not succeeded. The danger of favoring the emergence of drug resistance in this way was clearly recognized and, for this reason, priority was given to the development of combinations such as sulfonamides or sulfones with antifols, e.g., pyrimethamime. This is exactly the approach followed some years ago by Thompson and his colleagues who developed an injectable mixture of acedapsone and cycloguanil embonate (Elslager and Thompson, 1964). (This preparation unfortunately failed in field use for a variety of reasons, all of them probably avoidable.)

One means of prolonging the activity of a drug is to incorporate it into a slowly degraded carrier, biodegradable polymers currently being explored for this purpose (Wise *et al.*, 1976). Another alternative is to incorporate the compound into an implantable, nondegradable carrier, the advantage of this being that the material can be removed if adverse reactions result. Clearly, of course, implanting a drug has many practical disadvantages.

The problem of developing a new application form for primaquine so that a single dose can be given for the radical treatment of vivax malaria is one that appears soluble, particularly since it has been demonstrated that it is the total dose of this drug (Fig. 45) that is important to destroy secondary exoerythrocytic schizonts, rather than how much is given per day (Schmidt *et al.*, 1977c; Clyde and McCarthy, 1977).

B. Further Investigation of the Mode of Action of Existing Antimalarials and the Mechanisms of Drug Resistance

Rather than depend exclusively on *empirical drug screening* it has long been felt that the *rational approach* to drug development merits more attention. Surprisingly little is known about the mode of action even of such a compound as chloroquine and the ways in which malaria parasites become resistant to it. The recent advances in *in vitro* culture of the erythrocytic stages of *Plasmodium* should open the way to further studies on the fundamental biochemistry and host–parasite relationships of these parasites, a knowledge of which is fundamental to our learning how antimalarial drugs influence these functions. What is not

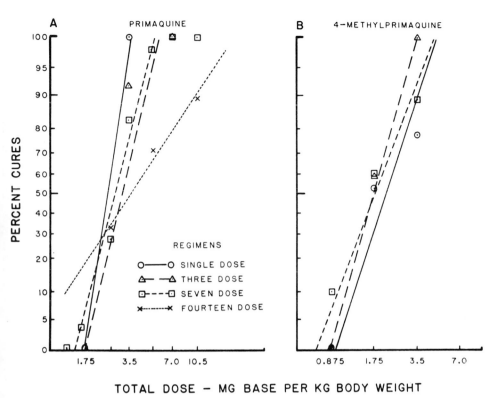

FIG. 45.   Plots of the capacities of single dose, 3-dose, and 7-dose courses of primaquine and 4-methylprimaquine and a 14-dose course of primaquine to effect radical cure of infections with the B strain of *P. cynomolgi.*

yet available, however, is a ready means of cultivating the exoerythrocytic stages of mammalian malaria parasites *in vitro,* the basic problem here being the difficulty of maintaining cell cultures of hepatocytes. It is not yet known even how a sporozoite enters a hepatocyte in order to commence its development, or the nature of the late tissue phases of relapsing infections such as *P. vivax* (Garnham, 1977).

In addition to the use of liver tissue cultures for this purpose, it may be useful to search for other, surrogate models in which to study the process of extra-erythrocytic development of *Plasmodium* or of *Plasmodium*-like hemoprotozoa. Landau and her colleagues (1976), for example, have made a close study of the host–parasite relationships of a variety of species of *Hepatocytis,* which may throw light on this question. They have also explored the nature of chronic tissue schizonts of *P. yoelii* (Landau *et al.,* 1975).

C. Development of New Models for Chemotherapy

There appear to be adequate animal models in which to screen potential new antimalarials, and it is likely that increasing use will now be made of such *in vitro* techniques as that published by Richards and Maples (1979). In order to evaluate compounds with inherently prolonged activity, modifications of the existing models are desirable, and such a model, in rodents, is currently being developed in our laboratory for the examination of both blood and tissue schizontocidal action.

It would be of obvious value if the target organisms, *P. falciparum, P. vivax,* and the other human malarias, could be adapted to surrogate hosts other than simians. With the currently accumulating knowledge of the importance and nature of erythrocyte surface receptors and host specificity (Miller and Carter, 1976), the biochemical factors concerned in the parasitization of red cells (Oelshlegel and Brewer, 1975), and methods for suppressing the host's immunological response, it should not be beyond the realms of possibility to adapt, say, *P. falciparum* to a rodent or a small avian host. Beaudoin *et al.* (1974), for example, have achieved the culture of avian exoerythrocytic stages of *P. lophurae* and *P. fallax* in embryonic mouse liver cultures. Hayes and Ward (1977) have shown the importance of dietary factors in adapting parasites to alien hosts, infecting *Aotus* liver with *P. falciparum* sporozoites by giving the animals supplementary DL-methionine. (This, interestingly, is the converse of the result achieved by Landau *et al.,* 1975, who slowed down the development of exoerythrocytic *P. yoelii* by giving the antimetabolite ethionine).

D. New Approaches to the Development of New Antimalarials

Among the interesting new approaches to the rational development of radically new antimalarials are the following.

1. Characterization of Parasite-Specific Metabolic Pathways and Synthesis of Selective Enzyme Inhibitors

This approach is a very obvious but, at the same time, very time-consuming one demanding much sophisticated enzymological research. That it may prove fruitful, however, is evidenced by success in other fields such as that of trypanosomiasis. Studies on the glycolytic pathways of *Trypanosoma brucei* have revealed that these protozoa utilize a special pathway that is absent from the mammalian host (Opperdoes and Borst, 1976). The application of glycerol together with salicylhydroxamic acid completely inhibits the further growth and survival of the trypanosomes in the blood of the host (Clarkson and Brohn, 1976).

2. Design of Receptor-Blocking Agents

The recognition that there are surface receptors on the erythrocyte to which the malaria merozoite attaches opens the way to the blocking of these receptors either by immunological or chemotherapeutic means. Until the chemical nature of these receptors is identified there is much to be gained by empirical study of the action of available drugs in blocking the penetration of merozoites into erythrocytes, using already available *in vitro* methods for maintaining the parasites and host cells.

The precise role of the histidine-rich protein in the rhoptries of the merozoite (Kilejian and Jensen, 1977) in the attachment to and penetration of new host erythrocytes has yet to be defined. However, in the meantime, the observation by Warhurst and Thomas (1975a) that mepacrine is concentrated in the rhoptries suggests that the interaction of antimalarials with the rhoptry contents also may be a fruitful avenue to explore *in vitro*.

3. Design of Lysosomotropic Agents

Recent investigations on the targetting of antiprotozoal agents against intracellular parasites support the suggestion by Trouet *et al.* (1977) that drugs should be designed aimed at exploiting the fact that certain compounds are selectively concentrated in lysosomes or can be modified in various ways so that they become lysosomotropic. Three groups, for example, have recently reported that organic antimonials are far more effective leishmanicidal agents when they are incorporated into liposomes, which are rapidly taken up by the macrophages in which *Leishmania donovani* develops, than when they are given alone in the classic manner (Black *et al.*, 1977; New *et al.*, 1978; Alving *et al.*, 1978). Since the exoerythrocytic stages of *Plasmodium* inhibit hepatocytes which are very rich in lysosomes, it seems possible that compounds could be directed at these parasites by ensuring their concentration in the host cells. On the other hand, experience with chloroquine indicates that the situation is not as simple as this, since chloroquine, like mepacrine, *is* in fact concentrated in hepatocytes, but neither drug is effective against the tissue schizonts. It is not yet known, however, whether these compounds are in fact present at a high concentration within hepatic schizonts, or for that matter whether they would have any effect on these stages even if they were present in them at a sufficiently high concentration.

As for the intraerythrocytic stages, it may be doubted whether the use of lysosomotropic agents would be of any value against parasites that live in cells that have few or no lysosomes. Indeed, there exists already a mechanism by which certain drugs, e.g., chloroquine, are highly concentrated in such intraerythrocytic parasites, although to date the precise nature of the high-affinity binding sites remains unidentified. Nevertheless it is theoretically possible to design liposome carriers that could blend with erythrocytes and perhaps, in this way, deliver an antimalarial agent to those that are parasitized.

E. Prevention of Drug Resistance

Almost the only way that has been discovered so far to slow down the rate at which malaria parasites become resistant to antimalarial drugs is either to limit their use or to use drug combinations (Peters, 1974b). So far the only successful ones in practical use are potentiating combinations of sulfonamides or sulfones and antifols. However, it is by no means unlikely that other fundamentally different potentiating pairs may be found. One such pair, the mechanism of which has not yet been adequately explored, is that exemplified by the combination of menoctone and cycloguanil, which Peters (1970b) demonstrated to have marked potentiating blood schizontocidal action against *P. berghei* in mice.

The urgent need to protect new compounds such as mefloquine *before* they are released for use on a wide scale has been stressed by a number of writers (e.g., Peters *et al.,* 1977b; Rieckmann *et al.,* 1974; Glew *et al.,* 1978). Even if compounds are not found that potentiate with this drug, it may be possible, by the judicious selection of a second compound, to minimize the rate at which malaria parasites become resistant to it. Peters *et al.* (1977b), for example, were able to achieve this experimentally by administering a sulfonamide or pyrimethamine or primaquine together with mefloquine. In no case were the drug pairs more than additive in their action. Primaquine with its potent gametocytocidal action appears to be a logical "mate" to consider for mefloquine, but it would clearly be necessary before using such a mixture in man to ensure that the two compounds do not potentiate each other's toxicity to the host. It will be recalled that another 8-aminoquinoline, pamaquine, was long ago found to potentiate the mammalian toxicity of mepacrine.

Probably the most important way to prevent the emergence of drug-resistant malaria is to remember the fundamental principle that any single method of controlling malaria, be it by chemotherapy, insecticide control of vectors, source reduction of vectors, immunization against malaria parasites, or whatever other means are devised, is highly unlikely to elminate the disease completely. In the future any concerted attack on malaria must exploit *all* available methods if real success in freeing man from this phoenixlike pestilence is to succeed.

ACKNOWLEDGMENTS

Original research of the writer to which reference has been made in this chapter has been supported by grants from the World Health Organization, the Medical Research Council of Great Britain, the U.S. Army Research and Development Command, and various pharmaceutical companies. The writer is particularly indebted to his former staff in the Department of Parasitology, Liverpool School of Tropical Medicine, to research students, past and present, for many years of fruitful collaborative research, and to colleagues at the Walter Reed Army Institute of Research for supplying numerous interesting compounds and invaluable dialogue. The manuscript was meticulously typed by Mrs. D. Steedman. Some of the illustrations were kindly provided by their original authors, and others were prepared by Mr. J. Brady and his staff at the Liverpool School of Tropical Medicine.

REFERENCES

Aikawa, M., and Beaudoin, R. L. (1968). Studies on nuclear division of a malarial parasite under pyrimethamine treatment. *J. Cell Biol.* **39**, 749–754.

Alving, A. S., Craige, B., Pullman, T. N., Whorton, C. M., Jones, R., and Eichelberger, L. (1948). Procedures used at Statesville Penitentiary for the testing of potential antimalarial agents. *J. Clin. Invest.* **27**, Suppl., 2–5.

Alving, C. R., Steck, E. A., Hanson, W. L., Loizeuaux, P. S., Chapman, W. L., and Waits, V. B. (1978). Improved therapy of experimental leishmaniasis by use of a liposome-encapsulated antimonial drug. *Life Sci.* **22**, 1021–1026.

Anonymous (1778). "The London Practice of Physic," 3rd ed., p. 34. G. Robinson, R. Baldwin, and J. Bew, London.

Anonymous (1927). "Malaria and Quinine." Bureau for Increasing the Use of Quinine, Amsterdam.

Bass, C. C., and Johns, F. M. (1912). The cultivation of malarial plasmodia (*Plasmodium vivax* and *Plasmodium falciparum*) in vitro. *J. Exp. Med.* **16**, 567–579.

Beale, G. H., Carter, R., and Walliker, D. (1978). Genetics. *In* "Rodent Malaria" (R. Killick-Kendrick and W. Peters, eds.), pp. 213–245. Academic Press, New York.

Beaudoin, R. L., and Aikawa, M. (1968). Primaquine-induced changes in morphology of exoerythrocytic stages of malaria. *Science* **160**, 1233–1234.

Beaudoin, R. L., Strome, C. P. A., and Clutter, W. E. (1969). A tissue culture system for the study of drug action against the tissue phase of malaria. *Mil. Med.* **134**, 979–983.

Beaudoin, R. L., Strome, C. P. A., and Clutter, W. G. (1974). Cultivation of avian malaria parasites in mammalian liver cells. *Exp. Parasitol.* **36**, 355–359.

Bishop, A. (1958). An analysis of the development of resistance to metachloridine in clones of *Plasmodium gallinaceum*. *Parasitology* **48**, 210–234.

Bishop, A. (1959). The production of drug resistance in clones of *Plasmodium gallinaceum*. *Proc. Int. Congr. Trop. Med. Malar., 6th, 1958* Vol. 7, pp. 86–90.

Bishop, A. (1962). An analysis of the development of resistance to proguanil and pyrimethamine in *Plasmodium gallinaceum*. *Parasitology* **52**, 495–518.

Black, C. D. V., Watson, G. J., and Ward, R. J. (1977). The use of Pentostam liposomes in the chemotherapy of experimental leishmaniasis. *Trans. R. Soc. Trop. Med. Hyg.* **71**, 550–552.

Black, R. H. (1946). The effect of antimalarial drugs on *Plasmodium falciparum* (New Guinea strains) developing *in vitro. Trans. R. Soc. Trop. Med. Hyg.* **40**, 163–170.

Black, R. H. (1973). Malaria in the Australian army in South Vietnam: Successful use of a proguanil-dapsone combination for chemoprophylaxis of chloroquine-resistant falciparum malaria. *Med. J. Aus.* **1**, 1265–1270.

Black, R. H., Bruce-Chwatt, L. J., Canfield, C. J., Clyde, D. F., Peters, W., and Wernsdorfer, W. (1980). "Manual on the Chemotherapy of Malaria." WHO, Geneva.

Brossi, A., Uskokovic, M., Gutzwiller, J., Krettli, A. U., and Brener, Z. (1971). Antimalarial activity of natural, racemic and unnatural dihydroquinone, dihydroquinidine and their various racemic analogs in mice infected with *Plasmodium berghei. Experientia* **27**, 1100–1101.

Bryson, V., and Szybalski, W. (1955). Microbial drug resistance. *Adv. Genet.* **7**, 1–46.

Burgess, R. W., and Young, M. D. (1959). The development of pyrimethamine resistance by *Plasmodium falciparum. Bull. W. H. O.* **20**, 37–46.

Canfield, C. J., Alstatt, L. B., and Elliott, V. B. (1970). An *in vitro* system for screening potential antimalarial drugs. *Am. J. Trop. Med. Hyg.* **19**, 905–909.

Canfield, C. J., and Rozman, R. S. (1974). Clinical testing of new antimalarial compounds. *Bull. W. H. O.* **50**, 203-212.

Carter, R. (1973). Enzyme variation in *Plasmodium berghei* and *Plasmodium vinckei. Parasitology* **66**, 297-307.

Center for Disease Control (1978). Chemoprophylaxis of malaria. *Morbid. Mortal. Wkly. Rep., Suppl.* **27**, 81-90.

Chance, M. L., Warhurst, D. C., Baggaley, V. C., and Peters, W. (1972). Preparation and characterisation of DNA from rodent malarias. *Trans. R. Soc. Trop. Med. Hyg.* **66**, 3-4.

Chance, M. L., Momen, H., Warhurst, D. C., and Peters, W. (1978). The chemotherapy of rodent malaria. XXIX. DNA relationships within the subgenus *Plasmodium (Vinckeia). Ann. Trop. Med. Parasitol.* **72**, 13-22.

Clarkson, A. B., and Brohn, F. H. (1976). Trypanosomiasis: An approach to chemotherapy by the inhibition of carbohydrate metabolism. *Science* **194**, 204-206.

Clyde, D. F. (1974). Treatment of drug-resistant malaria in man. *Bull. W. H. O.* **50**, 243-249.

Clyde, D. F., and McCarthy, V. C. (1977). Radical cure of Chesson strain vivax malaria in man by 7, not 14, days of treatment with primaquine. *Am. J. Trop. Med. Hyg.* **26**, 562-563.

Clyde, D. F., McCarthy, V. C., and Miller, R. M. (1974). Inactivity of RC-12 as a causal prophylactic and relapse inhibitor of *Plasmodium vivax* in man. *Trans. R. Soc. Trop. Med. Hyg.* **68**, 167-168.

Clyde, D. F., McCarthy, V. C., Miller, R. M., and Hornick, R. B. (1976). Suppressive activity of mefloquine in sporozoite-induced human malaria. *Antimicrob. Agents & Chemother.* **9**, 384-386.

Coatney, G. R. (1963). Pitfalls in a discovery: The chronicle of chloroquine. *Am. J. Trop. Med. Hyg.* **12**, 121-128.

Coatney, G. R., Cooper, W. C., Young, M. D., and McLendon, S. B. (1947). Studies in human malaria. I. The protective action of sulfadiazine and sulfapyrazine against sporozoite induced falciparum malaria. *Am. J. Hyg.* **46**, 84-104.

Coatney, G. R., Cooper, W. C., Eddy, N. B., and Greenberg, J. (1953). Survey of antimalarial agents. Chemotherapy of *Plasmodium gallinaceum* infections: toxicity, correlation of structure and action. *U.S., Public Health Serv., Public Health Monogr.* **9.**

Coatney, G. R., Collins, W. E., Warren, McW., and Contacos, P. G. (1971). "The Primate Malarias". US Govt. Printing Office, Washington, D.C.

Contacos, P. G., Coatney, G. R., Collins, W. E., Briesch, P. E., and Jeter, M. H. (1973). Five day primaquine therapy—An evaluation of radical curative activity against vivax malaria infection. *Am. J. Trop. Med. Hyg.* **22**, 693-695.

Contacos, P. G., Collins, W. E., Chin, W., Jeter, M. H., and Briesch, P. E. (1974). Combined chloroquine-primaquine therapy against vivax malaria. *Am. J. Trop. Med. Hyg.* **23**, 310-312.

Cook, M. K. (1958). The development of a pyrimethamine-resistant line of toxoplasma under *in vitro* conditions. *Am. J. Trop. Med. Hyg.* **7**, 400-402.

Covell, G., Coatney, G. R., Field, J. W., and Jaswant Singh (1955). Chemotherapy of malaria. *W.H.O. Monogr. Ser.* **27.**

Davey, D. G. (1946a). The use of avian malaria for the discovery of drugs effective in the treatment and prevention of human malaria. I. Drugs for clinical treatment and clinical prophylaxis. *Ann. Trop. Med. Parasitol.* **40**, 52-73.

Davey, D. G. (1946b). The use of avian amalaria for the discovery of drugs effective in the treatment and prevention of human malaria. II. Drugs for causal prophylaxis and radical cure of the chemotherapy of the exoerythrocytic forms. *Ann. Trop. Med. Parasitol.* **40**, 453-471.

Davidson, D. E., Johnsen, D. O., Tanticharoenyos, P., Hickman, R. L., and Kinnamon, K. E. (1976). Evaluating new antimalarial drugs against trophozoite induced *Plasmodium cynomolgi* malaria in rhesus monkeys. *Am. J. Trop. Med. Hyg.* **25**, 26-33.

Davidson, M. W., Griggs, B. G., Boykin, D. W., and Wilson, W. D. (1975). Mefloquine, a clinically useful quinolinemethanol antimalarial which does not significantly bind to DNA. *Nature (London)* **254**, 632–634.

Davies, E. E., Warhurst, D. C., and Peters, W. (1975). The chemotherapy of rodent malaria. XXI. Action of quinine and WR 122,455 (a 9-phenanthrene methanol) on the fine structure of *Plasmodium berghei* in mouse blood. *Ann. Trop. Med. Parasitol.* **69**, 147–155.

Davis, A. G., Huff, C. G., and Palmer, T. T. (1966). Procedures for maximum production of exoerythrocytic stages of *Plasmodium fallax* in tissue culture. *Exp. Parasitol.* **19**, 1–8.

Dempwolff, O. (1904). Bericht uber eine Malaria-Expedition nach Deutsche-Neu Guinea. *Z. Hyg. Infektionskr.* **47**, 81–132.

Diggens, S. M. (1970). 1. Single step production of pyrimethamine-resistant *P. berghei*. 2. Cloning erythrocytic stages of *P. berghei*. *Trans. R. Soc. Trop. Med. Hyg.* **64**, 9–10.

Diggens, S. M., Gutteridge, W. E., and Trigg, P. I. (1970). Altered dihydrofolate reductase associated with a pyrimethamine-resistant *Plasmodium berghei* produced in a single step. *Nature (London)* **228**, 579–580.

Doberstyn, E. B., Hall, A. P., Vetvutanapibul, K., and Sonkom, P. (1976). Single-dose therapy of falciparum malaria using pyrimethamine in combination with diformyldapsone or sulfadoxine. *Am. J. Trop. Med. Hyg.* **25**, 14–19.

Einheber, A., Palmer, D. M., and Aikawa, M. (1976). *Plasmodium berghei:* Phase contrast and electron microscopical evidence that certain antimalarials can both inhibit and reverse pigment clumping caused by chloroquine. *Exp. Parasitol.* **40**, 52–61.

Elslager, E. F., and Thompson, P. E. (1964). Repository antimalarial drugs. *Rep. 9th Med. Chem. Symp. Am. Chem. Soc.,* 6a–6z.

Fairley, N. H. (1945). Chemotherapeutic suppression and prophylaxis in malaria: An experimental investigation undertaken by medical research teams in Australia. *Trans. R. Soc. Trop. Med. Hyg.* **38**, 311–355.

Falco, E. A., Goodwin, L. G., Hitchings, G. H., Rollo, I. M., and Russell, P. B. (1951). 2:4-Diaminopyrimidines—A new series of antimalarials. *Br. J. Pharmacol. Chemother.* **6**, 185–200.

Ferone, R. (1970). Dihydrofolate reductase from pyrimethamine-resistant *Plasmodium berghei*. *J. Biol. Chem.* **245**, 850–854.

Ferone, R., Burchall, J. J., and Hitchings, G. B. (1969). *Plasmodium berghei* dihydrofolate reductase: Isolation, properties, and inhibition by antifolates. *Mol. Pharmacol.* **5**, 49–59.

Findlay, G. M. (1951). "Recent Advances in Chemotherapy," 3rd ed., Vol. 2. Churchill, London.

Fink, E. (1974). Assessment of causal prophylactic activity in *Plasmodium berghei yoelii* and its value for the development of new antimalarial drugs. *Bull. W. H. O.* **50**, 213–222.

Fink, E., and Dann, O. (1967). Eine Weiterentwicklung des Roehl-Test zur Prufung von Malariamitteln an *Plasmodium cathemerium* beim Kanarienvogel durch intravenose Verabreichung. *Z. Tropenmed. Parasitol.* **18**, 466–474.

Fink, E., and Kretschmar, W. (1970). Chemotherapeutische Wirkung von Standard-Malariamitteln in einem vereinfachten Prufverfahren an der *Plasmodium vinckei*-Infektion der NMRI-Maus. *Z. Tropenmed. Parasitol.* **21**, 167–181.

Fink, E., Nickel, P., and Dann, O. (1970). Neue gegen Malaria Wirksame 6-Amino-chinoline. *Arzneim. Forsch.* **20**, 1775–1777.

Fitch, C. D. (1969). Chloroquine resistance in malaria, a deficiency of chloroquine binding. *Proc. Natl. Acad. Sci. U.S.A.* **64**, 1181–1187.

Fitch, C. D., Chevli, R., and Gonzalez, Y. (1974). Chloroquine accumulation by erythrocytes: A latent capability. *Life Sci.* **14**, 2441–2446.

Fulton, J. D., and Grant, P. T. (1956). The sulphur requirements of the erythrocytic form of *Plasmodium knowlesi*. *Biochem. J.* **63**, 274–282.

Garnham, P. C. C. (1966). "Malaria Parasites and Other Haemosporidia." Blackwell, Oxford.

Garnham, P. C. C. (1977). The continuing mystery of relapses in malaria. *Protozool. Abstr.* **1**, 1–12.

Garrod, L. P., and O'Grady, F. (1971). "Antibiotic and Chemotherapy," 3rd ed. Livingstone, Edinburgh.

Gerberg, E. J. (1971). Evaluation of antimalarial compounds in mosquito test systems. *Trans. R. Soc. Trop. Med. Hyg.* **65**, 358–363.

Gerberg, E. J., Richard, L. T., and Poole, J. B. (1966). Standardized feeding of *Aedes aegypti* (L.) mosquitoes on *Plasmodium gallinaceum* Brumpt-infected chicks for mass screening of antimalarial drugs. *Mosq. News* **26**, 359–363.

Glew, R. H., Collins, W. E., and Miller, L. H. (1978). Selection of increased quinine resistance in *Plasmodium falciparum* in *Aotus* monkeys. *Am. J. Trop. Med. Hyg.* **27**, 9–13.

Goodman, L. S., and Gilman, A., eds. (1970). "The Pharmacological Basis of Therapeutics," 4th ed. Macmillan, New York.

Goodwin, L. G. (1949). Response of *Plasmodium berghei* to antimalarial drugs. *Nature (London)* **164**, 1133.

Greenberg, J. (1956). Differences in virulence between parent B1 strain of *Plasmodium gallinaceum* and substrains made resistant to pyrimethamine and metachloridine. *Am. J. Trop. Med. Hyg.* **5**, 377.

Greenberg, J., and Trembley, H. L. (1954). The apparent transfer of pyrimethamine resistance from the B1 strain of *Plasmodium gallinaceum* to the M strain. *J. Parasitol.* **40**, 667–672.

Gregory, K. G., and Peters, W. (1970). The chemotherapy of rodent malaria. IX. Causal prophylaxis. Part I. A method for demonstrating drug action on exoerythrocytic stages. *Ann. Trop. Med. Parasitol.* **64**, 15–24.

Guerra, F. (1977a). The introduction of cinchona in the treatment of malaria. Part 1. *J. Trop. Med. Hyg.* **80**, 112–118.

Guerra, F. (1977b). Theintroduction of chinchona in the treatment of malaria. Part 2. *J. Trop. Med. Hyg.* **80**, 135–139.

Guttman, P., and Ehrlich, P. (1891). Ueber die Wirkung des Methylenblau bei Malaria. *Berl. Klin. Wochenschr.* **28**, 953–956.

Hahn, F. E., O'Brien, R. L., Ciak, J., Allison, J. L., and Olenick, J. G. (1966). Studies on modes of action of chloroquine, quinacrine and quinine and on chloroquine resistance. *Mil. Med.* **131**, Suppl., 1071–1089.

Hall, A. P. (1976). The treatment of malaria. *Br. Med. J.* **1**, 323–328.

Hall, A. P. (1977). Sequential treatment with quinine and mefloquine or quinine and pyrimethamine-sulfadoxine for falciparum malaria. *Br. Med. J.* **1**, 1626–1628.

Hawking, F. (1963). History of chemotherapy. *Exp. Chemother.* **1**, 2.

Hawking, F. (1966). Chloroquine resistance in *Plasmodium berghei*. *Am. J. Trop. Med. Hyg.* **15**, 287–293.

Hayes, D. E., and Ward, R. A. (1977). Sporozoite transmission of falciparum malaria (Burma-Thau. strain) from man to *Aotus* monkey. *Am. J. Trop. Med. Hyg.* **26**, 184–185.

Haynes, J. D., Diggs, C. L., Hines, F. A., and Desjardins, R. E. (1976). Culture of human malaria parasites, *Plasmodium falciparum*. *Nature (London)* **263**, 767–769.

Hill, J. (1950). The schizontocidal effect of some antimalarials against *Plasmodium berghei*. *Ann. Trop. Med. Parasitol.* **44**, 291–297.

Hill, J. (1975). The activity of some antibiotics and long-acting compounds against the tissue stages of *Plasmodium berghei*. *Ann. Trop. Med. Parasitol.* **69**, 421–427.

Homewood, C. A., Warhurst, D. C., Peters, W., and Baggaley, V. C. (1972a). Lysosomes, pH, and the antimalarial action of chloroquine. *Nature (London)* **235**, 50–52.

Homewood, C. A., Warhurst, D. C., Peters, W., and Baggaley, V. C. (1972b). Electron transport in intraerythrocytic *Plasmodium berghei*. *Proc. Helminthol. Soc. Wash.* **39**, Suppl., 382–386.

Howells, R. E., Peters, W., and Fullard, J. (1970). The chemotherapy of rodent malaria. XIII. Fine structural changes observed in the erythrocytic stages of *Plasmodium berghei berghei* following exposure to primaquine and menoctone. *Ann. Trop. Med. Parasitol.* **64**, 203–207.

Howells, R. E., Peters, W., and Homewood, C. A. (1972). Physiological adaptability of malaria parasites. *In* "Comparative Biochemistry of Parasites" (H. Van den Bossche, ed.), pp. 235–246. Academic Press, New York.

James, R. (1749). "A Dissertation on Fevers and Inflammatory Distempers," 2nd ed. J. Newbury, London.

Jacobs, R. L., Alling, D. W. and Cantrell, W. F. (1963) An evaluation of antimalarial combinations against *Plasmodium berghei* in the mouse. *J. Parasitol.* **49**, 920–925.

Jaswant Singh, Nair, C. P., and Ray, A. P. (1954). Studies on Nuri strain of *P. knowlesi*. V. Acquired resistance to pyrimethamine. *Indian J. Malar.* **8**, 187–195.

Kilejian, A., and Jensen, J. B. (1977). A histidine-rich protein from *Plasmodium falciparum* and its interaction with membranes. *Bull. W. H. O.* **55**, 191–197.

Killick-Kendrick, R., and Peters, W., eds. (1978). "Rodent Malaria." Academic Press, New York.

Kopanaris, P. (1911). Die Wirkung von Chinin, Salvarsan und Atoxyl auf die Proteosoma- (*Plasmodium praecox*) Infektion des Kanarienvogels. *Arch. Schiffs- Trop.-Hyg.* **15**, 586–596.

Kretschmar, W. (1965). The effects of stress and diet on resistance to *Plasmodium berghei* and malarial immunity in the mouse. *Ann. Soc. Belge Med. Trop.* **45**, 325–344.

Ladda, R. (1966). Morphologic observations on the effect of antimalarial agents on the erythrocytic forms of *Plasmodium berghei in vitro*. *Mil. Med.* **131**, Suppl., 993–1008.

Landau, I., Boulard, Y., Miltgen, F., and Le Bail, O. (1975). Rechutes sanguines et modifications de la schizogonie pré-érythrocytaire de *Plasmodium yoelii* sous l'action de l'éthionine. *C. R. Hebd. Séances Acad. Sci., Sér. D* **280**, 2285–2288.

Landau, I., Miltgen, F., Yap, L.-F., and Bain, O. (1976). Hepatocystis de Malaisie. I. Redéscription d'*Hepatocystis malayensis* Field et Edeson 1950, parasite de Sciuridae. *Ann. Parasitol. Hum. Comp.* **51**, 271–286.

Laser, H. (1946). A method of testing the antimalarial properties of compounds *in vitro*. *Nature (London)* **157**, 301.

Laser, H., Kemp, P., Miller, N., Lander, D., and Klein, R. (1975). Malaria, quinine and red cell lysis. *Parasitology* **71**, 167–181.

Laveran, A. (1893). "Paludism." New Sydenham Society, London.

Lelijveld, J., and Kortmann, H. (1970). The eosin colour test of Dill and Glazko: A simple field test to detect chloroquine in urine. *Bull. W. H. O.* **42**, 477–479.

Macomber, P. B., Sprinz, H., and Tousimis, A. J. (1967). Morphological effects of chloroquine on *Plasmodium berghei* in mice. *Nature (London)* **214**, 937–939.

McCormick, G. J., and Canfield, C. J. (1972). *In vitro* evaluation of antimalarial drug combinations. *Proc. Helminthol. Soc. Wash.* **39**, Suppl., 292–297.

McCormick, G. J., Canfield, C. J., and Willet, G. P. (1974). *In vitro* antimalarial activity of nucleic acid precursor analogues in the simian malaria *Plasmodium knowlesi*. *Antimicrob. Agents & Chemother.* **6**, 16–21.

Maegraith, B. G., Deegan, T., and Sherwood-Jones, E. (1952). Suppression of malaria (*P. berghei*) by milk. *Br. Med. J.* **2**, 1382–1384.

Merkli, B., and Peters, W. (1976). A comparison of two different methods for the selection of primaquine resistance in *Plasmodium berghei berghei*. *Ann. Trop. Med. Parasitol.* **70**, 473–474.

Miller, L. H. (1977). Hypothesis on the mechanism of erythrocyte invasion by malaria merozoites. *Bull. W. H. O.* **55**, 157–162.

Miller, L. H., and Carter, R. (1976). Innate resistance in malaria. *Exp. Parasitol.* **40**, 132–146.

Miller, L. H., Wyler, D. J., Glew, R. H., Collins, W. E., and Contacos, P. G. (1974). Sensitivity of four Central American strains of *Plasmodium vivax* to primaquine. *Am. J. Trop. Med. Hyg.* **23,** 309–310.

Morgan, S. (1974). The genetics of malaria parasites: Studies on pyrimethamine resistance. Ph.D. Thesis, Edinburgh University.

Most, H., and Montuori, W. A. (1975). Rodent systems (*Plasmodium berghei-Anopheles stephensi*) for screening compounds for potential causal prophylaxis. *Am. J. Trop. Med. Hyg.* **24,** 179–182.

Most, H., Nussenzweig, R. S., Vanderberg, J., Herman, R., and Yoeli, M. (1966). Susceptibility of genetically standardised (JAX) mouse strains to sporozoite-and blood-induced *Plasmodium berghei* infections. *Mil. Med.* **131,** Suppl., 915–918.

Most, H., Herman, R., and Schoenfeld, C. (1967). Chemotherapy of sporozoite- and blood-induced *Plasmodium berghei* infections with selected antimalarial agents. *Am. J. Trop. Med. Hyg.* **16,** 572–575.

New, R. R. C., Chance, M. L., Thomas, S. C., and Peters, W. (1978). Antileishmanial activity of antimonials entrapped in liposomes. *Nature (London)* **272,** 55–56.

Nodiff, E. A., Tanabe, K., Seyfriend, C., Matsuura, S., Kondo, Y., Chen, E. H., and Tyagi, M. P. (1971). Antimalarial phenanthrene aminoalcohols. 1. Fluorine-containing 3- and 6-substituted 9-phenanthrenemethanols. *J. Med. Chem.* **14,** 921–925.

Oelshlegel, F. J., and Brewer, G. J. (1975). Parasitism and the red blood cell. *In* "The Red Blood Cell" (D. MacN. Surgenor, ed.), 2nd ed., Vol. 2, pp. 1263–1302. Academic Press, New York.

Ohnmacht, C. J., Patel, A. R., and Lutz, R. E. (1971). Antimalarials. 7. Bis(trifluoromethyl)-*a*-(2-piperidyl)-4-quinolinemethanols. *J. Med. Chem.* **14,** 926–928.

Omar, M. S., and Collins, W. E.)1974). Studies on the antimalarial effects of RC-12 and WR 14,997 on the development of *Plasmodium cynomolgi* in mosquitoes and rhesus monkeys. *Am. J. Trop. Med. Hyg.* **23,** 339–349.

Omar, M. S., Collins, W. E., and Contacos, P. G. (1973). Gametocytocidal and sporontocidal effects of antimalarial drugs on malaria parasites. I. Effect of single and multiple doses of primaquine on *Plasmodium cynomolgi*. *Exp. Parasitol.* **34,** 229–241.

Omar, M. S., Collins, W. E., and Contacos, P. G. (1974). Gametocytocidal and sporontocidal effects of antimalarial drugs on malaria parasites. II. Action of the folic reductase inhibitors, chlorguanide, and pyrimethamine against *Plasmodium cynomolgi*. *Exp. Parasitol.* **36,** 167–177.

Opperdoes, F. R., and Borst, P. (1976). The effect of salicylhydroxamic acid on the glycerol-3-phosphate oxidase (GPO) of *Trypanosoma brucei:* Its influence on a *T. brucei* model infection and the intracellular localization of GPO. *In* "Biochemistry of Parasites and Host-parasite Relationships" (H. Van den Bossche, ed.), pp. 509–517. North-Holland Publ., Amsterdam.

Osdene, T. S., Russell, P. B., and Rane, L. (1967). 2,4,7-Triamino-6-ortho-substituted arylpteridines: A new series of potent antimalarial agents. *J. Med. Chem.* **10,** 431–434.

Pearlman, E. J., Thiemanun, W., and Castaneda, B. F. (1975). Chemosuppressive field trials in Thailand. II. The suppression of *Plasmodium falciparum* and *Plasmodium vivax* parasitaemias by a diformlyldapsone-pyrimethamine combination. *Am. J. Trop. Med. Hyg.* **24,** 901–909.

Pelletier, P. J., and Caventou, J. B. (1820). Recherche chimiques sur les quinquinas. *Ann. Chim. Phys.* **15,** 289–318 and 337–365.

Peters, W. (1965a). Drug resistance in *Plasmodium berghei* Vincke and Lips, 1948. I. Chloroquine resistance. *Exp. Parasitol.* **17,** 80–89.

Peters, W. (1965b). Morphological and physiological variations in chloroquine-resistant *Plasmodium berghei,* Vincke and Lips, 1948. *Ann. Soc. Belge Med. Trop.* **45,** 365–368.

Peters, W. (1968a). The chemotherapy of rodent malaria. V. Dynamics of drug resistance. Part I. Methods for studying the acquisition and loss of resistance to chloroquine by *Plasmodium berghei*. *Ann. Trop. Med. Parasitol.* **62,** 277–287.

Peters, W. (1968b). The chemotherapy of rodent malaria. VII. The action of some sulphonamides alone or with folic reductase inhibitors against malaria vectors and parasites. Part 2. Schizontocidal action in the albino mouse. *Ann. Trop. Med. Parasitol.* **62,** 488–494.

Peters, W. 1970a). "Chemotherapy and Drug Resistance in Malaria," Academic Press, New York.

Peters, W. (1970b). A new type of antimalarial drug potentiation. *Trans. R. Soc. Trop. Med. Hyg.* **64,** 462–464.

Peters, W. (1974a). Recent advances in antimalarial chemotherapy and drug resistance. *Adv. Parasitol.* **12,** 69–114.

Peters, W. (1974b). Prevention of drug resistance in rodent malaria by the use of drug mixtures. *Bull. W. H. O.* **51,** 379–383.

Peters, W., and Howells, R. E. (1978). Chemotherapy, *In* "Rodent Malaria" R. Killick-Kendrick, and W. Peters, eds., pp. 345–391. Academic Press, New York.

Peters, W., Portus, J. H., and Robinson, B. L. (1973). The chemotherapy of rodent malaria. XVII. Dynamics of drug resistance. Part 3: Influence of drug combinations on the development of resistance to chloroquine in *P. berghei. Ann. Trop. Med. Parasitol.* **67,** 143–154.

Peters, W., Portus, J. H., and Robinson, B. L. (1975a). The chemotherapy of rodent malaria. XXII. The value of drug-resistant strains of *P. berghei* in screening for blood schizontocidal activity. *Ann. Trop. Med. Parasitol.* **69,** 155–171.

Peters, W., Davies, E. E., and Robinson, B. L. (1975b). The chemotherapy of rodent malaria. XXIII. Causal prophylaxis. Part II. Practical experience with *Plasmodium yoelii nigeriensis* in drug screening. *Ann. Trop. Med. Parasitol.* **69,** 311–328.

Peters, W., Howells, R. E., Portus, J. H., Robinson, B. L., Thomas, S. C., and Warhurst, D. C. (1977a). The chemotherapy of rodent malaria. XXVII. Studies on mefloquine (WR 142,490). *Ann. Trop. Med. Parasitol.* **71,** 407–418.

Peters, W., Portus, J. H., and Robinson, B. L. (1977b). The chemotherapy of rodent malaria. XXVIII. The development of resistance to mefloquine (WR 142,490). *Ann. Trop. Med. Parasitol.* **71,** 419–427.

Peters, W., Chance, M. L., Lissner, R., Momen, H., and Warhurst, D. C. (1978). The chemotherapy of rodent malaria. XXX. The enigmas of the "NS lines" of *P. berghei. Ann. Trop. Med. Parasitol.* **72,** 23–36.

Polett, H. (1966). *In vitro* cultivation of erythrocytic forms of *Plasmodium knowlesi* and *Plasmodium berghei. Mil. Med.* **131,** Suppl., 1026–1031.

Porter, M., and Peters, W. (1976). The chemotherapy of rodent malaria. XXV. Antimalarial activity of WR 122,455 (a 9-phenanthrenemethanol) *in vivo* and *in vitro. Ann. Trop. Med. Parasitol.* **70,** 259–270.

Powell, R. D., and Berglund, E. M. (1974). Effects of chloroquine upon the maturation of asexual erythrocytic forms of *Plasmodium vivax in vitro. Am. J. Trop. Med. Hyg.* **23,** 1007–1014.

Powers, K. G., Aikawa, M., and Nugent, K. M. (1976). *Plasmodium knowlesi:* Morphology and course of infection in rhesus monkeys treated with clindamycin and its *N*-demethyl-4'-pentyl analog. *Exp. Parasitol.* **40,** 13–24.

Ramakrishnan, S. P., and Satya Prakash (1961). A note on the rapid selection of primaquine-resistant strain of *Plasmodium knowlesi* in *Macaca mulatta. Bull. Natnl. Soc. India Malar.* **9,** 261–265.

Ramakrishnan, S. P., Satya Prakash, and Sen Gupta, G. P. (1956). Studies on *Plasmodium berghei,* Vincke and Lips, 1948. XXIII. Isolation of and observations on a "milk-resistant" strain. *Indian J. Malar.* **10,** 175–182.

Ramakrishnan, S. P., Basu, P. C., Singh, H., and Singh, N. (1962). Studies on the toxicity and action of diaminodiphenylsulphone (DDS) in avian and simian malaria. *Bull. W. H. O.* **27,** 213–221.

Ramkaran, A. E., and Peters, W. (1969a). Infectivity of chloroquine resistant *Plasmodium berghei* to *Anopheles stephensi* enhanced by chloroquine. *Nature (London)* **223,** 635–636.

Ramkaran, A. E., and Peters, W. (1969b). The chemotherapy of rodent malaria. VIII. The action of some sulphonamides alone or with folic reductase inhibitors. Part 3. The action of sulphormethoxine and pyrimethamine on the sporogonic stages. *Ann. Trop. Med. Parasitol.* **63,** 449–454.

Rane, L., and Rane, D. S. (1972). A screening procedure, based on mortality, with sporozoite-induced *Plasmodium gallinaceum* malaria in chicks. *Proc. Helminthol. Soc. Wash.* **39,** Spec. Issue, 283–287.

Richards, W. H. G. (1966). Antimalarial activity of sulphonamides and a sulphone, singly and in combination with pyrimethamine against drug resistant and normal strains of laboratory plasmodia. *Nature (London)* **212,** 1494–1495.

Richards, W. H. G., and Maples, B. K. (1979). Studies on *Plasmodium falciparum* in continuous cultivation. I. The effect of chloroquine and pyrimethamine on parasite growth and viability. *Ann. Trop. Med. Parasitol.* **73,** 99–108.

Richards, W. H. G., and Williams, S. G. (1973). Malaria studies *in vitro.* II. The measurement of drug activities using leucocyte-free blood-dilution cultures of *Plasmodium berghei* and ^{3}H-leucine. *Ann. Trop. Med. Parasitol.* **67,** 179–190.

Richards, W. H. G., and Williams, S. G. (1975). Malaria studies *in vitro.* III. The protein synthesising activity of *Plasmodium falciparum in vitro* after drug treatment *in vivo. Ann. Trop. Med. Parasitol.* **69,** 135–140.

Richardson, A. P., Hewitt, R. I., Seager, L. D., Brooke, M. M., Martin, F., and Maddux, H. (1946). Chemotherapy of *Plasmodium knowlesi* infections in *Macaca mulatta* monkeys. *J. Pharmacol.* **87,** 203–213.

Rieckmann, K. H. (1971). Determination of the drug-sensitivity of *Plasmodium falciparum. J. Am. Med. Assoc.* **217,** 573–578.

Rieckmann, K. H., McNamara, J. V., Frischer, H., Stockert, T. A., Carson, P. E., and Powell, R. D. (1968a). Gametocytocidal and sporontocidal effects of primaquine and of sulfadiazine with pyrimethamine in a chloroquine-resistant strain of *Plasmodium falciparum. Bull. W. H. O.* **38,** 625–632.

Rieckmann, K. H., McNamara, J. V., Frischer, H., Stockert, T. A., Carson, P. E., and Powells, R. D. (1968b). Effects of chloroquine, quinine, and cycloguanil upon maturation of asexual erythrocytic forms of two strains of *Plasmodium falciparum in vitro. Am. J. Trop. Med. Hyg.* **17,** 661–671.

Rieckmann, K. H., Trenholme, G. M., Williams, R. L., Carson, P. E., Frischer, H., and Desjardins, R. E. (1974). Prophylactic activity of mefloquine hydrochloride (WR 142,490) in drug-resistant malaria. *Bull. W. H. O.* **51,** 375–377.

Rieckmann, K. H., Campbell, G. H., Sax, L. J., and Mrema, J. E. (1978). Drug sensitivity of *Plasmodium falciparum:* An *in vitro* technique. *Lancet* **1,** 22–23.

Rosario, V. E. (1976). Genetics of chloroquine resistance in malaria parasites. *Nature (London)* **261,** 585–586.

Rosario, V. E., Walliker, D., Hall, R., and Beale, G. H. (1978). Persistence of drug-resistant malaria parasites. *Lancet* **1,** 185–187.

Rossan, R. N., and Baerg, D. C. (1975). Development of falciparum malaria in a Panamanian subspecies of howler monkey. *Am. J. Trop. Med. Hyg.* **24,** 1035–1036.

Rossan, R. N., Young, M. D., and Baerg, D. C. (1975). Chemotherapy of *Plasmodium vivax* in *Saimiri* and *Aotus* models. *Am. J. Trop. Med. Hyg.* **24,** 168–173.

Schmidt, L. H. (1973). Infections with *Plasmodium falciparum* and *Plasmodium vivax* in the owl monkey—Model systems for basic biological and chemotherapeutic studies. *Trans. R. Soc. Trop. Med. Hyg.* **67,** 446–474.

Schmidt, L. H., and Genther, C. S. (1953). The antimalarial properties of 2,4-diamino-5-*p*-chlorophenyl-6-ethylpyrimidine (Daraprim). *J. Pharmacol. Exp. Ther.* **107,** 61–91.

Schmidt, L. H., Rossan, R. N., Fradkin, R., Woods, J., Schulemann, W., and Kratz, L. (1966). Studies on the antimalarial activity of 1,2-dimethoxy-4-(bidiethylaminoethyl)-amino-5-bromo-benzene. *Bull. W. H. O.* **34,** 783–788.

Schneider, J. (1954). *Plasmodium berghei* and chemotherapy. *Indian J. Malar.* **8,** 275–279.

Schneider, J., Decourt, Ph., and Montézin, G. (1949). Sur l'utilisation d'un nouveau plasmodium (*Pl. berghei*) pour l'étude et la recherche de médicaments antipaludiques. *Bull. Soc. Pathol. Exot.* **42,** 449–452.

Schmidt, L. H., Cramer, D. V., Rossan, R. N., and Harrison, J. (1977a). The characteristics of *Plasmodium cynomolgi* infections in various Old World primates. *Am. J. Trop. Med. Hyg.* **26,** 356–372.

Schmidt, L. H., Fradkin, R., Harrison, J., and Rossan, R. N. (1977b). Differences in the virulence of *Plasmodium knowlesi* for *Macaca irus (fascicularis)* of Philippine and Malayan origins. *Am. J. Trop. Med. Hyg.* **26,** 612–622.

Schmidt, L. H., Fradkin, R., Vaughan, D., and Rasco, J. (1977c). Radical cure of infections with *Plasmodium cynomolgi:* A function of total 8-aminoquinoline dose. *Am. J. Trop. Med. Hyg.* **26,** 1116–1128.

Schnitzer, R. J., and Hawking, F., eds. (1963). "Experimental Chemotherapy," Vol. 1. Academic Press, New York.

Sen Gupta, G. P., Sharma, G. K., Singh, H., and Ray, A. P. (1958). Screening of compound 377C54 against avian and simian malaria parasites. *Indian J. Malar.* **12,** 247–252.

Smalley, M. E., and Sinden, R. E. (1977). *Plasmodium falciparum* gametocytes: Their longevity and infectivity. *Parasitology* **74,** 1–8.

Strube, R. E. (1975). The search for new antimalarial drugs. *J. Trop. Med. Hyg.* **78,** 171–185.

Sucharit, P., Harinasuta, T., Chongsuphajaisiddhi, T., Tongprasroeth, N., and Kasemsuth, R. (1977). *In vivo* and *in vitro* studies of chloroquine-resistant malaria in Thailand. *Ann. Trop. Med. Parasitol.* **71,** 401–405.

Terzian, L. A. (1947). A method for screening antimalarial drugs in the mosquito host. *Science* **106,** 449–450.

Thompson, P. E., and Werbel, L. M. (1972). "Antimalarial Agents: Chemistry and Pharmacology." Academic Press, New York.

Thompson, P. E., Olszewski, B., Bayles, A. and Waitz, J. A. (1967). Relations among antimalarial drugs. Results of studies with cycloguanil-, sulfone-, or chloroquine-resistant *Plasmodium berghei* in mice. *Am. J. Trop. Med. Hyg.* **16,** 133–145.

Thurston, J. P. (1950). The action of antimalarial drugs in mice infected with *Plasmodium berghei*. *Br. J. Pharmacol. Chemother.* **5,** 409–416.

Thurston, J. P. (1951). Morphological changes in *Plasmodium berghei* following proguanil, sulphadiazine and mepacrine therapy. *Trans. R. Soc. Trop. Med. Hyg.* **44,** 703–706.

Thurston, J. P. (1953). The chemotherapy of *Plasmodium berghei*. I. Resistance to drugs. *Parasitology* **43,** 246–252.

Trager, W., and Jensen, J. B. (1976). Human malaria parasites in continuous culture. *Science* **193,** 673–675.

Trenholme, G. M., Williams, R. L. Desjardins, R. E., Frischer, H., Carson, P. E., and Rieckmann, K. H. (1975). Mefloquine (WR 142,490) in the treatment of human malaria. *Science* **190,** 792–794.

Trigg, P. I. (1975). "Parasite Cultivation in Relation to Research on the Chemotherapy of Malaria," Cyclostyled Doc. TDR/CM/WP/75.6. WHO, Geneva.

Trigg, P. I., and Gutteridge, W. E. (1971). A minimal medium for the growth of *Plasmodium knowlesi* in dilution cultures. *Parasitology* **62,** 113–123.

Trouet, A., Deprez de Campeneere, D., Maldague, P., Jadin, J. M., and Van Hoof, F. (1977). The concept of lysosomotropic chemotherapy: Applications to neoplastic and parasitic diseases. *Drug. Des. Adverse React. Proc. Alfred Benzon Symp. 10th, 1977* p. 77–88.

Vivona, S., Brewer, G. J., Conrad, M., and Alving, A. S. (1961). The concurrent weekly administration of chloroquine and primaquine for the prevention of Korean vivax malaria. *Bull. W. H. O.* **25**, 267–269.

von Wasiliewski, T. (1908). "Studien und Mikrophotogramme zur Kentniss der Pathogenen Protozoen," Vol. 2, pp. 131–133. Barth, Leipzig.

Wan, Y.-P., Porter, T. R., and Folkers, K. (1974). Antimalarial quinones for prophylaxis based on a rationale of inhibition of electron transfer in *Plasmodium. Proc. Natl. Acad. Sci. U.S.A.* **71**, 952–956.

Warhurst, D. C. (1973). Chemotherapeutic agents and malaria research *In* "Chemotherapeutic Agents in the Study of Parasites" (A. E. R. Taylor and R. Muller, eds.), pp. 1–28. Blackwell, Oxford.

Warhurst, D. C., and Folwell, R. O. (1968). Measurement of the growth rate of the erythrocytic stages of *Plasmodium berghei* and comparisons of the potency of inocula after various treatments. *Ann. Trop. Med. Parasitol.* **62**, 349–360.

Warhurst, D. C., and Hockley, D. J. (1967). Mode of action of chloroquine on *Plasmodium berghei* and *P. cynomolgi. Nature (London)* **214**, 935–936.

Warhurst, D. C., and Thomas, S. C. (1975a). Localisation of mepacrine in *Plasmodium berghei* and *Plasmodium falciparum* by fluorescence microscopy. *Ann. Trop. Med. Parasitol.* **69**, 417–420.

Warhurst, D. C., and Thomas, S. C. (1975b). Pharmacology of the malaria parasite—A study of dose-response relationships in chloroquine-induced autophagic vacuole formation in *Plasmodium berghei. Biochem. Pharmacol.* **24**, 2047–2056.

Warhurst, D. C., and Thomas, S. C. (1978). The chemotherapy of rodent malaria. XXXI. The effect of some metabolic inhibitors upon chloroquine-induced pigment clumping (CIPC) in *Plasmodium berghei. Ann. Trop. Med. Parasitol.* **72**, 203–211.

Warhurst, D. C., and Williamson, J. (1970). Ribonucleic acid from *Plasmodium knowlesi* before and after chloroquine treatment. *Chem. Biol. Interact.* **2**, 89–106.

Warhurst, D. C., Homewood, C. A., Peters, W., and Baggaley, V. C. (1972). Pigment changes in *Plasmodium berghei* as indicators of activity and mode of action of antimalarial drugs. *Proc. Helminthol. Soc. Wash.* **39**, Suppl., 271–278.

Warhurst, D. C., Homewood, C. A., and Baggaley, V. C. (1974). The chemotherapy of rodent malaria, XX. Autophagic vacuole formation in *Plasmodium berghei in vitro. Ann. Trop. Med. Parasitol.* **68**, 265–281.

Wellde, B. T., Briggs, N. T., and Sudan, E. H. (1966). Susceptibility to *Plasmodium berghei:* Parasitological, biochemical and haematological studies in laboratory and wild mammals. *Mil. Med.* **131**, Suppl., 859–869.

Wilkinson, R. N., Noeypatimanondh, S., and Gould, D. J. (1976). Infectivity of falciparum patients for anopheline mosquitoes before and after chloroquine treatment. *Trans. R. Soc. Trop. Med. Hyg.* **70**, 306–307.

Williams, S. G., and Richards, W. H. G. (1973). Malaria studies *in vitro*. I. Techniques for the preparation and culture of leucocyte-free blood-dilution cultures of *Plasmodia. Ann. Trop. Med. Parasitol.* **67**, 169–178.

Wise, D. L., McCormick, G. J., Willet, G. P., and Anderson, L. C. (1976). Sustained release of an antimalarial drug using a copolymer of glycolic/lactic acid. *Life Sci.* **19**, 867–874.

Wiselogle, F. Y. (1946). "A Survey of Antimalarial Drugs 1941–1945," Vol. 1. Edwards, Ann Arbor, Michigan.

Woodward, R. B., and Doering, W. E. (1944). The total synthesis of quinine. *J. Am. Chem. Soc.* **66**, 849.

World Health Organization (1973). Chemotherapy of malaria and resistance to antimalarials. Report of a WHO Scientific Group. *W. H. O., Tech. Rep. Ser.* **529.**

World Health Organization (1976a). "Report of the First Meeting of the Task Force on Chemotherapy of Malaria," Cyclostyled Rep. No. TDR/CM/76.1. WHO, Geneva.

World Health Organization (1976b). Information on the world malaria situation. *Wkly. Epidemiol. Rec.* **51,** 181–200.

Yoeli, M., Upmanis, R. S., and Most, H. (1969). Drug resistance transfer among rodent plasmodia. I. Acquisition of resistance to pyrimethamine by a drug-sensitive strain of *P. berghei* in the course of its concomitant development with a pyrimethamine resistant *P. vinckei* strain. *Parasitology* **59,** 429–447.

Young, M. D. (1957). Resistance of *Plasmodium malariae* to pyrimethamine (Daraprim). *Am. J. Trop. Med. Hyg.* **6,** 621–624.

Young, M. D., and Burgess, R. W. (1959). Pyrimethamine resistance in *Plasmodium vivax* malaria. *Bull. W. H. O.* **20,** 27–36.

Young, M. D., Baerg, D. C., and Rossan, R. N. (1975). Parasitological review: Experimental monkey hosts for human plasmodia. *Exp. Parasitol.* **38,** 136–152.

Morphology of Plasmodia

Masamichi Aikawa and Thomas M. Seed

I. INTRODUCTION

In both clinical and basic malaria research a thorough understanding of parasite morphology is often a critical prerequisite and of fundamental importance. For example, the taxonomy and systematics of plasmodia are based largely on morphology. Since Laveran's initial observations in 1880 of the intraerythrocytic ameboid movement of human malarial parasites in wet mount preparations, a mass of morphological information has accumulated. The early morphological work was affected by the limited resolving power of the optical light microscope and failed to reveal many of the detailed structures now known to exist. The first reports of electron microscopy of malarial parasites were published in 1942 by the German workers Emmel, Jakob, and Golz (1942 a and b). Since these pioneering efforts, numerous studies have been reported which have greatly advanced our knowledge of the biology of plasmodia.

Malaria, Vol. 1
Copyright © 1980 by Academic Press, Inc.
All rights of reproduction in any form reserved.
ISBN 0-12-426101-9

In this chapter we will describe the salient morphological features of malarial parasites as a group. Major morphological differences among mammalian, avian, and reptilian species will be emphasized, based on correlated light and electron microscopic observations. The subject of host–parasite interaction with induced host cell alterations will be discussed in the context of ultrastructural features.

II. HISTORICAL REVIEW

The observation by early nineteenth century researchers (e.g., Shutz in 1846 and Merkel in 1847) of malarial pigment within internal organs of diseased individuals at autopsy provided the first real clue to the etiology of malaria. Laveran (1880) is credited with the first morphological description of malarial parasites as distinct microbial entities. Following the introduction, in 1892, of the improved Romanowsky's method for staining blood smears, various new species were identified, as were various stages of the complex life cycle. Since then numerous types of preparative techniques and optical equipment have been successfully utilized, which have provided new information concerning the parasite's biology. Although the electron microscope had been utilized as early as 1942 to examine blood forms (Emmel *et al.*, 1942 a and b), it was not until 1956 that Fulton and Flewett applied electron microscopy to the study of the relation of *Plasmodium berghei* and *P. knowlesi* to host erythrocytes and reported that they were intracellular. Their finding was accepted by most investigators and, for the most part, ended the long-standing controversy as to whether or not malarial parasites were indeed intracellular or simply surface-adherent. Fulton and Flewett's (1956) pioneering study of malarial parasites by the thin-sectioning technique was limited, however, by the lack of structural detail obtained; this was due to technical difficulties encountered in specimen preparation. As the technology of electron microscopy has improved, more detailed electron microscopic observations of various species of malarial parasites have been made. Recently, scanning electron microscopy has become available for the study of parasites, making possible three-dimensional views with high magnification. Freeze-fracture and etching techniques have also extended our knowledge of the morphology of the parasites.

III. MORPHOLOGY, TAXONOMY, AND SYSTEMATICS

Parasite morphology and species of host infected are primary attributes considered in the taxonomy of plasmodia. The principal tool used in assigning morphological descriptors has been the light microscope. Over the past two decades, however, the electron microscope with its capacity for detecting fine-structural detail has become increasingly important to the systematist. The existence of common fine-structural features in the various stages of the many plasmodial species has certainly strengthened the concept of *Plasmodium* as a distinct taxonomic group with characteristic morphological affinities.

There are basically three classes of morphological descriptors: direct, indirect, and relative characteristics. Direct characteristics include the parasite's size and shape, number of nuclei, number and size of progeny, pigmentation (form, color, density, and distribution), ratio of asexual to sexual forms, and gametocyte sex ratio. Indirect characteristics include the nature and extent of host cell distortion and the degree and site of parasite involvement in tissues. The useful relative characteristics include host cell type, intracellular parasite position, and relative size (Ayala, 1977). The sum of these features, when properly analyzed, can aid in the assigning of a given parasite to a characteristic phenotype for either speciation or for general biological experimental consideration. Other factors such as the ecological niche of the host, the blood picture, and the stage of infection influence parasite morphology and fine structure. These factors must be considered along with the morphological differences related to species, host, and life cycle stage.

Based to a large extent on morphological considerations, malarial parasites are taxonomically placed within the suborder Haemosporina, which is characterized by a heteroxenous life cycle with schizogony occurring in the vertebrate host and sporogony in the invertebrate. Distinctive characteristics of the sexual forms identify, in part, the suborder. Microgametocytes produce, singularly and independently, flagellated microgametes. Sexual fusion of gametes yields a motile zygote. Sporozoites of plasmodia, in spite of their name, do not reside in spores and are not sporelike, but naked. They are, however, the stages which correspond to the forms found in spores in the monoxenous coccidia.

There are about 12 subgenera of plasmodia; 3 occur in mammals, 4 in birds, and 5 in reptiles. Garnham (1966) recognized 3 reptilian subgenera, whereas Ayala (1978) suggested a grouping of 5. The mammalian subgenera are *Plasmodium, Laverania,* and *Vinckeria.* The subgenus *Plasmodium* is morphologically characterized by round gametocytes and large exoerythrocytic schizonts. Host species are always primates above the lemuroid level (Garnham, 1966), like those of the *Laverania* plasmodia. The latter have distinctive elongate gametocytes and large exoerythrocytic schizonts. Vinckeria-type plasmodia are found in rodents and other lower mammals. These parasites have round gametocytes and small exoerythrocytic stages.

The avian subgenera include *Haemamoeba, Giovannolaia, Novyella,* and *Huffia.* Species having round gametocytes are grouped within the *Haemamoeba.* Species having elongate gametocytes and schizogony in primitive red cells are considered to belong to the subgenus *Huffia. Giovannolaia* species have elongate gametocytes, large asexual forms, and schizogony within well-differentiated red cells. Species of the *Novyella* group are similar to those of the *Giovannolaia* group; however, the asexual stages are relatively small.

There are considered to be five subgenera of reptilian malaria parasites (Ayala, 1978): *Carinamoeba* are characterized by tiny schizonts which produce approximately 4 merozoites. Gametocytes are large and round. The *Telfordi* group has larger schizonts, producing 6–15 merozoites. Gametocytes may be round, oval, or elliptical and are approximately equal in size to the host cell nuclei. Members of the *Tropiduri* group have still larger segmenters; 8–25 merozoites are produced. Gametocytes are considerably larger than the host cell nuclei. Host cells may include leukocytes as well as red cells. The fourth group, *Mexicanum*, has large schizonts which produce 8–30 merozoites. Gametocytes are generally large, round, and elongate. Like those of the *Tropiduri* group, parasites of this group will invade leukocytes. Members of the fifth group, the *Sauramoeba*, produce large numbers of merozoites ($\cong 100$) from massive, round, elongate schizonts. Gametocytes are also quite large and are round or elongate.

IV. LIGHT MICROSCOPY OF TYPE SPECIES

A. Mammalian Species

1. Primate Species

Garnham (1966) lists 20 species within the subgenus *Plasmodium*. Only 3 of these species infect humans (namely, *P. vivax, P. malariae,* and *P. ovale*). The others infect subhuman primates. Each can be readily identified by light microscopy in stained blood films and in combination with the clinical manifestations of the infection. *Plasmodium vivax* will serve as the type species. *Plasmodium vivax* infections are globally distributed, with the greatest incidence in temperate climates. It is not prevalent in areas where summer isotherms fall below 15°C as sporogony is inhibited at these lower temperatures (Coatney *et al.,* 1971), and infections by this organism are absent from West Africa—the indigenous black population appears highly refractory to this species (Young *et al.,* 1955; Coatney *et al.,* 1971). *Plasmodium* as a subgenus is characterized by a complex parasite life cycle involving a sexual and sporogonic mode of reproduction in the anopheline mosquito and an asexual reproductive mode involving two schizogonic cycles in the primate host. The first of these occurs in the parenchymal cells of the liver; massive numbers of merozoites (i.e., >10,000) are produced in successive generations. The second asexual cycle occurs in the blood. Intraerythrocytic growth forms ingest hemoglobin and deposit a pigmented by-product, hemozoin. Blood infection with *P. vivax* is seen approximately 8 days following sporozoite inoculation.

Characteristic features of *P. vivax* in its bloodstream phase include a preferential attack of reticulocytes, prominent stippling (Schüffner's dots), enlargement and loss of color of the infected red cell with growth of the parasite, and sluggish movement of the earliest intracellular forms followed by the development of progressively active ameboid growth forms. (A micrograph of an enlarged and stippled host cell infected with the primate malarial parasite *P. simium* is shown in Fig. 1.) After 36–42 hours of intracellular growth the large oval or horseshoe-shaped nucleus begins to divide, producing in four mitotic cycles a schizont with 16 nuclei. With cytoplasmic segmentation the typical "daisy" configuration (budding daughter cells surrounding a central mother residue) becomes apparent and occupies much of the enlarged (e.g., >10 μm), infected host cell.

The sexual forms of *P. vivax* are distinguishable by a compact, spherical appearance, a lack of ameboid movement, and a lack of cytoplasmic vacuoles. The macrogametocyte of *P. vivax* has a characteristic grayish-blue cytoplasm and a large granule-containing, pink nucleus which appears to comprise about one-half the area of the parasite. The sex ratio of the circulating gametocytes approaches two macrogametocytes per microgametocyte. The maturation time required for both these forms is approximately twice that of the sexual stages.

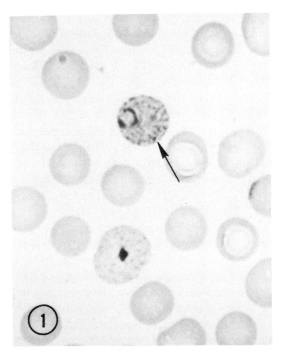

FIG. 1.   Light micrograph of rhesus erythrocytes infected with *P. simium*. Prominent stippling is seen in the erythrocyte cytoplasm (arrow). × 150.

Upon feeding of the susceptible anopheline mosquito on an infected individual and passage of mature gametocytes into its gut, the active sexual processes begin. The formation of the eight motile microgametes is an exceedingly exuberant process as observed in wet mount preparations by light microscopy. This is true not only for vivax-type parasites but for all malarial parasites. Pigment streams rapidly back and forth within the microgametocyte as points along its surface bulge out and retract with the sudden ejection at the surface of long hairlike fibers. Concomitantly, the nucleus begins to divide with newly formed chromatin condensates migrating into the bulbous surface regions. After cytoplasmic segmentation, the eight newly formed microgametes measure 20–25 μm; the microgametes of *P. vivax* appear somewhat more active than those of other species (Garnham, 1966). The total process of "exflagellation," as assessed *in vitro,* takes about 10 minutes. During this period the macrogamete sheds its host cell and awaits attachment by the microgamete to a discernible surface protrusion. At this point, the microgamete is drawn inside. Initially both nuclei can be seen, but in several hours the two fuse. The resultant zygote (i.e., the ookinete) is a pear-shaped organism (approximately 15 μm at its anterior and 22 μm at its posterior), exhibiting complex patterns of mobility including gliding, bending, and peristaltic contractions. One to two days following the blood meal, the formed ookinete penetrates the epithelium of the midgut. The encysted organism initiates a reduction division miotic cycle; two diploid chromosomes, one dot and one rod-shaped, line up at the equatorial plate at metaphase and migrate polarly at telophase, resulting in the production of two haploid nuclei (Bano, 1949). Further mitotic divisions occur. At this early stage (e.g., 3 days) the oocysts range from 11 to 14 μm in diameter; several days later (e.g., day 6) they are 20–30 μm; and finally when sporogony is complete, they are over 50 μm in diameter (Shute and Maryon, 1952). Oocyst growth and development are highly variable and dependent on a multitude of host relationships and environmental factors. Temperature is one critical factor; at 30°C complete oocyst maturation takes only 7–8 days. At 20°C, it takes 16 days, and at 17°C approximately 30 days. Below 15°C sporogony is totally blocked. Mature *P. vivax* oocysts yield 1000–10,000 sporozoites which are narrow and slender with pointed ends (the posterior end appears more pointed) and are, when wet, approximately 14 μm long. There appear to be several modes of sporozoite motility; these include wavelike constrictions and movement associated with posterior end secretions. By light microscopy, the centrally placed nucleus commonly appears segmented in this species. The stained mass at the anterior end is associated with specialized organelles of the anterior, involved in host cell penetration. At the time the mosquito bites, sporozoites are injected into the bloodstream, circulate for a short period ($\cong$ 1 hour), and enter the liver. Here they penetrate the parenchymal cells and begin an asexual growth cycle. This exoerythrocytic cycle, a prepatent period, lasts approximately 8 days in humans with *P. vivax* infection. Up to

10,000 infective merozoites are produced by each tissue schizont. Pockets of viable, but latent, organisms in the liver appear to be responsible for relapses of blood infection following quiescent periods. Tissue schizonts generally double in size from the fourth to the seventh day following sporozoite infection. The cytoplasm of early stages stains dark blue with some local granulation and contains large vacuoles with faint yellow globules. With maturity the vacuoles and cytoplasmic clumping disappear.

In contrast to other species, the exoerythrocytic stages of *P. vivax* at maturity fail to show any definite patterning of nuclei or cytoplasm; they assume an irregular sometimes hourglass or lobulated shape. Mature, oblong schizonts measure approximately 60×40 μm. Cytoplasm with dotlike structures condenses about the tightly packed segmented nuclei, which at this time are strongly Feulgen-positive. Secondary exoerythrocytic forms of *P. vivax* are morphologically similar to primary stages; this is in contrast to those of some other species such as *P. cynomolgi* whose secondary tissue schizonts appear to have distinctive crinkled surfaces (Garnham, 1966).

Plasmodium falciparum is the only species within the *Laverania* subgenus which infects humans. *Plasmodium reichenowi,* the second species in the group, is a parasite of the chimpanzee. Both species have strong biological and morphological similarities. There is a marked 48-hour period in the asexual growth cycle of the blood phase parasite. Clinically the infections are quite severe, producing a relatively high mortality rate. Distinctive subgeneric features include crescent-shaped gametocytes, very small ring stages with "ringapplique" patterns in multiple infections, an appreciable lack of parasite ameboidicity, asymmetric schizonts which produce 8–20 merozoites, and host cell stippling (Maurer's dots). The last-mentioned characteristic is related to parasite development and, in turn, is thought to be responsible for the phenomenon of "deep vascular schizogony" and the absence of the more mature forms in the peripheral blood. Exoerythrocytic tissue stages of *Laverania* type species differ from those of other *Plasmodium* type species (e.g., *P. ovale* and *P. vivax*) in that a massive single generation of merozoites is produced by primary schizonts. Exoerythrocytic stages are characterized by a pronounced tendency to lobate, i.e., to appear "misshapen" (Coatney *et al.,* 1971); the latter presumably is indicative of pseudocytomere and subsequent merozoite formation.

Morphological aspects of the cycle of *P. falciparum* in the insect are typical of those in other mammalian species. Four to six microgametes are produced during exflagellation, each measuring 16–25 μm in length (Garnham, 1966). The crescent-shaped macrogamete rounds up as it sheds the host red cell. The ookinete of *P. falciparum* is generally more slender than that of *P. vivax* and measures 11–13 μm in length (Garnham, 1966). In typical fashion, one end of the ookinete is truncated and the other rounded and more bulbous; the two poles appear light yellow and pink, respectively, in Giemsa-stained preparations. The nucleus is irregular in shape and slightly acentric. The cytoplasm is uneven, appearing pigmented and at times striated because of the presence of the anterior organelles. Oocyst development requires approximately 10 days; this varies, however, depending on the species of anopheline mosquito infected and on an assortment of environmental conditions. At maturity, oocyst diameters range from 8 to 60 μm (Shute and Maryon, 1952; Coatney *et al.*, 1971). The distribution of coarse, black pigment granules (10–20), in semicircular rows or chains, is somewhat characteristic of the species. The processes of nuclear division and cytoplasmic segmentation into sporoblastic islands are morphologically similar to those in other species. Sporozoites of *P. falciparum* are typical of those of mammalian-type species; i.e., they are long (10–12 μm) and slender (~0.8 μm wide) and often sickle-shaped. The oblong nucleus, ≅1.2 μm in length, is centrally positioned and extends the width of the body. The anterior end is generally more pointed than the posterior, and its cytoplasm more dense.

2. Rodent Species

The subgenus *Vinckeria* encompasses a rather heterogeneous group of malaria parasites. Members of the subgenus *Vinckeria* have as natural hosts a variety of lower mammals largely indigenous to the tropical forests of Africa. The biology of many of the *Vinckeria* species remains ill-defined. The malaria parasites of African murine rodents are certainly the best understood within the *Vinckeria* subgenus, since a number of species have been extensively utilized as laboratory models of human malaria. Four distinct species are recognized within this group: *P. berghei*, *P. yoelii*, *P. vinckei*, and *P. chabaudi*. Each of these except *P. berghei*, has several subspecies based mainly on morphological features of blood and exoerthryocytic parasites and on oocysts and sporozoites. The salient biological features of many of these species are described in the rather comprehensive review by Carter and Diggs (1977). *Plasmodium berghei*, as it infects white rats, mice, and hamsters, will be used here as the type species. The asexual cycle in the blood requires 22–25 hours and, in terms of the total parasite population, is asynchronous. In contrast, *P. vinckei* and *P. chabaudi* infections in laboratory mice are generally synchronous. Reticulocytes and immature red cells are preferentially infected. Host cell hypertrophy is common in infected reticulocytes, but less so when mature red cells are involved. With special stains slight stippling of infected cells can be demonstrated. Small, round forms, lacking vacuoles, develop into larger, round, vacuole-containing trophozoites. The morphology of malarial pigment varies depending on the cell type infected; i.e., fine black pigment granules are associated with infected reticulocytes, while larger brown aggregates are seen in the more mature, hemoglobinized red cell. Twelve to 18 merozoites are produced by mature schizonts. The morphology of the schizont, which can range from large and plump to small and ragged rosettes, and its merozoite yield are dependent, in part, on the host species and on whether the infection was sporozoite or blood-induced.

Gametocytes are large (8–9 μm) and spherical. Upon maturation the host cell is completely filled. The host cell always seems to be a mature erythrocyte. As is typical of other plasmodial species, the macrogametocyte's cytoplasm stains dark blue, there is a scattering of fine dark pigment granules, and the red nucleus which has a pink veil is pushed to one side. The microgametocyte, in contrast, stains a light steel gray. The differences between the microgametocyte and macrogametocyte are attributed to differences in ribosomal densities.

Exoerythrocytic stages are found exclusively in the liver and appear to be solely the product of sporozoite invasion. The primary growth and division cycle may be as short as 43 hours, resembling in this respect tissue stages of avian species. The initial exoerythrocytic body is round, measuring 13 μm, and usually contains multiple nuclei (two to five). At maturity the smooth-contoured schizont, having undergone rapid nuclear division and cytoplasmic segmentation, measures 24–28 μm and contains about 8000–20,000 small infective merozoites, each measuring approximately 1.5 μm. It is of interest that early trophic stages appear to lack functional cytostomes; pinocytosis has been suggested as the principal nutritional mechanism. Other characteristic structures such as microtubules and the pellicular labyrinth appear to be lacking as well (Desser *et al.*, 1972).

The cycle of *P. berghei* in the anopheline mosquito is similar to that of other mammalian species. Exflagellation is rapid, occurring in 10–15 minutes at 27°C. Four to eight microgametes are formed, each measuring 15 μm. Large numbers of sexual matings can occur as evidenced by the observation, at times, of massive numbers of ookinetes (e.g., 1000) in the gut. The ookinete is generally "banana-shaped" (10–12 μm) and has a slightly bulbous posterior. Oocyst development commonly occurs in 8 days, with meiotic division taking place after 48 hours. The mean diameter of fully mature oocytes under optimal conditions is 45 μm (Carter and Diggs, 1977). Bano (1959) has described four beadlike diploid chromosomes. Golden-brown pigment granules arranged in single or double curved lines are characteristic features. *Plasmodium berghei* sporozoites are of the typical mammalian type, i.e., very slender, often sickle-shaped, and 11–12 μm in length. In Giemsa-stained preparations the nucleus often appears segmented. In wet mounts, sporozoites move in a gliding, bending fashion. Certain rodent species have morphologically distinctive sporozoites (e.g., *P. chabaudi* sporozoites are less slender and have blunter ends).

B. Avian Species

The avian plasmodial subgenera effectively maintain a worldwide distribution through the migratory patterns of their many host species. There are about 25 species presently recognized (Seed and Manwell, 1977). This is, however, many fewer species than are recognized in the mammalian group. Some of the distinguishing characteristics of this major group are: the host red blood cell is nucleated; exoerythrocytic stages are found in mesodermal tissues and not in the liver; the primary tissue cycle occupies a minimum of three reproductive generations, with schizonts yielding less than 1000 merozoites each. Parasites produced in these generations are called cryptozoites, metacryptozoites, and phanerozoites, respectively.

The subgenus *Giovannolaia* is characterized by elongated gametocytes and moderate to large blood schizonts. There are approximately seven species found in game birds and two in passerine birds. *Plasmodium circumflexum* is a natural type species for the latter group. Distinguishing characteristics in its bloodstream phase include preferential invasion of immature erythrocytes with multiple invasion common, oval to elongate parasites lacking appreciable ameboidicity although pseudopodial processes are apparent, a polar clumping of hemozoin, and little distortion of the host cell nucleus. The gametocytes are large and elongate, curving about the host cell nucleus and often distorting it. Hemozoin is randomly scattered throughout the gametocyte's cytoplasm.

Species of the *Haemamoeba* subgenus infect both galliform (e.g., *P. gallinaceum, P. durae,* and *P. griffithei*) and passerine birds (e.g., *P. relictum, P. matutinum, P. cathemerium,* and *P. giovannolai*). *Plasmodium gallinaceum* infection of the domestic hen (*Gallus gallus*) serves as an appropriate example of the galliform group, since it has been used extensively as a laboratory model of human malaria. Young birds are generally more susceptible than mature birds; females are generally more severely infected than males, with shorter prepatent periods and higher parasitemias. Blood infections, which are moderately synchronous, are characterized by the presence of large numbers of merozoites, multiply infected erythrocytes, and enlargement of the host cell with nuclear displacement especially within gametocyte-infected cells. The parasite retains a spherical or oval shape (Fig. 2). Mature schizonts are approximately 8 μm in diameter and upon full maturation will yield 16–20 merozoites (Fig. 3). Black pigment with a golden luster remains aggregated near the center of the schizont. In sporozoite-induced infection the primary site of exoerythrocytic schizogony is in wandering macrophages of the skin, initially near the site where the mosquito took the blood meal. Several hundred elongate cryptozoites and metacryptozoites are produced by large schizonts in two successive generative cycles within a 72-hour period. Secondary sites of exoerythrocytic schizogony are established via the circulation in distant organs (e.g., spleen, lungs, and brain). Progeny observed from these secondary sites are called phanerozoites and have a distinctive morphology. A number of variations in the nature of the cytoplasmic division of the maturing schizont have been described (Huff *et al.,* 1960; Huff, 1969); all involve an apparent segmentation of cytoplasm into islands or pseudocytomeres during merozoite formation. There is considerable variation in size, in shape, and in the staining properties of tissue merozoites; the extreme variants have dark-blue cytoplasm with large bright-red nuclei or a lightly stain-

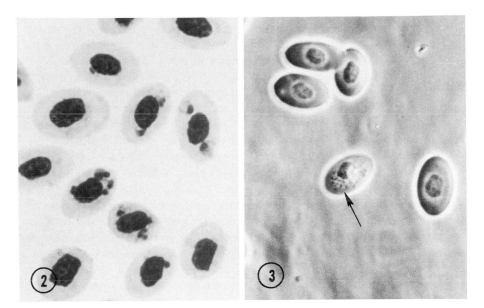

FIG. 2. Light micrograph of chicken erythrocytes infected with *P. gallinaceum*. Enlargement of host cells with nuclear displacement is prominent. ×150.

FIG. 3. Light micrograph of chicken erythrocytes with multiple merozoites (arrow). ×150.

ing cytoplasm and smaller nuclei. Exoerythrocytic merozoites are about 0.8 μm in diameter, which is not significantly different from merozoites of schizonts in blood cells (Huff, 1969). Phanerozoites, when viewed by combined cinemicrography–phase-contrast microscopy, are highly active forms (Huff *et al.*, 1960; Huff, 1969). They emerge explosively through the peripheral membrane of the schizont. The active movement of these newly born daughters is highlighted by a trailing, thin, rotating filament. Initially this filament was thought to be functional in host cell attachment and in subsequent cell penetration; however, this does not appear to be the case. The structure appears viscous, unstructured, and posteriorly located. Electron microscopic examination of phanerozoites has failed to reveal this structure, which is apparently lost during the specimen-processing steps. The material may have an immunological and chemotactic reactivity, since there appears to be a phanerozoite-induced response by wandering phagocytes which are potential host cells. Host cell penetration by phanerozoites is very rapid and is completed in a few seconds (Huff, 1969). Other features of living exoerythrocytic parasites were described by Huff and co-workers (1960; Huff, 1969) and included rather dramatic mitochondrial movements within trophozoites, typical protozoan-type nuclear division requiring approximately 24 minutes, and interior migration and posterior anchoring of the newly formed daughter cells to the mother bud residue during the terminal phases of pseudocytomere formation.

Immunity is rapidly gained in immunologically competent birds to the exoerythrocytic schizogony which occurs primarily within the cells of the reticuloendothelial cell system. This immunity confines the infection to the blood by limiting the duration and extent of secondary exoerythrocytic schizogony (Huff, 1969). In contrast to mammalian malaria parasites, avian blood parasites can reinitiate exoerythrocytic schizogony.

It has been reported that blood gametocytes arise directly from both exoerythrocytic and blood stage merozoites (Lumsden and Bertram, 1940; Huff, 1969). Mature gametocytes are generally spherical to oval in shape and range in size from 8 to 9 μm. The host cell nucleus is most often pushed to one end of the cell. The Romanowsky staining patterns are typical of those of most plasmodia; i.e., the macrogametocyte's cytoplasm is grayish blue, and the nucleus is light pink, irregular in shape, and polarly located; the microgametocyte's cytoplasm is faintly stained, and its nucleus is diffuse, having a single dense dot. Malarial pigment is found randomly scattered throughout the cytoplasm in both forms.

Once the blood meal has been taken and the pH, temperature, carbon dioxide concentration, etc., are appropriate, exflagellation ensues with the formation of eight flagellated microgametes, each 11–15 μm in length.

The newly formed *P. gallinaceum* zygotes are tiny 3-μm bodies speckled with black pigment; these transform into elongate ($\cong 16$ μm in length), often banana-shaped organisms which are slightly bulbous posteriorly. Mature ookinetes (at approximately 30 hours after a blood meal) have a single centrally placed or slightly anterior nucleus, associated vacuoles, and coarse granules, some of which appear crystalloid by electron microscopy. A thick, gelatinous surface material is associated with the ookinete's posterior, which resembles that on sporozoites.

Once the *P. gallinaceum* ookinete has penetrated the gut wall, apparently by direct passage through the epithelial cells of the peritrophic membrane, oocyst development begins. This occurs about 48 hours after a blood meal. Initially the oocyst is approximately 8 μm long and contains a single diploid nucleus and a scattering of black pigment granules which later become clumped and eventually obscured during the sporogonic process. Several hours later, the processes of reduction division occur as the two dot and two rodlike chromosomes polarly segregate, yielding a binucleate oocyst (Bano, 1959). After several mitotic cycles, multinucleated forms are seen in which the nuclei are generally peripherally arranged. With proper microenvironmental conditions, oocysts of *P. gallinaceum* grow to approximately four times their original size in 10 days at 25°C (Shute and Maryon, 1952). *Plasmodium gallinaceum* sporozoites are elongate, often bow-shaped organisms 0.7 μm in width and approximately 9–10 μm in length. They appear quite plump in comparison to the more slender sporozoites of the plasmodia of mammals. There is a centrally placed, slightly oblong nucleus which often is segmented. Anterior dense structures which are the apical organelle complex, may be clearly seen in stained preparations. A thick, trailing surface slime is often present at the sporozoite's posterior end. Although devoid of obvious locomotor organelles, sporozoites move with a slow, gliding, twisting motion.

Plasmodium relictum, which naturally infects a wide range of passerine birds, is a representative species of the *Haemamoeba* subgenus. Garnham (1966) lists about 140 avian species as natural hosts of *P. relictum.* Characteristic features include a fairly synchronous blood cycle, 30–36 hours in length and with peak segmentation occurring early in the morning. The small, compact trophozoites have little pigment and are only slightly ameboid. With intracellular growth and development there is significant displacement and distortion of the host cell nucleus. Mature schizonts segment and yield approximately 8–15 merozoites depending on the stage of infection and the host species. Gametocytes are generally large and spherical in shape and consistently displace the host cell nucleus.

Exoerythrocytic schizogony first occurs in the mesodermal cells of the skin, with several generative cycles occurring over approximately 3 days. Subsequently other organs such as the spleen, lung, and brain become infected; after about 4–5 days the blood becomes infected. Thirty-six hours after sporozoite infection the primary exoerythrocytic schizont, which infects a macrophage in the skin, is a small, round body (5–6 μm) with several nuclei. In Giemsa-stained sections they appear as vacuolated, dark-blue bodies. These primary segmenters produce approximately 30 small (2 μm), oval to elongate cryptozoites. Secondary exoerythrocytic parasites have an affinity for endothelial cells of such organs as the brain, liver, and spleen and have more strongly stained nuclei than the primary forms. Garnham (1966) and others also claim that the secondary forms are larger than the primary ones.

The sexual stages in the insect appear to be similar to those of other avian species. Microgametocytes yield approximately six microgametes under proper stimulation. The ookinete is a long, curved body with prominent vacuoles, an irregular nucleus, and large brown-black granules. Oocyst development begins 32 hours postfeeding. At 5 days the average oocyst is 18 μm in diameter, at 6 days 20 μm, and at 8 days 32 μm. Sporozoites are typically banana-shaped, are 14–16 μm in length, and have centrally placed nuclei.

The *Novyella* group is the third subgenus of avian malarial parasites. *Plasmodium vaughani* is the type species for this group; a natural host is the American robin in which the course of infection is generally short and seldom lethal. The blood phase parasites are small and have some ameboid activity. The schizogonic cycle is approximately 26 hours in length and has a low degree of synchrony. Irregularly shaped schizonts yield four to eight merozoites. There is a preferential invasion of immature erythrocytes. In contrast to *P. relictum, P.*

vaughani causes little host cell enlargement and minimal nuclear displacement. The gametocytes are elongated bodies, irregular in outline and vacuolated. The exoerythrocytic stages occur in the macrophages of the lung, bone marrow, spleen, and kidney. Schizonts are approximately 20 μm in diameter and yield approximately 50 merozoites with exceptionally large nuclei. Stages in the mosquito are not known.

The fourth subgenus is *Huffia* which has only two species, *P. elongatum* and *P. huffia.* Culex mosquitoes are the most likely vectors. Oocytes range in size from 15 to 36 μm at maturity. Sporozoites tend to be straighter than is normal for most bird malarias with one blunt end and the other more pointed. The primary exoerythrocytic cycle takes 9–12 days. During later exoerythrocytic generations there is invasion of the bone marrow and infection of free hemopoietic cells. In Giemsa-stained sections the parasites have bright-blue cytoplasm and cherry-red nuclei. Mature schizonts are approximately 11 μm in diameter and upon segmentation yield 20–30 merozoites which are typically elongated bodies with spherical nuclei. The infection in the blood is fairly synchronous and has a 24-hour cycle. *Plasmodium elongatum* are typically small parasites which rarely distort the host cell nucleus. They preferentially infect the more primitive hemopoietic cells. *Plasmodium huffia,* unlike *P. elongatum,* have an affinity for lymphoid elements as well as erythroid ones. Multiple infections are common. Young trophozoites are oval to elongate with ragged edges and appear more ameboid than those of many avian species. Typical rings are rare. Schizonts often appear fanlike, as the six newly formed nuclei are seen near the edge of the parasite, giving it a scalloped appearance. Gametocytes are distinctive in that they are found in mature red cells. They are strikingly elongate but do not envelope the host cell nucleus. Just beneath the limiting membrane is an irregular border which most likely corresponds to the peculiar surface complex of the gamont described with electron microscopy.

Because of the strong affinity these *Huffia* species exhibit for hemopoietic tissues, a characteristic they share with the reptilian species, it has been suggested that they are the most primitive of the avian plasmodia.

C. Reptilian Species

There is some debate concerning the number of reptilian subgenera. Garnham (1966) suggests two subgenera, namely, *Sauramoeba* characterized by large schizonts, and *Carinamoeba* with small schizonts. Ayala (1977) considers that there are an additional three subgenera: the *Telfordi, Tropiduri,* and *Mexicanum* groups, with intermediate-sized schizonts and other differentiating characteristics. Garnham (1966) further suggests that the single species found in snakes, *P. wenyonii,* should be separated taxonomically into a distinct subgenus,

Ophidiella. In contrast to avian and mammalian malaria parasites, reptilian parasites appear to lack fixed morphological traits, thus complicating the grouping of species into subgenera. The geographical distribution of reptilian species is quite unlike that of primate plasmodial species. Reptilian species are prevalent in the Americas, the East Indies, the Pacific islands, tropical Africa, and Australia. The distributions of the various species both within and among these geographical regions are quite restricted; this is in all probability due to the limited mobility of the host populations. The exception to this is *P. minasense (carinii)* which is found in several locales. The most common vertebrate hosts for these parasites are iguanids, aganids, and skinks (Garnham, 1966). The vectors for almost all these species are unknown, although the blood-sucking nocturnal Diptera (e.g., ceratopogonids, phlebotomids, and culicid mosquitoes) have been implicated. Like that of avian species, especially the *Huffia* species, exoerythrocytic schizogony occurs in both the fixed and wandering mesodermal tissues, and the exoerythrocytic parasites exhibit strong affinity for hemopoietic elements.

Species of the subgenus *Carinamoeba* have small schizonts which yield few merozoites and have round to oval gametocytes. The New World species *P. minasense* is a good example of the group. This species is, however, somewhat unique in that its geographical range is greater than that of other species. In natural hosts, infections are generally mild and highly synchronous (Garnham, 1966). Small rings (4 μm) transform into larger pleomorphic, often spindle-shaped growth forms which lack appreciable amounts of malarial pigment. As is characteristic of the *Carinamoeba* group, *P. minasense* has small (4–5 μm) fan-shaped schizonts which yield four pyriform merozoites each measuring 2 μm in length. Mature gametocytes are generally ovoid in shape and are approximately 8–9 μm in length. The macro- and microgametocytes have typical cytological characteristics. The host cell nucleus is only slightly displaced, if at all.

Species of the subgenus *Sauramoeba* (e.g., *P. diploglossi*) are easily identified by the very large schizonts they produce, which yield large numbers of daughter cells. Parasites of this subgenus have very large round or elongate gametocytes. *Plasmodium diploglossi* in its natural host, the American lizard, produces asynchronous blood infections. Because of the large size of the mature blood forms, there is marked swelling and deformity of the host cell and its nucleus. Small rings develop into large trophozoites which tend to curl around the host cell nucleus. Malarial pigment tends to aggregate polarly during schizogony. Upon completion of schizogony approximately 48 merozoites are formed. Gametocytes are also quite large and cause significant host cell distortion. The mature microgametocyte may completely encircle the host cell nucleus. It has a delicate nuclear network and a pale-staining cytoplasm. The macrogametocyte's nucleus and cytoplasm, in contrast, are much more dense.

The type species of the *Carinamoeba* and *Sauramoeba* subgenera are clearly distinguishable on the basis of the differences in schizont and gametocyte size. Many reptilian species have schizonts of intermediate size, however, making them difficult to place in either of these two groups. Ayala (1977) accordingly has suggested grouping of these intermediate-sized species into additional groups with distinguishable morphological characteristics, namely, *Telfori, Tropiduri,* and *Mexicanum.*

Plasmodia of the *Tropiduri* group are somewhat more variable in their morphology than plasmodia of the other reptilian groups. Schizonts of the *Tropiduri* group are larger than those in species of the *Telfordi* or *Carinamoeba* group; the patterns of segmentation vary from fan- to daisy-type configurations. The extent of host cell and nuclear distortion is highly variable, as is the host cell preference exhibited by the different species within this group. For example, in a number of the species (e.g., *P. mabuyi, P. tupinambi, P. modesta, P. simplex,* etc.) schizogony occurs predominantly, if not exclusively, in leukocytes (Ayala, 1977). Still other species appear to lack the characteristic traits which distinguish the *Plasmodium* genus itself, namely, production of the pigment hemozoin and the presence of schizonts as well as gametocytes in the circulating blood cells. Gametocytes are generally spherical to oval in shape and are slightly larger than the host cell nucleus. However, there are many exceptions to this; e.g., *P. acumination* has spindle-shaped gametocytes and *P. clelandi* has very large, elongated, hooked gametocytes. Such variability occurs within individual species and is probably a function of both intrinsic host factors and extrinsic factors such as environmental conditions.

Ayala (1977) places *P. mexicanum* within the *Tropiduri* group. This species has large ($\cong 8$ μm), round to oval schizonts which yield 8–25 elongate, fusiform merozoites. With *P. mexicanum,* as with all plasmodia of the saurian group, exoerythrocytic schizogony occurs in both the fixed mesoderm of the spleen, in the capillary endothelium, and in the hemopoietic elements.

The sporogonic cycle for most of the reptilian species, including those of the *Tropiduri* group, is unknown. Nocturnal, blood-sucking Diptera are the probable vectors. In the few reptilian species studied, the processes of microgametocyte exflagellation appear typical of other plasmodial species, with eight flagellated microgametes being formed within an hour after the blood meal. Ayala (1977) points out that ookinete penetration of the stomach in certain of the suspected dipteran vectors can be so extensive as to cause death. Sporogonic processes in *P. mexicanum* are typical of the genus. Initially a large sporoblast is formed by peripheralization of the nuclei, cytoplasmic infolding, and island formation, with eventual sporozoite formation. The mature oocytes of *P. mexicanum* in sandflies are 30–40 μm in diameter and contain about 1000 sporozoites (Ayala, 1977). Reptilian sporozoites, like their avian counterparts, are highly elongate, often banana-shaped organisms with centrally placed nuclei.

V. ULTRASTRUCTURAL FEATURES

Plasmodium species, as a group, share many common morphological and ultrastructural features. Structural differences do exist, however, especially among reptilian-, avian-, and mammalian-type parasites. Similarly, the various stages in the malarial parasite's life cycle exhibit both common and distinct patterns of structural organization.

A. Erythrocytic Stages

1. Merozoites

The merozoite is oval in shape, 1.5 μm in length, and 1 μm in diameter, possesses a nucleus and various cytoplasmic organelles, and is bounded by a pellicular complex (Figs. 4 and 5).

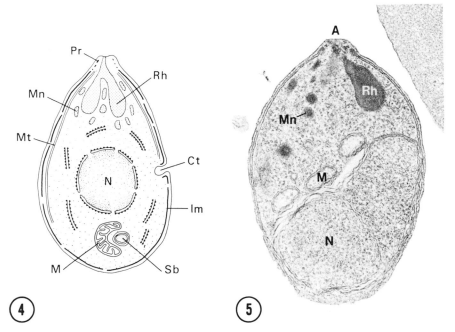

FIG. 4.   Schematic drawing of an erythrocytic merozoite. Ct, Cytostome; Im, inner membrane; M, mitochondria; Mn, micronemes; Mt, subpellicular microtubules; N, nucleus; Pr, polar rings; Rh, rhoptries; Sb, spherical body.

FIG. 5.   Electron micrograph of an erythrocytic merozoite of *P. knowlesi* showing the apical end (A), rhoptry (Rh), micronemes (Mn), nucleus (N), mitochondria (M), and surface coat. ×47,000.

The pellicle of the merozoite is composed of an outer and two closely aligned inner membranes (Aikawa, 1966; Ladda, 1969; Scalzi and Bahr, 1968; Seed *et al.*, 1973). The outer membrane, i.e., the plasma membrane, is about 7.5 nm thick. The inner membrane is about 15 nm thick and has fenestrations. Face-on, in negatively stained or freeze-cleaved preparations, this inner membrane appears labyrinthine (Aikawa, 1967; Seed *et al.*, 1971). This structure generally appears more prominent in avian parasites and less pronounced in those of mammalian species. Beneath this inner membrane, there is a row of subpellicular microtubules which originate from the distal polar ring of the apical complex and radiate posteriorly (Figs. 4 and 6). On the lateral side of the pellicle there is a circular structure called a cytostome through which ingestion of host cell cytoplasm may occur in the later stages (Fig. 7).

The cytostome of avian and reptilian parasites has an inner diameter of 170–200 nm. The cytostome of mammalian parasites is smaller than that of avian parasites, being only 60–100 nm in diameter (Aikawa *et al.*, 1966 a and b). The size of the cytostome appears to be correlated with the size of the food vacuole formed.

It has been suggested that the inner membrane and microtubular structure

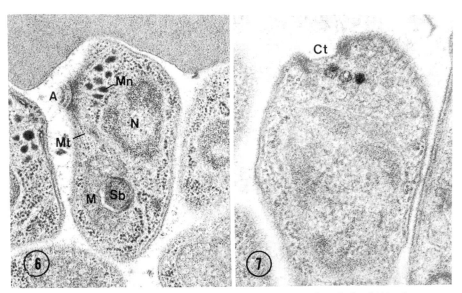

FIG. 6. An erythrocytic merozoite of *P. cathemerium* showing the apical end (A), micronemes (Mn), nucleus (N), mitochondrion (M), spherical body (Sb), and subpellicular microtubules (Mt). ×38,000. (Reproduced from Aikawa, 1977 with permission of the author and publisher.)

FIG. 7. An erythrocytic merozoite of *P. elongatum* showing a cytostome (Ct). ×51,000.

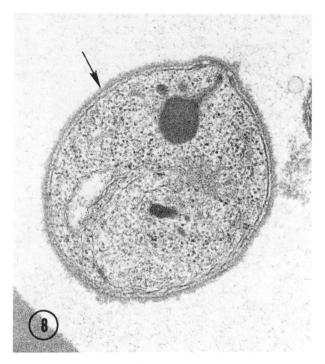

FIG. 8.   An erythrocytic merozoite of *P. knowlesi* after incubation with immune serum. Note the thick surface coat (arrow). ×45,000.

functions as a cytoskeleton, giving rigidity to the merozoite (Aikawa, 1966). The merozoite's outer membrane is covered with a surface coat ≅20 nm thick when the merozoite is outside the host cell (Fig. 5). The coat is electron-dense, compact, and fibrillar. It appears to be proteinaceous in nature, since it can be removed by trypsin (Miller *et al.*, 1975a). The surface coat does not appear to be present on schizont-derived merozoites located within intact erythrocytes; however, exteriorized merozoites and those situated within hemolyzed erythrocytes do exhibit a surface coat. It seems likely, therefore, that the coat is formed or at least increases in density when the merozoite interacts with substances within the plasma. Although the function of the surface coat is still not fully understood, it appears to play a role in the parasite's response to the immune reactions of the host (Fig. 8) (Miller *et al.*, 1975a; Brooks and Kreier, 1978).

The nucleus of the erythrocytic merozoite is a large, round, centrally located body. The chromatin is clumped at the periphery, and small, dense particles and fine fibrils are loosely scattered in the nucleoplasm. There is no report of the presence of distinct nucleoli in the erythrocytic merozoites of any species; the significance of this is not clear. Typically structured nuclear pores are present along the nuclear envelope.

The apical end of the erythrocytic merozoite is a truncated, cone-shaped projection demarcated by three polar rings (Fig. 5). Two electron-dense rhoptries and several micronemes are present in this region (Figs. 4 and 5). A ductule extends from each rhoptry and forms a common duct which extends to the tip of the apical end. The rhoptries and micronemes appear to play a role in the entry of malarial parasites into host cells (Kilejian, 1976). A detailed discussion of the function will be presented in Section VI,A.

Typical protozoan-type mitochondria are seen in the posterior portion of both avian and reptilian parasites (Fig. 6). They are composed of outer and inner membranes and microtubular cristae formed by invaginations of the inner membrane. Cristate mitochondria have also been observed in certain mammalian malarial parasites such as *P. falciparum, P. malariae, P. brasilianum, P. inui, P. vivas, P. cynomolgi,* and *P. berghei* (Sterling *et al.,* 1972). However, cristae are fewer in the mitochondria of mammalian parasites than in those of other parasites (Fig. 5). Some mammalian parasites lack structures that can be identified as mitochondria; instead, they have double-membrane-bounded structures considered to be equivalent to mitochondria. The evidence suggesting that these structures are equivalent to mitochondria comes from cytochemical studies that have shown them to contain cytochrome oxidase. Cytochemical studies have demonstrated succinic dehydrogenase activity in cristate mitochondria, whereas no such activity has been found in acristate mitochondria (Howells *et al.,* 1969). This suggests that malarial parasites with cristate mitochondria utilize a Krebs cycle, while it not clear whether the Krebs cycle is used by parasites with mitochondria without cristae.

A spherical body measuring about 310 nm in diameter is located close to the mitochondrion and is partially surrounded by it (Figs. 4 and 6). The matrix is granular and is bounded by several layered membranes. It has been suggested that the close association of the spherical body with the mitochondrion indicates that the spherical body is an energy reservoir (Aikawa, 1966). Mitochondria are known to be located near a readily available supply of substrates. Since the erythrocytic merozoite is motile, although sluggish, extra energy may be required for this movement.

Ribosomes are abundant in the merozoite cytoplasm, although little endoplasmic reticulum is observed. Golgi complexes are inconspicuous in erythrocytic merozoites.

2. Uninucleate Trophozoites

The fine structure of the erythrocytic trophozoites has been extensively studied by many investigators, because this form is more prevalent than the others in the blood samples of the malaria-infected host. Many species of malarial parasites have been studied by electron microscopy, but the most common subjects for study are *P. gallinaceum, P. berghei, P. falciparum, P. cynomolgi,* and *P. knowlesi.*

Merozoites can be seen by light microscopy to round up upon entry into a new red blood cell (Fig. 9). This phenomenon has been observed in detail by electron microscopy. The round-up process appears to be caused by the rapid degradation of the inner membrane and microtubules of the pellicular complex (Fig. 9) (Aikawa, 1966). After completion of the breakdown of these structures, the trophozoite is surrounded by only a single plasma membrane in addition to the parasitophorous vacuole membrane which originated from the host cell (Fig. 10). Apical end organelles such as polar rings, rhoptries, micronemes, and spherical bodies also break down.

The trophozoite becomes irregular in shape. This supports the supposition that the inner membrane and microtubules serve as a cytoskeleton. Some trophozoites, particularly those of primate parasites, show prominent ameboid movement. This ameboid activity produces tortuous extensions and invaginations of the parasite cytoplasm. Ring forms seen in the early stages of trophozoite development appear to result from these extensions of the cytoplasm (Fig. 10).

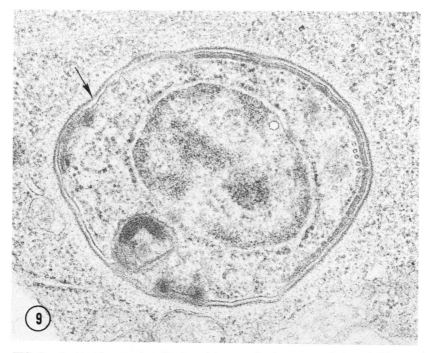

FIG. 9. A uninucleate trophozoite situated in a parasitophorous vacuole (arrow). The parasite has rounded up, and the organelles specific to the merozoite have started to break down. ×59,000. (Reproduced from Aikawa, *et al.,* 1967, with permission of the author and publisher.)

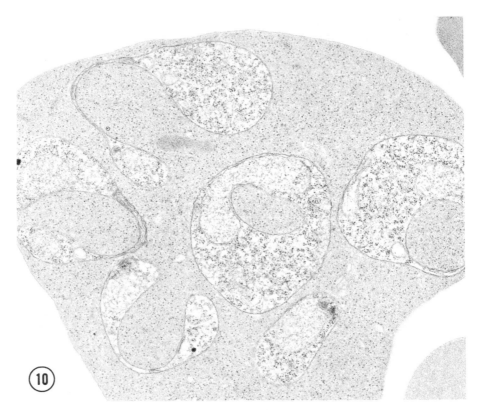

(10)

FIG. 10.   Several uninucleate trophozoites in a reticulocyte. The parasites become irregular in shape at this stage. ×33,000. (Reproduced from Aikawa and Sterling, 1974, with permission of the author and publisher.)

In recent observations made on freeze-etch replicas of *P. knowlesi* and *P. gallinaceum* (McLaren *et al.*, 1977; T. M. Seed, unpublished observations) the limiting plasma membranes of the host cell and of the parasite can be readily distinguished by the arrangement of intramembranous particles. Intramembranous particles (8.5 nm) of the erythrocyte's plasmalemma are randomly dispersed with a high particle density. The outer face (extracellular) is quite smooth and particle- free (Fig. 11). In contrast, the interior of the parasitophorous membrane (the P face) is characterized by a reticular array of aggregated particles. Clear, particle-free areas occur between particle aggregates. Again the exterior face appears smooth (Fig. 11) (Seed *et al.*, 1973). There is some question, however, as to whether or not the pebbled appearance of the parasite's plasmalemma is real or simply a heat-induced artifact. Other workers (Meszoely *et al.*, 1972), utilizing similar techniques, have not observed these striking differences in membrane

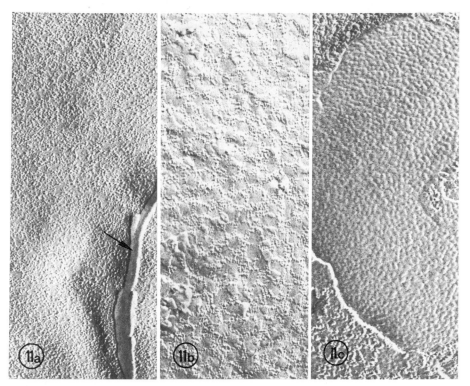

FIG. 11. Electron micrographs of freeze-fractured *P. gallinaceum* trophozoites. (a) Replica of the P fractured face of the erythrocyte plasmalemma with intramembranous particles. The extracellular face is smooth and particle-free (arrow). (b) Replica of the P fractured face of the parasitophorous membrane showing a reticular array of aggregated intramembranous particles. (c) Replica of the P fractured face of the plasmalemma of a *P. gallinaceum* erythrocytic trophozoite. ×60,000.

structure between host cell and parasite. Nevertheless, if the cobbled appearance of the parasite's limiting membrane is artifactual, still the selective deformation by heat of a particular membrane type within the sample suggests a major difference in membrane structure. The high-phospholipid, low-carbohydrate content of parasite membranes, compared to that of host cell membranes, might be responsible for such membrane deformation and might support the hypothesis that selective deformation reflects differences in membrane structure (Seed and Kreier, 1972; 1976; Seed *et al.*, 1974).

The trophozoite is the stage in which ingestion of host cell cytoplasm and growth of the parasite occur. Rudzinska and Trager in 1957 and 1959 reported the ingestion of host cell cytoplasm by the trophozoites of *P. berghei* and *P. lophurae*. Since they observed a large area of engulfed erythrocyte cytoplasm, they interpreted this as phagocytic ingestion of host cell cytoplasm by the parasites and termed this process phagotrophy. In a series of papers, Aikawa *et al.* (1966a,b) demonstrated that ingestion of host cytoplasm occurred through the circular structure in the pellicle (Fig. 12), and they named this structure the cytostome because of its function (Fig. 12). Recently, Langreth (1976) showed that, in culture, the cytostome of free trophozoites is the only place through which ferritin particles are taken up.

The exact process of ingestion of erythrocyte cytoplasm through the cytostome differs among species of plasmodia. In *P. cathemerium*, *P. fallax*, *P. gallinaceum*, *P. lophurae*, *P. knowlesi*, and *P. cynomolgi*, erythrocyte cytoplasm appears to be pinched off from the wall of the enlarged cytostomal cavity. On the other hand, in *P. elongatum* (Aikawa *et al.*, 1967), the bulge of host cell cytoplasm in the cytostomal cavity is pinched off at the cytostomal orifice together with the cytostomal wall, creating a small food vacuole with the same diameter as the cytostomal orifice (Aikawa *et al.*, 1967). As soon as a food vacuole is formed, the orifice of the cytostome is sealed by a membrane. At this stage the two dark, short segments of the lateral wall of the cytostome remain at the original site. In the next stage the protrusion of the host cell cytoplasm through the cytostome again occurs, and the cytostome repeats the same process, forming several food vacuoles.

The digestion of host cell cytoplasm occurs within the food vacuoles (Figs. 13

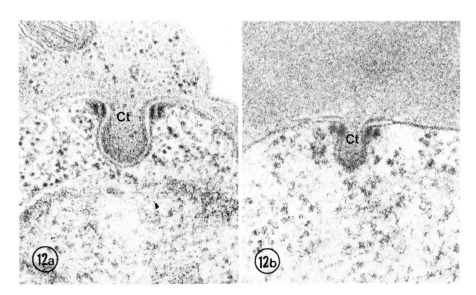

FIG. 12. (a) *Plasmodium cathemerium* trophozoite ingesting host cell cytoplasm through a cytostome (Ct). ×73,000 (b) *Plasmodium knowlesi* trophozoite ingesting host cell cytoplasm through a cytostome (Ct). ×73,000.

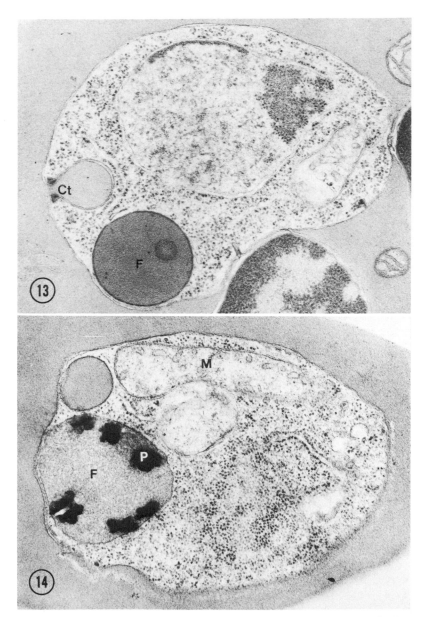

FIG. 13. *Plasmodium gallinaceum* trophozoite showing a cytostome (Ct) and a food vacuole (F). ×45,000. (Reproduced from Aikawa, *et al.*, 1966, with permission of the author and publisher.)

FIG. 14. Food vacuoles (F) with malarial pigment particles (P) and cristate mitochondria (M). ×37,000. (Reproduced from Aikawa, *et al.*, 1966, with permission of the author and publisher.)

and 14). The process of digestion is indicated by the formation of malarial pigment particles or hemozoin (Fig. 14) and the subsequent decreased density of the host cell cytoplasm within the food vacuoles. The amounts of malarial pigment and the density of erythrocyte cytoplasm in the food vacuoles are inversely related.

The malarial pigment particles in avian and reptilian malarial parasites are uniformly electron-dense and do not have a clear, crystalloid appearance. On the other hand, the malarial pigment particles seen in mammalian malarial parasites are crystalloid and rectangular in shape. When sections of mammalian parasites are stained with a high-pH solution, such as lead citrate, the malarial pigment particles are dissolved, leaving a clear area where they were previously located. Hemozoin of avian parasites is not dissolved under similar conditions (Aikawa, 1972). This difference may be due to the differences in the composition of avian and mammalian hemoglobin ingested by the parasite. The food vacuole of avian and reptilian parasites is larger than that of mammalian parasites. This appears to be related to the size of the cytostomal orifice.

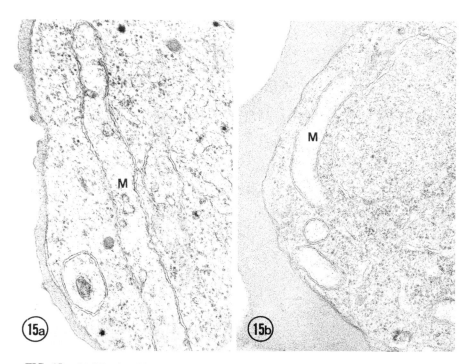

FIG. 15. (a) Mitochondria (M) of *P. brasilianum* with typical protozoan-type cristae (arrow). ×43,000. (b) Mitochondria (M) of *P. knowlesi* without cristae. ×31,000. (Reproduced from Aikawa and Sterling, 1974, with permission of the author and publisher.)

Several mitochondria are present in each erythrocytic trophozoite of avian and reptilian malarial parasites. They are composed of outer and inner membranes which invaginate to form microtubular cristae (Fig. 14). Although cristate mitochondria are also seen in some mammalian malarial parasites, others lack organelles which can be positively identified as mitochondria (Fig. 15). Instead, they have double-membrane-bounded structures considered mitochondrial equivalents.

Ribosomes are abundant in the erythrocytic trophozoites. Many of them are of the free type. Both monomeric and polymeric ribosomes also occur. Study of isolated ribosomes from the erythrocytic stages of *P. knowlesi* has shown that most monomers are of the 80 S variety and are approximately 36 nm in length and 25 nm in width (Cook *et al.*, 1971). They are composed of a large and a small subunit separated by a narrow groove (Fig. 16). Polyribosomes are often composed of four to six monomers arranged linearly. These features of ribosomes are similar to those observed in typical eukaryotic cells. The endoplasmic reticulum is scanty and is composed mostly of small, vesicular or short, canalicular forms lined with ribosomes. Smooth-surfaced endoplasmic reticulum is rare. The Golgi apparatus is inconspicuous in malarial parasites and is composed of small vesicles loosely associated with the endoplasmic reticulum.

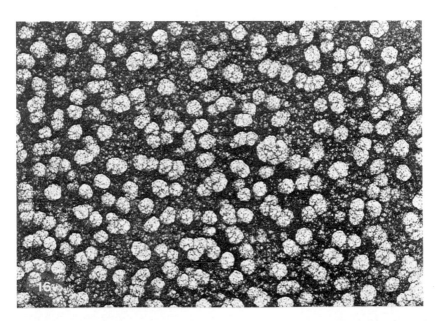

FIG. 16. Electron micrographs of ribosomes of *P. knowlesi* prepared by the shadow-casting technique. The ribosomes have a cleft dividing the monomers into two subunits. ×140,000. (Reproduced from Aikawa and Cook, 1971, with permission of the author and publisher.)

The nucleus of the trophozoite contains more finely granular and filamentous chromatin materials than the nucleus of the merozoite. The presence of abundant euchromatin in the nucleus of the trophozoite suggests that the nucleus is undergoing preparation for nuclear division. Although nucleoli have been described in erythrocytic trophozoites in the past, they are not conspicuous and are often lacking.

3. Schizonts

The schizont is defined as a parasite possessing more than one nucleus. The schizont is larger than either the merozoite or uninucleate trophozoite. During

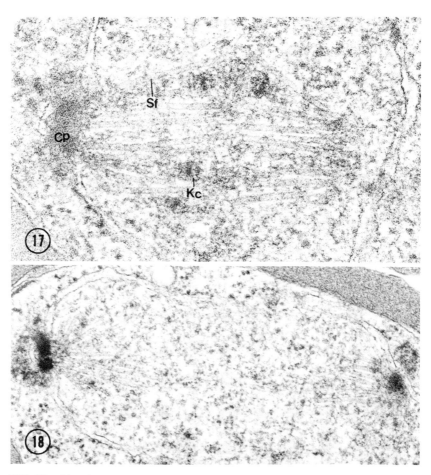

FIG. 17. Metaphase nucleus of *P. gallinaceum* showing centriolar plaques (Cp), spindle fibers (Sf), and kinetochores (Kc). ×100,000. (Reproduced from Aikawa and Beaudoin, 1968, with permission of the author and publisher.)

FIG. 18. Telophase nucleus of *P. gallinaceum.* ×69,000.

schizogony, nuclear division and differentiation of the cytoplasmic organelles occur.

In the schizont, nuclear division is accompanied by considerable morphological change. One of the first changes is the appearance of spindle fibers in the nucleus. Bundles of microtubules radiate in a fan-shaped fashion from a poorly delineated electron opaque region located on the nuclear membrane and at the midway point of the nucleus meet with other microtubules originating from the opposite pole (Fig. 17). The electron-opaque region has

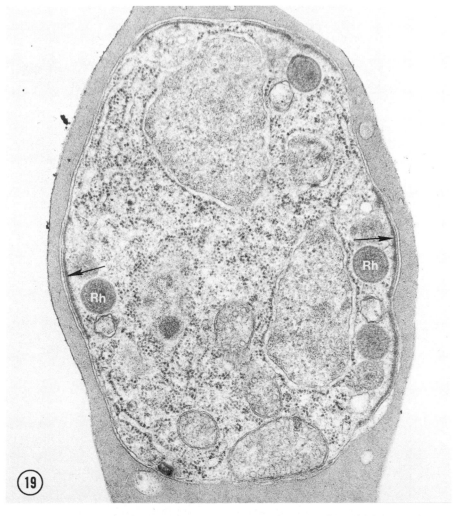

FIG. 19. Beginning of schizogony of *P. cathemerium*. Segments of the thick inner membranes (arrows) together with rhoptries (Rh) appear along with parasite plasmalemma. ×48,000. (Reproduced from Aikawa and Sterling, 1974, with permission of the author and publishers.)

been referred to as a centriolar plaque or centriole equivalent (Aikawa, 1972). At the end of the microtubules are minute electron-dense structures with subunits. These structures appear to be kinetochores instead of chromosomes, since they cannot be extracted by DNase. Between the kinetochores are ill-defined electron-dense zones that can be extracted with DNase and may, therefore, be chromosomes (Aikawa *et al.*, 1972). As nuclear division progresses, the nucleus becomes dumbbell-shaped (Fig. 18). A nucleolus appears at the narrow isthmus, and eventually the microtubules disappear. Finally two daughter nuclei are formed. During nuclear division, the nuclear membrane remains, except at the place where the centriolar plaque is located.

While nuclear division is taking place, the cytoplasmic organelles also change. Mitochondria increase in size and become irregular, forming several buds. Fi-

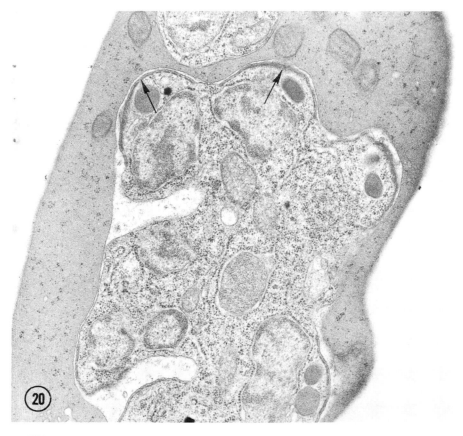

FIG. 20. Advanced stage of schizogony of *P. cathemerium*. The areas covered by segments of thick membrane protrude outward, forming new merozoites (arrows). ×28,000. (Reproduced from Aikawa, 1966, with permission of the author and publisher.)

nally they undergo fission, yielding many mitochondria. The cytoplasmic organelles which had disappeared at the beginning of trophozoite development reappear (Fig. 19). The organelles first noted in the parasite are randomly distributed segments of the inner membrane of the merozoite pellicle and are usually seen opposite the centriolar plaque. Subpellicular microtubules and rhoptry precursors appear beneath the inner membrane. The rhoptry precursors become more dense as the process of merozoite formation progresses. The area covered by the inner membrane begins to protrude outward into the parasitophorous vacuole space to form new merozoites, while areas not covered by the inner membrane do not protrude to form new merozoites (Fig. 20).

With the progression of merozoite budding, various organelles, including a nucleus, mitochondria, spherical bodies together with endoplasmic reticulum, and ribosomes migrate into the developing merozoites from the schizont. As the merozoites develop and grow, the size of the original schizont decreases until finally only a residual body with malarial pigment particles remains.

B. Exoerythrocytic Stages

The fine-structure study of the exoerythrocytic stages of malarial parasites has lagged behind that of the erythrocytic stages. The sparseness of the exoerythrocytic stages in the hosts is mainly responsible for the difficulty of electron microscopy study. This difficulty was partly overcome by the use of tissue culture systems developed by Davis *et al.* (1966).

Although the morphological similarity between the exoerythrocytic and erythrocytic stages of malarial parasites is apparent, there are several structural differences between them. These include the (1) shape of the merozoites, (2) number of micronemes, (3) ingestion process, and (4) presence or absence of food vacuoles.

The exoerythrocytic merozoite is more elongate than the erythrocytic merozoite and is 3–4 μm in length and 1–2 μm in width (Fig. 21). There are more micronemes in the exoerythrocytic stages, and the rhoptries appear to be more elongated. The feeding process of the exoerythrocytic stages appears to be somewhat different from that of the erythrocytic stages. Cytostomal ingestion of host cell cytoplasm similar to that occurring in the erythrocytic stages has been reported to occur in exoerythrocytic stages of *P. elongatum* (Aikawa *et al.*, 1967), *P. gallinaceum* (Aikawa *et al.*, 1968), and *P. lophurae* (Beaudoin and Strome, 1972). On the other hand, it is still questionable whether the cytostome is involved in the ingestion of host cell cytoplasm in the exoerythrocytic stages of *P. fallax* (Hepler *et al.*, 1966). Since there is no direct evidence for cytoplasmic function in the exoerythrocytic stages of *P. fallax*, Hepler *et al.* (1966) has suggested that the cytostome of the exoerythrocytic stages of *P. fallax* does not ingest host cell cytoplasm and that the simple diffusion of nutrients through the host cell and parasite membrane supplies the exoerythrocytic parasites with nutrients necessary for their metabolic activity.

The food vacuoles of the erythrocytic stages of malarial parasites are easily detected, because of the electron-dense nature of erythrocytic cytoplasm. On the other hand, the cytoplasms of the exoerythrocytic stages and of their host cells are morphologically similar, and it is difficult to identify ingested host cell cytoplasm within the parasite. Vacuoles seen near the cytostome have been reported to be the food vacuoles of the exoerythrocytic stages. Beaudoin and Strome (1972) has reported that food vacuoles seen in the exoerythrocytic stages are small and electron-transparent, with a granular matrix. No pigment particles can be found in the food vacuoles.

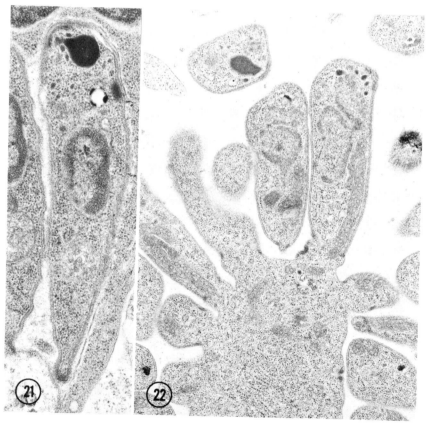

FIG. 21.   An exoerythrocytic merozoite of *P. elongatum.* ×31,000.

FIG. 22.   Budding of exoerythrocytic merozoites of *P. gallinaceum.* ×27,000. (Reproduced from Aikawa *et al.,* 1968, with permission of the author and publisher.)

The structures of the exoerythrocytic stages of mammalian parasites such as *P. berghei* (see Fig. 26) and *P. cynomolgi* have been found to be similar to those of avian parasites, although more vacuoles are seen at the periphery of the cytoplasm of *P. cynomolgi*. Sodeman *et al.* (1970) have noted two types of cytoplasmic vacuoles. One is round and electron-translucent, and the other smaller and more electron-dense. These vacuoles appear to coalesce and form clefts subdividing the cytoplasm of the exoerythrocytic stages of *P. cynomolgi*. Although similar vacuoles are observed in the cytoplasm of *P. berghei,* they are not so prominent as in *P. cynomolgi*. No typical mitochondria are found in the exoerythrocytic stages of these mammalian parasites. The processes of merozoite budding in exoerythrocytic schizonts are similar to those of the erythrocytic stages, although more merozoites are formed from an exoerythrocytic schizont than from an erythrocytic one (Fig. 22).

C. Mosquito Stages

1. Ookinetes and Oocysts

After ingestion of a blood meal infected with malarial parasites by a mosquito, microgametes mate with macrogametes to form zygotes. As the zygote develops, it becomes a motile ookinete which penetrates the intestinal wall of the mosquito. The ookinete enters the mosquito midgut wall through the epithelium and reaches the outer layer of the midgut wall which is in contact with the epithelial basal lamina (Garnham *et al.,* 1962). There it becomes an oocyst. By sporogony, the oocyst produces a large number of sporozoites through an intermediary form, the sporoblast.

The structure of the ookinete is similar to that of merozoites and sporozoites (Fig. 23). The ookinete is surrounded by a pellicular complex composed of an outer and an inner membrane and a row of microtubules. The anterior end of the ookinete is a truncated cone shape and contains many electron-dense micronemes similar to those seen in merozoites and sporozoites (Fig. 24). However, no rhoptries have been observed. A nucleus is located in the center of the ookinete. The nucleus contains patchy, granular structures. A nucleolus has been reported to be present in *P. gallinaceum* ookinetes (Garnham *et al.,* 1962). A few mitochondria are present in ookinetes of *P. gallinaceum* and *P. cynomolgi*. An aggregate of particles measuring 35 μm has been reported to be present in the posterior of the ookinete (Fig. 25). Garnham *et al.* (1962) has pointed out the morphological similarity between these particles and virus particles. Terzakis (1972) has also reported similar bodies in the ookinete of *P. gallinaceum*. The particles are regularly arranged in a hexagonal pattern and are embedded in a amorphous low-density matrix. Terzakis has reported that these viruslike parti-

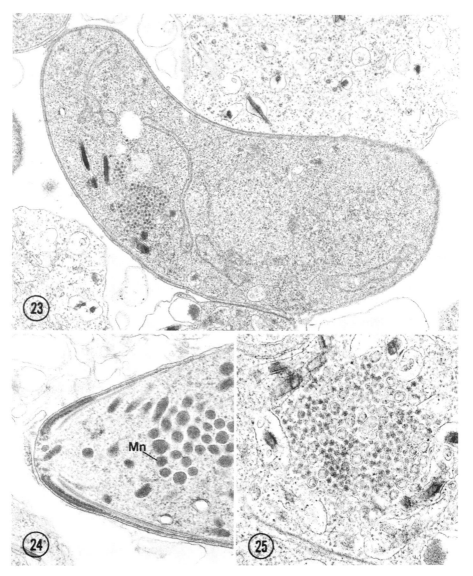

FIG. 23.   An ookinete of *P. berghei*. ×18,000.

FIG. 24.   Apical end of an ookinete of *P. berghei* showing micronemes (Mn). ×31,000.

FIG. 25.   Viruslike inclusion in an ookinete. ×38,000.

cles also occur in the cytoplasm of the oocyst, indicating that these aggregations of particles are not specific to the ookinete.

The process of penetration of the midgut of the mosquito by the ookinete has been described by Garnham *et al.* (1962). With its anterior end the ookinete pushes aside the microvilli of the epithelial cells of the mosquito gut and enters the epithelial cells. Garnham *et al.* has suggested that proteolytic substances are

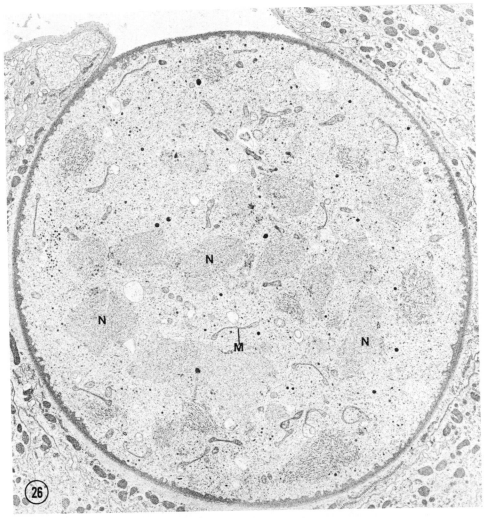

FIG. 26. Oocyst of *P. berghei* in *Aedes aegypti* mosquito gut epithelium. Nucleus (N); Mitochondria (M). ×8000. (Reproduced from Aikawa and Sterling, 1974, with permission of the author and publisher.)

secreted by the micronemes, which aid the entry of the ookinete. There are no descriptions of the migration of the ookinete in the gut wall, nor is it known how it reaches the basement membrane of the gut and becomes an oocyst at the external border of the gut.

The fine structure of oocysts of malarial parasites (Fig. 26) has been described by several investigators. The oocyst is surrounded by a thick electron-dense capsule 1 μm thick. Initially the oocyst is a solid structure containing abundant

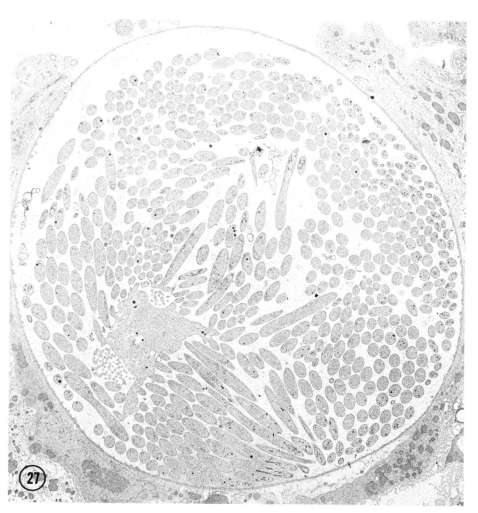

FIG. 27.   Advanced stage of *P. berghei* sporozoite formation in an oocyst. ×5000. (Reproduced from Aikawa and Sterling, 1974, with permission of the author and publisher.)

ribosomes, a nucleus, mitochondria, and spherical inclusions of a dense material, presumably pigment. This solid form originally possesses a single nucleus, but eventually nuclear division takes place, forming several nuclei. The nuclear division process is similar to that occurring in other stages of plasmodia (Terzakis *et al.*, 1967).

As the oocyst grows, vacuoles appear beneath the oocyst capsule. The vacuoles enlarge, coalesce, and form large clefts that subdivide the oocyst cytoplasm into several sporoblasts. From the sporoblasts, sporozoites develop in a fashion similar to that by which merozoites are formed. During cleft formation, the internal surface of the capsule becomes irregular, and small globules of capsular material appear to discharge into the clefts. Some workers have suggested that these capsular materials are nutrients for the sporoblasts (Vanderberg *et al.*, 1967). The fine structure of sporoblasts resembles that of erythrocytic and exoerythrocytic schizonts (Fig. 27). Resemblances include the appearance of segments of inner membrane together with microtubules along the outer membrane of the sporoblasts. Along the inner membrane precursors of rhoptries are apparent. The areas covered by segments of the inner membrane protrude outward, and by a budding process sporozoites emerge from the sporoblasts.

2. Sporozoites

There are many descriptions of the fine structure of the sporozoites of many plasmodial species including *P. bastianellii, P. berghei, P. basilianum, P. cathemerium, P. falciparum, P. gallinaceum, P. ovale, P. relictum, P. vivax,* and *P. cynomolgi.*

The sporozoites are more elongated than either erythrocytic or exoerythrocytic merozoites (Figs. 28 and 29). They measure about 11 μm in length and 1.0 μm in diameter. The organelles found in the sporozoites are essentially the same as those of the merozoites (Terzakis *et al.*, 1967; Vanderberg *et al.*, 1967). The pellicle is composed of an outer membrane, a double inner membrane, and a row of subpellicular microtubules. Freeze-fracture of the sporozoites of *P. cynomolgi, P. knowlesi,* and *P. berghei* similarly shows the two membranes (Aikawa *et al.*, 1979). The two internal faces of the plasma membrane possess randomly distributed intramembranous particles (Fig. 30). One face (P) of the inner membrane complex shows intramembranous particles aligned in very distinct rows conforming to the long axis of the sporozoites (Fig. 31). These aligned particles may correspond to the underlying subpellicular microtubules. The other fracture face (E) has very few intramembranous particles (Fig. 32). Cross sections of the sporozoites of *P. berghei* show 15–16 microtubules arranged around two-thirds of the periphery of the sporozoite in addition to a single tubule in the remaining one-third (Fig. 32). On the other hand, Garnham *et al.* (1963) have reported that the sporozoites of *P. gallinaceum* possess an 11 + 1, P.

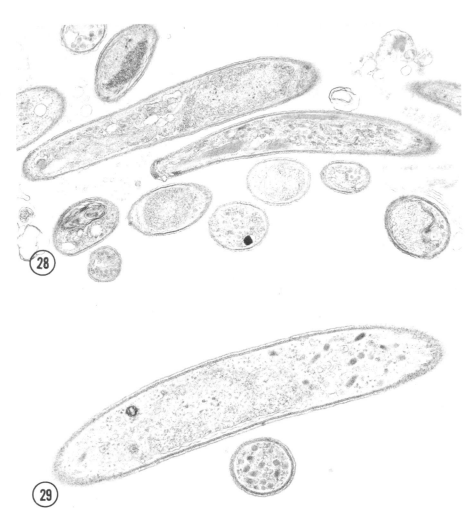

FIG. 28. Sporozoite of *P. cynomolgi*. ×20,000. (Reproduced from Cochrane, A. *et al.*, 1976, with permission of the author and publisher.)

FIG. 29. Sporozoite of *P. cynomolgi* incubated in normal serum. ×28,000. (Reproduced from Cochrane *et al.*, 1976, with permission of the author and publisher.)

FIG. 30. Electron micrograph of a freeze-fractured *P. cynomolgi* sporozoite. The P face (P1) of the plasma membrane is uniformly covered by intramembranous particles, whereas they are fewer on the E face (E2) of the intermediate membrane. ×45,000. (Reproduced from Aikawa *et al.*, (1979), with permission of the author and publisher.)

FIG. 31. Electron micrograph of a freeze-fractured *P. knowlesi* sporozoite showing intramembranous particles aligned with the long axis of the sporozoite on the P face (P3) of the inner pellicular membrane. ×60,000 (Reproduced from Aikawa *et al.*, 1979, with permission of the author and publisher.)

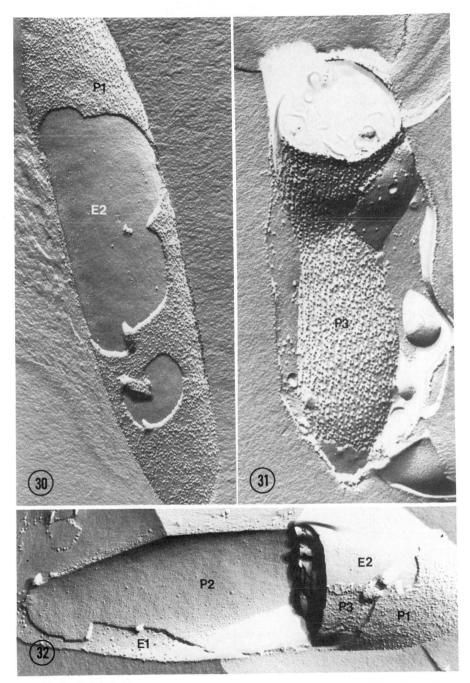

FIG. 32. A freeze-fractured *P. knowlesi* sporozoite showing the P (P1) and E (E1) faces of the plasma membrane, the P (P2) and E (E2) faces of the intermediate membrane and the P (P3) face of the inner membrane. ×51,000. (Reproduced from Aikawa *et al.*, 1979, with permission of the author and publisher.)

brasilianum an 10 + 1, and *P. ovale* an 12 + 1 pattern of tubule distribution.

Sporozoites are reported to possess a very thin (15 nm) surface coat of fibrillar material surrounding the outer sporozoite membrane. The surface coat appears to play a role in the sporozoite's response to the immune reactions of the host (Cochrane *et al.*, 1976). The circumsporozoite precipitation (CSP) reaction seen in sporozoites incubated with immune serum is a result of the formation of an electron-dense coat along the surface of the sporozoite (Figs. 33, 34, and 36). Pretreatment of sporozoites with mouse antisporozoite serum followed by incubation with rabbit anti-mouse IgG conjugated to hemocyanin has revealed hemocyanin particles on the sporozoite's surface (Fig. 35). Scanning electron microscopy of sporozoites incubated with immune serum has shown that they are considerably different in surface configuration from parasites incubated with normal serum (Cochrane *et al.*, 1976). Sporozoites incubated in normal serum have a relatively smooth outline (Fig. 37). Sporozoites incubated in immune serum are considerably thicker and have a highly irregular contour along most of their surfaces (Fig. 38). The anterior end of the sporozoite incubated in immune serum remains relatively unaltered and free of deposited material, while the posterior end is covered with a thick coat with a taillike precipitate. These observations indicate that immunoglobulins participate in the formation of the thick surface coat of sporozoites incubated in immune serum.

Cytostomes have been observed in sporozoites and appear similar to these structures in the erythrocytic stages. Originally it was thought that the sporoplasm of the sporozoite was extruded outward from this structure when the sporozoite infected the vertebrate host. However, this has never been demonstrated. Current opinion holds that the cytostome of the sporozoite is structurally and functionally similar to the organelle of erythrocytic forms.

The rhoptries are extremely long and extend from the apical end to the midportion of the sporozoite. Mitochondria are present in the posterior end of the sporozoite. Mitochondria with microtubular cristae are found in the sporozoites of mammalian malarial parasites that do not possess such mitochondria in the erythrocytic stage in the vertebrate host. The transformation of mitochondria without cristae to those with cristae apparently occurs with the change in host (Sterling *et al.*, 1972). A spherical body always associated with a mitochondrion in the erythrocytic and exoerythrocytic stages has not been found in the sporozoites of mammalian plasmodia.

FIG. 33.   Sporozoite of *P. cynomolgi* incubated in immune serum. The surface is covered with a thick coat which is more abundant around the posterior portion. ×19,000. (Reproduced from Cochrane *et al.*, 1976, with permission of the author and publisher.)

FIG. 34.   Sporozoite of *P. cynomolgi* incubated in immune serum. Note cytoplasmic vacuolization (V) and separation of the plasma membrane (arrow). ×25,000. (Reproduced from Cochrane *et al.*, 1976, with permission of the author and publisher.)

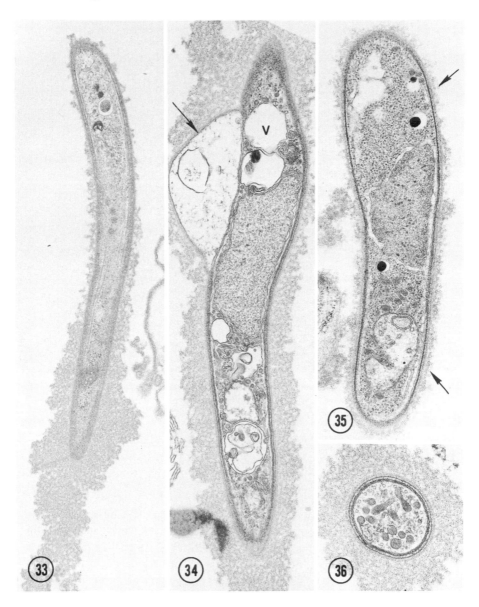

FIG. 35.   Sporozoite of *P. berghei* incubated with immune serum and with rabbit anti-mouse immunoglobulin conjugated with hemocyanin (arrows). ×40,000. (Reproduced from Cochrane *et al.*, 1976, with permission of the author and publisher.)

FIG. 36.   Cross section of sporozoite of *P. cynomolgi* incubated in immune serum. ×29,000. (Reproduced from Cochrane *et al.*, 1976, with permission of the author and publisher.)

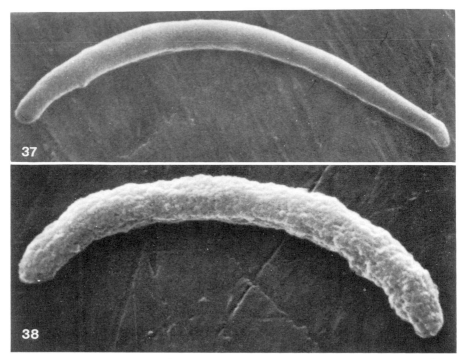

FIG. 37. Scanning electron micrograph of *P. cynomolgi* sporozoite. Note the smooth surface. ×21,000. (Reproduced from Cochrane *et al.*, 1976, with permission of the author and publisher.)

FIG. 38. Scanning electron micrograph of *P. cynomolgi* sporozoite incubated in immune serum. ×19,000. (Reproduced from Cochrane *et al.*, 1976, with permission of the author and publisher.)

D. Sexual Forms

The sexual forms or gametocytes arise from erythrocytic merozoites. Two gametocyte forms, macrogametocytes and microgametocytes, can be readily recognized by electron microscopy (Figs. 39 and 40). The parasite identifiable as a gametocyte, by electron microscopy, is a uninucleate parasite surrounded by three membranes (Fig. 40). These membranes are particularly pronounced in the gametocytes of avian and reptilian malarial parasites but are not quite so apparent in mammalian parasites (Aikawa *et al.*, 1969). The outer of the three membranes appears to be the host cell membrane of the parasitophorous vacuole. The gametocyte's pellicle is, therefore, actually composed of two membranes. The inner membrane is 15–18 nm in thickness and appears as two unit membranes in apposition. In the gametocytes of some species, a row of several subpellicular microtubules is observed. This observation has led to a hypothesis that the

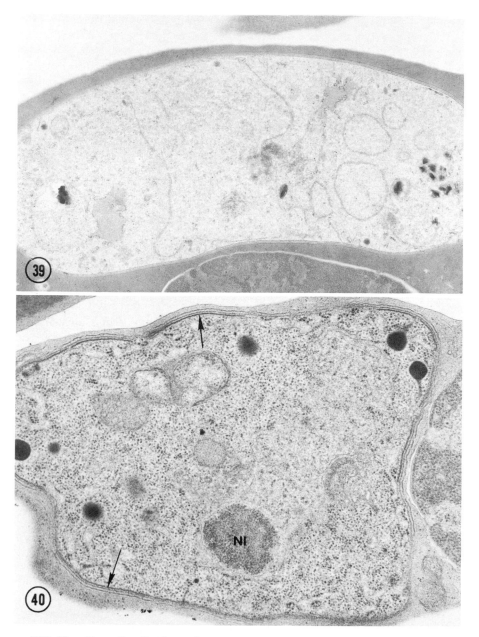

FIG. 39. *Plasmodium floridense* microgametocyte characterized by few ribosomes and poorly developed endoplasmic reticulum. ×18,000. (Reproduced from Aikawa and Jordan, 1968, with permission of the author and publisher.)

FIG. 40. The macrogametocyte of *P. floridense* showing more ribosomes than the microgametocyte. Note three distinct membranes surrounding the parasite (arrows). Nucleolus, (Nl). ×27,000. (Reproduced from Aikawa and Jordan, 1968, with permission of the author and publisher.)

gametocyte originates from a merozoite that has failed to break down the inner membrane after infecting a new erythrocyte (Aikawa *et al.*, 1969).

Cytostomes are a prominent feature of the pellicle of micro- and macrogametocytes. Erythrocyte cytoplasm is ingested through the cytostome of gametocytes, as it is in the asexual erythrocytic stages. Food vacuoles formed through the cytostome are surrounded by a single membrane, and malarial pigment particles can be present in the vacuoles. Clusters of small vesicles which appear to be derived from the endoplasmic reticulum and which may be the Golgi complex are present near the nucleus. Electron-dense spherules are often associated with the Golgi complex and with food vacuoles and may be primary lysosomes. Other electron-dense structures, "osmiophilic bodies," also are observed in the cytoplasm near the pellicle (Fig. 40). They are surrounded by a single membrane and frequently have narrow ductules extending to the inner membrane of the pellicle. These osmiophilic bodies may have a function similar to that of the rhoptries and micronemes of the merozoites and sporozoites. They are more frequently present in the macrogametocyte than in the microgametocyte. Mitochondria possess prominent tubular cristae, but some mammalian parasite gametocytes only possess acristate mitochondria. Dense granules are occasionally observed within the mitochondrial matrix. These mitochondria are located near the nucleus.

The cytoplasm of mature macrogametocytes is filled with ribosomes, while microgametocytes contain fewer ribosomes (Figs. 39 and 40). This difference accounts for the basophilic character of the Romanowsky stained cytoplasm of macrogametocytes.

A dense nucleus is found in macrogametocytes (Fig. 40), whereas a large diffuse nucleus is seen in microgametocytes. A distinct nucleolus is found in the nucleus of the mature macrogametocyte, but it is lacking in the microgametocyte. The presence of a definite nucleolus in macrogametocytes and its absence from microgametocytes correlates with the ribosome concentrations in macro- and microgametocytes. In mature gametocytes, centrioles are seen near the nucleus (Aikawa *et al.*, 1969; Sinden *et al.*, 1976). Each centriole has a cartwheel appearance and is composed of one central and nine single radial microtubules. Arms connect the central and radial microtubules.

In the gut of mosquitoes, the gametocytes leave their host cells and become gametes. During microgametogenesis, the outmost membrane (the parasitophorous membrane) is lost and the double inner membrane becomes interrupted. Nuclear division occurs by a process similar to that in the asexual stages. Kinetosomes are seen near centriolar plaques located at the nuclear membrane. Condensation of chromatin occurs at the periphery of the nucleus. The nucleus becomes irregular in shape with long projections. Concurrently kinetosome–axoneme complexes appear from the kinetosomes. Each axoneme has the 9 + 2 arrangement of microtubules typical of eukaryotic flagella (Fig. 41).

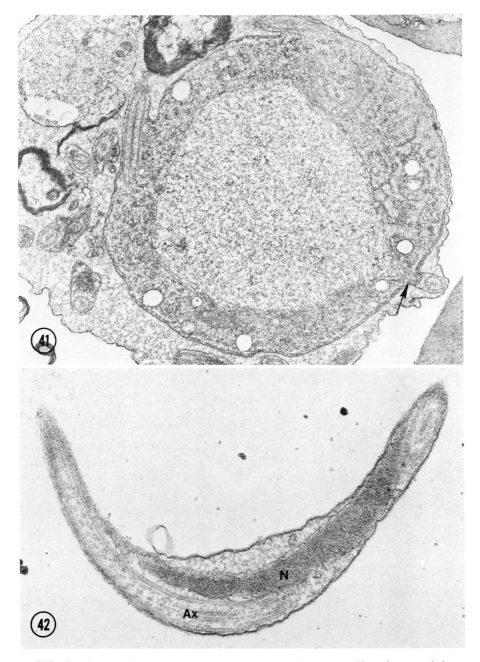

FIG. 41. Intracellular microgametocyte with budding microgametes. Note close association between the nucleus and axoneme (arrow). ×41,000.

FIG. 42. Microgamete with a nucleus (N) and an axoneme (Ax). ×44,000.

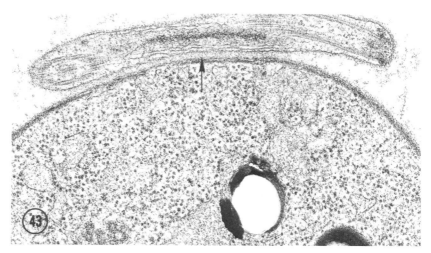

FIG. 43. Adhesion of a microgamete and a macrogamete (arrow). Note fibrillar material between them. ×43,000.

The nuclear membrane remains intact during chromatin segregation, but nuclear budding occurs. These nuclear buds become closely associated with the kinetosome–axoneme complexes (Fig. 41). The kinetosome–axoneme complex and attached nuclear chromatin migrate to the surface of the microgametocyte and participate in the formation of microgametes. The gametes are reported to slide off tangentially from the surface of the microgametocyte after the tail of the microgamete protrudes (Sinden *et al.*, 1976).

A free microgamete consists of a single axoneme, a kinetosome, dense spheres, and a nucleus intertwined with the axoneme (Fig. 42). At fertilization of a macrogamete with a microgamete, the latter approaches the surface of the macrogamete and fusion occurs (Fig. 43). At first a microgamete with an axoneme and a nucleus can be observed in the fertilized macrogamete, but soon the nucleus disappears, leaving eventually only the axoneme (Sinden *et al.*, 1976).

VI. HOST CELL INTERACTION

A. Host Cell Entry by *Plasmodium*

The mechanism of invasion of host erythrocytes by malarial merozoites has been studied by several investigators, but the invasion of other host cells by other development stages has not been studied. Therefore, in this section only the interaction between erythrocytes and erythrocytic merozoites will be discussed.

Erythrocyte entry by merozoites has been studied extensively since Ladda *et al.* (1969) described the invasion of erythrocytes by merozoites of *P. berghei* and *P. gallinaceum*. They established that merozoites entered by invagination of the erythrocyte membrane rather than by penetrating it. Dvorak *et al.* (1975) used interference phase-contrast microscopy to study the invasion of erythrocytes by *P. knowlesi* and observed that the invasion consisted of attachment of the apical end of the parasite to the erythrocyte, deformation of the erythrocyte, and entry of the merozoite by invagination of the erythrocyte membrane.

Electron microscopic studies of erythrocyte invasion by *Plasmodium* were hindered by sampling problems. However, Dennis *et al.* (1975) recently reported a new method for the collection of large quantities of free, viable merozoites of *P. knowlesi* which could invade erythrocytes. By applying this method, several new findings on invasion processes have come to light (Aikawa *et al.*, 1978). The invasion of erythrocytes by merozoites of *Plasmodium* involves a number of distinct steps. They include (1) recognition and attachment of the merozoite to the erythrocyte membrane, (2) invagination of the erythrocyte membrane around the merozoite to form a parasitophorous vacuole, and (3) sealing of the parasitophorous vacuole after completion of merozoite invasion. Evidence for the presence of host recognition sites on *Plasmodium* comes from observations that, for successful endocytosis, the parasite must come in contact with the host cell in a particular orientation. Endocytosis of a *Plasmodium* merozoite is initiated only when it attaches to the host cell by the apical end (Fig. 44). However, it is not known what makes the exposed elements on the apical end different from the rest of the surface of the merozoite. Alteration of host plasma membrane by proteases has been shown specifically to abolish attachment of *Plasmodium*. Trypsinization of human erythrocytes reduces their susceptibility to penetration by *P. falciparum* but does not alter penetration by a monkey parasite, *P. knowlesi* (Miller *et al.*, 1978). Chymotrypsin treatment of erythrocytes blocks infection by *P. knowlesi* but has no effect on infection by *P. falciparum* (Miller *et al.*, 1978). Miller and his associates (1975b) have reported that initial recognition and attachment of *P. vivax* merozoites to erythrocytes is probably mediated by Duffy blood group-related antigens.

When a merozoite contacts an erythrocyte with its apical end, the erythrocyte membrane at the point of the interaction is slightly raised initially (Fig. 44), but eventually a depression is created in the erythrocyte membrane (Fig. 45). The erythrocyte membrane to which the merozoite is attached becomes thickened and forms a junction with the merozoite plasma membrane. However, no junction is formed between the *P. vivax* merozoite and Duffy-negative human erythrocytes, which are the only human erythrocytes refractory to invasion by *P. vivax* malarial parasites. Instead, the Duffy-negative erythrocyte is connected to the merozoite by thin filaments of 3 to 5-nm thickness (Fig. 46). The filaments originate from the edge of the truncated, cone-shaped apical end, such that two

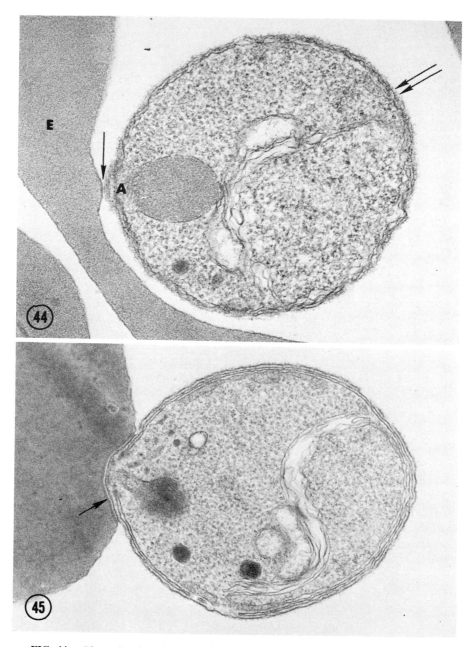

FIG. 44. *Plasmodium knowlesi* merozoite at the initial contact (arrow) between the merozoite's apical end (A) and an erythrocyte (E). The merozoite surface is covered with a surface coat (double arrow). ×50,000. (Reproduced from Aikawa *et al.*, 1978b, with permission of the author and publisher.)

FIG. 45. *Plasmodium knowlesi* merozoite contacting an erythrocyte. The erythrocyte membrane becomes thickened at the attachment site (arrow). ×47,000.

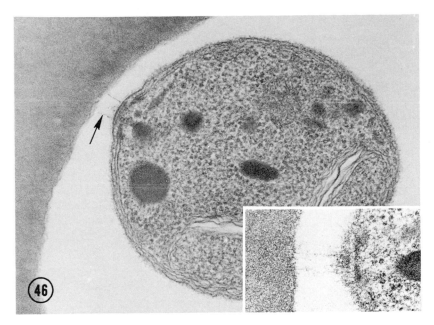

FIG. 46. *Plasmodium knowlesi* merozoite is connected with a Duffy-negative erythrocyte by fine filaments (arrow). The erythrocyte membrane is unaltered. ×50,000. Inset: High-magnification micrograph showing fine fibrils connecting the apical ends of a merozoite and a Duffy-negative erythrocyte. ×78,000. (Reproduced from Miller *et al.*, 1978, with permission of the author and publisher.

distinct filaments can be seen in thin sections. Trypsin treatment of Duffy-negative erythrocytes makes them susceptible to invasion by *P. vivax* merozoites and permits junction formation with the merozoites. The absence of junction formation with Duffy-negative erythrocytes may indicate that the Duffy-associated antigen acts as a second receptor for junction formation or, alternatively, a determinant on Duffy-negative erythrocytes blocks junction formation (Miller *et al.*, 1978).

There is increasing evidence that, following attachment, some product from the apical organelles of the merozoite, i.e., the rhoptries and micronemes, initiates invagination of the host cell membrane and participates in invagination of the host cell plasmalemma. A ductule runs from the rhoptries to the apical end of the merozoite, which is the point of initial attachment between the merozoite and erythrocyte (Fig. 45). Throughout invasion, the apical end remains in contact with the erythrocyte membrane. An electron-dense band appears between the tip of the apical end of the merozoite and the erythrocyte and is continuous with the common duct of the rhoptries (Fig. 49). The low electron density in the ductule during invasion suggests a release of rhoptry contents. Histochemical studies

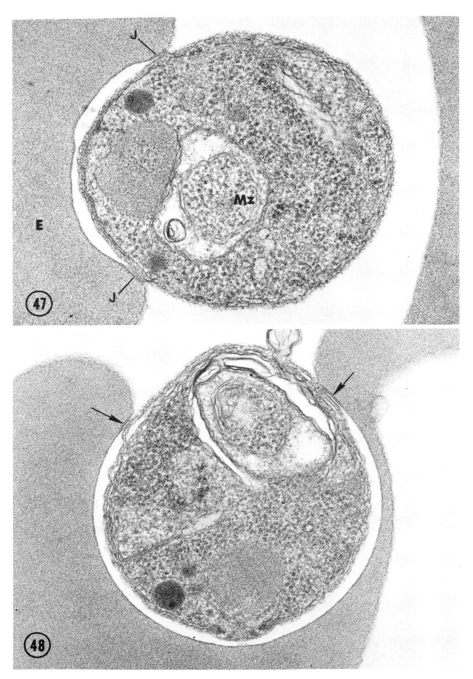

FIG. 47. An advanced stage of erythrocyte (E) entry by a merozoite (Mz). The invagination of the erythrocyte is created by the merozoite. Note a junctional attachment (J) on each side of the entry orifice. ×54,000. (Reproduced from Aikawa *et al.*, 1978, with permission of the author and publisher.)

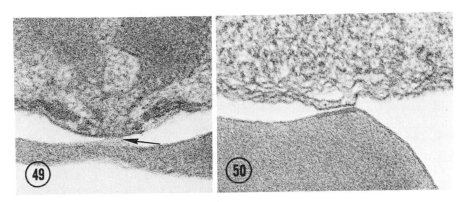

FIG. 49. An electron-opaque projection (arrow) connecting the rhoptry (R) and the erythrocyte membrane. ×120,000.

FIG. 50. High-magnification micrograph of the junction showing the thickened erythrocyte membrane and fine fibrils between the two parallel membranes. ×120,000.

indicate the presence of protein and carbohydrate in rhoptries (Kilejian, 1976). Indirect experimental evidence suggests that a histidine-rich protein isolated from *P. lophurae* may be a component of the apical organelles of this malarial parasite; the protein was shown to cause invagination of erythrocyte membranes *in vitro*.

As invasion progresses, the depression in the erythrocyte deepens and conforms to the shape of the merozoite (Figs. 47 and 48). At this time, the thickened, electron-dense zone on the erythrocyte is no longer observed at the point of the initial attachment but now appears at the orifice of the merozoite-induced invagination of the erythrocyte membrane (Fig. 47). The thickened area of the erythrocyte membrane is about 15 nm in thickness and about 250 nm in length and appears to be a thickening of the inner leaflet of the bilayer (Fig. 50). The thickened erythrocyte membrane forms a junction with the merozoite. The gap between these two membranes is about 10 nm, and fine fibrils extend between these two parallel membranes. The junction appears to form a circumferential interaction at the orifice of the invaginated erythrocyte membrane (Aikawa *et al.*, 1978), since it is always located on each side of the orifice regardless of the plane through which the section passes.

The events occurring during invasion appear to be somewhat similar to endocytotic processes by which phagocytic cells ingest inert particles, other cells, and microorganisms. In 1975, Griffin and his associates proposed a hypothesis for endocytosis of inert particles. This hypothesis proposed specific attachment

FIG. 48. A very advanced stage of erythrocyte entry by a merozoite. The junction (arrows) is always located at the orifice of erythrocyte entry. ×48,000. (Reproduced from Aikawa *et al.*, 1978, with permission of the author and publisher.)

triggering endocytosis and zippering. However, this hypothesis does not explain fully the invasion by *Plasmodium* merozoites. Aikawa *et al.* (1978), therefore, proposed the following models for the invasion of erythrocytes by *Plasmodium* merozoites. (1) Movement of the junction at the level of the membrane, which may be related to the lateral displacement of the junction by the agency of membrane flow, and (2) an attachment–detachment (modified zippering) model which prescribes that the junction itself may be capable of migrating on the surface of a relatively stable plasma membrane.

Cytochalasin B is known to affect microfilaments (Wessells *et al.*, 1971), glucose transport, and possibly other functions. When merozoites are treated with cytochalasin B, they can attach to the erythrocyte membrane but do not invade the erythrocyte (Fig. 51) (Miller *et al.*, 1978).

The merozoite is covered with a uniform surface coat 10 nm in thickness (Aikawa *et al.*, 1978; Miller *et al.*, 1975a) (Fig. 5). During host cell entry, no surface coat is visible on the portion of the merozoite within the erythrocyte invagination, whereas the surface coat, on the portion of the merozoite remaining outside the erythrocyte, appears to be similar to that seen on free merozoites. Ladda *et al.* (1969) reported the accumulation of a surface coat at the orifice, however, no accumulation of the surface coat was seen at the orifice of the entry

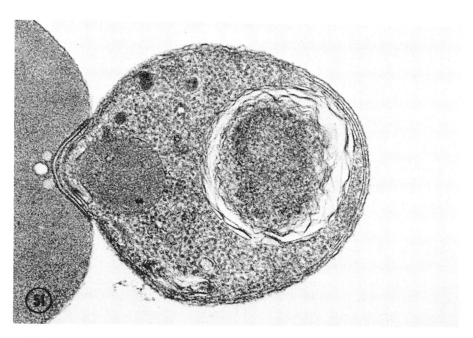

FIG. 51. The attachment between a cytochalasin B-treated merozoite and an erythrocyte. ×50,000. (Reproduced from Miller *et al.*, 1978, with permission of the author and publisher.)

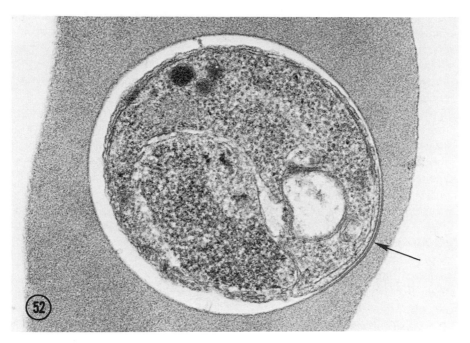

FIG. 52.   A merozoite inside an erythrocyte. However, the posterior end of the merozoite is still attached (arrow) to the thickened erythrocyte membrane. ×50,000. (Reproduced from Aikawa *et al.*, (1978b), with permission of the author and publisher.)

site of the erythrocyte by the merozoite in more recent work (Aikawa *et al.*, 1978). The surface coat beyond the junction appears to be unaltered in density. Therefore, simple capping does not seem to fit the observations. The significance of the surface coat in invasion must be further explored.

There are few reports on the closure of the parasitophorous vacuole membrane after completion of interiorization of the merozoite. When entry is completed, the junction appears to fuse at the posterior end of the merozoite (Fig. 52), closing the orifice in the fashion of an iris diaphragm (Aikawa *et al.*, 1978). The merozoite still remains in close apposition to the thickened erythrocyte membrane at the point of final closure. After completion of the host cell entry, the merozoite is surrounded by the membrane of the parasitophorous vacuole that originated from the erythrocyte membrane.

B. Host Cell Alterations

The parasitophorous vacuole membrane that originated from the erythrocyte membrane expands with the developing parasite and is retained until formation of the next generation of merozoites. Changes in the molecular organization of this parasitophorous vacuole membrane are apparent very early in development. Freeze-fracture studies have shown major differences in the distribution of intramembranous particles of erythrocyte membranes and the vacuole membrane (McLaren *et al.*, 1977) (Fig. 11). Cytochemical studies also indicated differences in surface charge (Seed *et al.*, 1974), glycoprotein, and enzyme distribution (Langreth, 1977) between these two membranes.

Malarial parasites also influence host cell plasma membranes. Scanning electron microscopy of erythrocytes infected with malarial parasites shows pits on the surface (Fig. 53). Dramatic changes are seen in erythrocytes infected by some species of malarial parasites. The structures that occur in infected erythrocytes and that can be seen by light microscopy have been given various names: Schüffner's dots, Maurer's clefts, Zieman's stippling, and Stinton's and Mulligan's stippling. Schüffner's dots seen in erythrocytes infected by vivax-type and ovale-type malarial parasites were demonstrated by electron microscopy to be caveola–vesicle complexes along the erythrocyte plasma membrane (Aikawa *et al.*, 1975) (Fig. 54). They consist of caveolae surrounded by small vesicles arranged in an alveolar fashion (Fig. 55). Horseradish-peroxidase-labeled immunoglobulin from monkeys infected with *P. vivax* has been shown to bind to the vesicle membrane, indicating the presence of malarial antigens within them. After incubation of viable parasitized erythrocytes with ferritin, ferritin particles

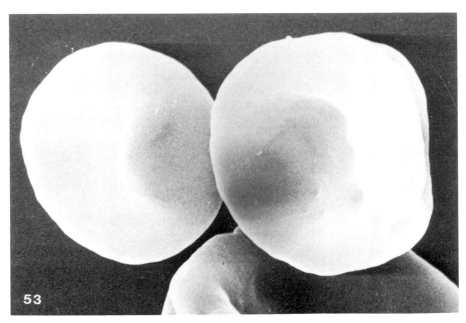

FIG. 53.   Scanning electron micrograph of erythrocytes infected with *P. berghei*. Note several pits on the surface. ×26,000.

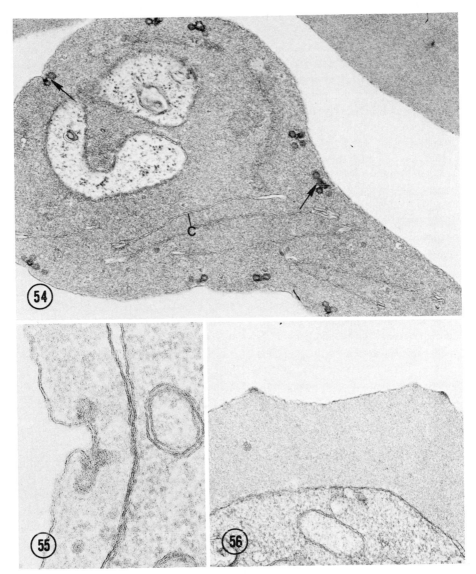

FIG. 54. Erythrocyte infected with *P. vivax,* showing caveola–vesicle complexes (arrow) and clefts (C). ×33,000. (Reproduced from Aikawa *et al.,* 1975, with permission of the author and publisher.)

FIG. 55. High-magnification micrograph showing a caveola–vesicle complex. ×100,000. (Reproduced from Aikawa *et al.,* 1977, with permission of the author and publisher.)

FIG. 56. Excrescences along the membrane of an erythrocyte infected with *P. simiovale.* ×32,000. (Reproduced from Aikawa *et al.,* 1977, with permission of the author and publisher.)

appear within the vesicles, indicating that these vesicles are pinocytotic in origin (Aikawa *et al.*, 1975; Seed *et al.*, 1976). Maurer's clefts seen by light microscopy appear to correspond to narrow slitlike structures in the cytoplasm that could be extrusions of the parasitophorus vacuole membrane. Another prominent change in infected erythrocytes is the development of excrescences on the erythrocyte plasmalemma (Fig. 56). These excrescences form focal junctions with the membranes of endothelial cells or with excrescences on other erythrocytes, suggesting that they are responsible for the sequestration of infected erythrocytes in the deep organs. Some of these changes are species-specific, and others are not. Erythrocytes infected by vivax- and ovale-type parasites show caveola–vesicle complexes and cytoplasmic clefts, while those infected by malariae-type parasites exhibit excrescences and cytoplasmic clefts. Erythrocytes infected by falciparum-type parasites show excrescences and cytoplasmic clefts. In addition, caveolae without vesicles are seen in erythrocytes infected with *P. fragile* and *P. coatneyi,* while *P. falciparum*-infected erythrocytes lack caveolae. It is still not known why a given group of malarial parasites produces changes in the erythrocytes specific to that given group.

Exoerythrocytic malarial parasites also produce changes in the host cell. The host cell increases in size and becomes distorted when the parasitophorous vacuole containing the parasite enlarges. However, the organelles of the host cell do not show any significant changes. These observations may indicate that the host cell changes are due to the presence of malarial parasites as foreign bodies and not to "toxic effects" of the parasites. There are no reports on the fine-structural changes in host cells in mosquitoes infected with malarial parasites.

ACKNOWLEDGMENTS

This work was supported in part by research grants AI-10645 and AI-13366 by the U.S. Public Health Service, by the U.S. Army R & D Command (DADA-17-70-C-0006) and by the U.S. Department of Energy.

The submitted manuscript has been authored by a contractor of the U.S. Government under contract No. W-31-109-ENG-38. Accordingly, the U.S. Government retains a nonexclusive, royalty-free license to publish or reproduce the published form of this contribution or allow others to do so for the U.S. Government.

REFERENCES

Aikawa, M., (1966). The fine structures of the erythrocytic stages of three avian malarial parasites, *Plasmodium fallax, P. lophurae* and *P. cathemerium. Am. J. Trop. Med. Hyg.* **15,** 449–471.
Aikawa, M., (1967). Ultrastructure of the pellicular complex of *Plasmodium fallax. J. Cell Biol.* **35,** 103–113.
Aikawa, M., (1972). Parasitological review. *Plasmodium:* The fine structure of malarial parasites. *Ex. Parasitol.* **30,** 284–320.

Aikawa, M. (1977), Variations in structure and function during the life cycle of malarial parasites. *Bull. W.H.O.* **55**, 137–154.

Aikawa, M., and Beaudoin, R. (1968). Studies on nuclear division of a malarial parasite under pyrimethamine treatment. *J. Cell Biol.* **39**, 749–754.

Aikawa, M., and Cook, R. T. (1971). Ribosomes of the malarial parasite, *Plasmodium knowlesi*. II ultrastructural features. *Comp. Biochem. Physiol. B* **39**, 913–917.

Aikawa, M., and Jordan, H. (1968). Fine structure of reptilian malarial parasites. *J. Parasitol.* **54**, 1023–1033.

Aikawa, M., and Sterling, C. (1974). "Intracellular Parasitic Protozoa." Academic Press, New York.

Aikawa, M., Hepler, P. K., Huff, C. G., and Sprinz, H. (1966a). Feeding mechanisms of avian malarial parasites. *J. Cell Biol.* **28**, 355–373.

Aikawa, M., Huff, C. G., and Sprinz, H.(1966b). Comparative feeding mechanisms of avian and primate malarial parasites. *Mil. Med.* **131**, 969–983.

Aikawa, M., Huff, C. G., and Sprinz, H. (1967). Fine structure of the asexual stages of *Plasmodium elongatum*. *J. Cell Biol.* **34**, 229–249.

Aikawa, M., Huff, C. G., and Sprinz, H. (1968). Exoerythrocytic stages of *Plasmodium gallinaceum* in chick-embryo liver as observed electron microscopically. *Am. J. Trop. Med. Hyg.* **17**, 156–169.

Aikawa, M., Huff, C. G., and Sprinz, H. (1969). Comparative fine structure study of the gametocytes of avian, reptilian and mammalian malarial parasites. *J. Ultrastruct. Res.* **26**, 316–331.

Aikawa, M., Sterling, C. R., and Rabbege, J. (1972). Cytochemistry of the nucleus of malarial parasites. *Proc. Helminthol. Soc. Wash.* **39**, 174–194.

Aikawa, M., Miller, L. H., and Rabbege, J. (1975). Caveola-vesicle complexes: The plasmalemma of erythrocytes infected by *Plasmodium vivax* and *Plasmodium cynomolgi*: Unique structure related to Schüffner's dots. *Am. J. Pathol.* **79**, 285–300.

Aikawa, M., Hsieh, C. L. and Miller, L. H. (1977). Ultrastructural changes of the erythrocyte membrane in ovale-type malarial parasites. *J. Parasitol.* **63**, 152–154.

Aikawa, M., Cochrane, A. H., and Nussenzweig, R. S. (1979). Freeze fracture study on normal and antibody-treated malarial sporozoites. *J. Protozool.* **26**, 273–279.

Aikawa, M., Miller, L. H., Johnson, J., and Rabbege, J.(1978). Erythrocyte entry by malarial parasites: A moving junction between erythrocyte and parasite. *J. Cell Biol.* **77**, 72–82.

Ayala, S. C. (1977). Plasmodia of reptiles. In "Parasitic Protozoa" (J. P. Kreier, ed.), Vol. 3, pp. 267–309. Academic Press, New York.

Ayala, S. C. (1978). Check list, host index and annotated biography of the plasmodia of reptiles. *J. Protozool.* **25**, 87–100.

Bano, L. (1959). A cytological study of the early oocysts of seven species of *Plasmodium* and the occurrence of post-zygotic mitosis. *Parasitology* **49**, 559–585.

Beaudoin, R. L., and Strome, C. P. A. (1972). The feeding process in the exoerythrocytic stages of *Plasmodium lophurae* based upon observations with the electron microscope. *Proc. Helminthol. Soc. Wash.* **39**, 163–173.

Brooks, C., and Kreier, J. P. (1978). Role of surface coat in *in vitro* attachment and phagocytosis of *Plasmodium berghei* by peritoneal macrophages. *Infect. Immun.* **20**, 827–835.

Carter, R., and Diggs, C. L. (1977). Plasmodia of rodents. In "Parasitic Protozoa" (J. P. Kreier, ed.), Vol. 3, pp. 359–465. Academic Press, New York.

Coatney, G. R., Collins, W. E., Warren, N. W., and Contacos, P. G. (1971). "The Primate Malarias". US Govt. Printing Office, Washington, D.C.

Cochrane, A. H., Aikawa, M., Jeng, M., and Nussenzweig, R. S. (1976). Antibody-induced ultrastructural changes of malarial sporozoites. *J. Immunol.* **116**, 859–867.

Cook, R. T., Rock, R. C., Aikawa, M., and Fournier, M. J. (1971). Ribosomes of the malarial parasite, *Plasmodium knowlesi*. I. Isolation, activity and sedimentation velocity. *Comp. Biochem. Physiol. B* **39**, 897–911.

Davis, A. G., Huff, C. G., and Palmer, T. T. (1966). Procedure for maximum production of exoerythrocytic stages of *Plasmodium fallax* in tissue culture. *Exp. Parasitol.* **19**, 1–8.

Dennis, E. D., Mitchell, G. H., Butcher, G. A., and Cohen, S. (1975). *In vitro* isolation of *Plasmodium knowlesi* merozoite using polycarbon sieves. *Parasitology* **71**, 475–481.

Desser, S. S., Well, I., and Yoeli, M. (1972). An ultrastructural study of the pre-erythrocytic development of *Plasmodium berghei* in the tree rat. *Can. J. Zool.* **50**, 821–825.

Dvorak, J. A., Miller, L. H., Whitehouse, W. C., and Shiroishi, T. (1975). Invasion of erythrocytes by malarial merozoites. *Science* **187**, 748–750.

Emmel, L., Jakob, A., and Golz, G. (1942a). Elektronenoptische Untersuchungen an malarial Sporozoiten und Beobachtungen an Kulturformen von *Leishmania donovani*. *Dtsch. Tropenmed. Z.* **46**, 344–348.

Emmel, L., Jakob, A., and Golz, G. (1942b). Elektronenoptische Untersuchungen an malarial Sporozoiten. *Dtsch. Tropenmed. A.* **46**, 573–575.

Fulton, J. D., and Flewelt, T. H. (1956). The relation of *Plasmodium berghei* and *P. knowlesi* to their respective red cell hosts. *Trans. R. Soc. Trop. Med. Hyg.* **50**, 150–156.

Garnham, P. C. C. (1966). "Malaria Parasites and Other Haemosporidia." Blackwell, Oxford.

Garnham, P. C. C., Bird, R. G., and Baker, J. R. (1962). Electron microscope studies of motile stages of malarial parasites. III. The ookinetes of *Haemamoeba* and *Plasmodium*. *Trans. R. Soc. Trop. Med. Hyg.* **56**, 116–120.

Garnham, P. C. C., Bird, R. G., and Baker, J. R. (1963). Electron microscope studies of motile stages of malarial parasites. IV. The fine structure of the sporozoite of four species of *Plasmodium*. *Trans. R. Soc. Trop. Med. Hyg.* **61**, 58–68.

Griffin, F. M., Griffin, J. A., Leider, J. E., and Silverstein, S.C. (1975). Studies on the mechanisms of phagocytosis. I. Requirements for circumferential attachment of particle-bound ligands to specific receptors on the macrophage plasma membrane. *J. Exp. Med.* **142**, 1263–1282.

Hepler, P. K., Huff, C. G., and Sprinz, H. (1966). The fine structure of the exoerythrocytic stages of *Plasmodium fallax*. *J. Cell Biol.* **30**, 333–358.

Howells, R. E., Peters, W., and Fullard, J. (1969). Cytochrome oxidase activity in a normal and some drug-resistant strains of *Plasmodium berghei*—A cytochemical study. I. Asexual erythrocytic stages. *Mil. Med.* **134**, 893–915.

Huff, C. G. (1969). Exoerythrocytic stages of avian and reptilian malarial parasites. *Exp. Parasitol.* **24**, 383–421.

Huff, C. G., Pipkin, A. C., Weathersby, A. B., and Jensen, D. V. (1960). The morphology and behavior of living exoerythrocytic stages of *Plasmodium galinaceum* and *P. fallax* and their host cells. *J. Biophys. Biochem. Cytol.* **7**, 93–102.

Kilejian, A. (1976). Does a histadine-rich protein from *Plasmodium lophurae* have a function in merozoite penetration? *J. Protozool.* **23**, 272–277.

Ladda, R. L. (1969). New insights into the fine structure of rodent malarial parasites. *Mil. Med.* **134**, 825–864.

Ladda, R. L., Aikawa, M., and Sprinz, H. (1969). Penetration of erythrocytes by merozoites of mammalian and avian malarial parasites. *J. Parasitol.* **55**, 633–644.

Langreth, S. G. (1976). Feeding mechanisms in extracellular *Babesia microti* and *Plasmodium lophurae*. *J. Protozool.* **23**; 215–223.

Langreth, S. G. (1977). Electron microscope cytochemistry of host-parasite membrane interactions with malaria. *Bull. W.H.O.* **55**, 171–178.

Lumsden, W. H. R., and Bertram, D. S. (1940). Observations on the biology of *Plasmodium gallinaceum* Bumpt, 1935, in the domestic fowl, with special reference to the production of gametocytes and their development in *Aedes aegypti* (L). *Ann. Trop. Med. Parasitol.* **34**, 135–160.

McLaren, D. J., Bannister, L. H., Trigg, P. I., and Butcher, G. A. (1977). A freeze-fracture study on the parasite erythrocyte interrelationship in *Plasmodium knowlesi* infections. *Bull. W.H.O.* **55**, 199–203.

Meszoely, C. A. M., Steere, R. L., and Bahr, G. F. (1972). Morphologic studies on the freeze-etched avian malarial parasite *Plasmodium gallinaceum*. *Proc. Helminthol. Soc. Wash.* **39**, 149–162.

Miller, L. H., Aikawa, M., and Dvorak, J. A. (1975a). Malaria (*Plasmodium knowlesi*) merozoites: Immunity and the surface coat. *J. Immunol.* **114**, 1237–1242.

Miller, L. H., Mason, S. J., Dvorak, M., McGinniss, H., and Rothman, I. K. (1975b). Erythrocyte receptors for (*Plasmodium knowlesi*) malaria: Duffy blood group determinants. *Science* **189**, 561–562.

Miller, L. H., Aikawa, M., Johnson, J., and Shiroishi, T. (1978). Interaction between cytochalasin B-treated malarial parasites and red cells: Attachment and junction formation. *J. Exp. Med.* **149**, 172–184.

Rudzinska, M. A., and Trager, W. (1957). Intracellular phagotrophy by malarial parasites: An electron microscope study of *Plasmodium lophurae*. *J. Protozool.* **4**, 190–199.

Rudzinska, M. A., and Trager, W. (1959). Phagotrophy and two new structures in the malaria parasite, *Plasmodium berghei*. *J. Biophys. Biochem. Cytol.* **6**, 103–112.

Scalzi, H. A., and Bahr, G. H. (1968). An electron microscopic examination of erythrocytic stages of two rodent malarial parasites. *Plasmodium chabaudi* and *Plasmodium vinckei*. *J. Ultrastruc. Res.* **24**, 116–133.

Seed, T. M., and Kreier, J. P. (1972). *Plasmodium gallinaceum:* Erythrocyte membrane alterations and associated plasma changes induced by experimental infection. *Proc. Helminthol. Soc. Wash.* **39**, 387–411.

Seed, T. M., and Kreier, J. P. (1976). Surface properties of extracellular malaria parasites: Electrophoretic and lectin-binding characteristics. *Infect. Immun.* **14**, 1339–1347.

Seed, T. M., and Manwell, R. D. (1977). Plasmodia of birds. In "Parasitic Protozoa" (J. P. Kreier, ed.), Vol. 3, pp. 311–357. Academic Press, New York.

Seed, T. M., Pfister, R., Kreier, J. P., and Johnson, A. (1971). *Plasmodium gallinaceum:* Fine structure by freeze-etch technique. *Exp. Parasitol.* **30**, 73–81.

Seed, T. M., Aikawa, M., Prior, R. B., Kreier, J. P., and Pfister, R. M. (1973). *Plasmodium sp:* Topography of intra- and extracellular parasites. *Z. Tropenmed. Parisitol.* **24**, 525–535.

Seed, T. M., Aikawa, M., Sterling, C., and Rabbege, J. (1974). Surface properties of extracellular malaria parasites: Morphological and cytochemical study. *Infect. Immun.* **9**, 750–761.

Seed, T., Sterling, C. R., Aikawa, M., and Rabbege, J. (1976). *Plasmodium simium:* Ultrastructure of erythrocytic phase. *Exp. Parasitol.* **39**, 262–276.

Shute, P. G., and Maryon, M. (1952). A study of human malaria oocysts as an aid to species diagnosis. *Trans. R. Soc. Trop. Med. Hyg.* **46**, 272–292.

Sinden, R. E., Canning, E. V., and Spain, B. (1976). Gametogenesis and fertilization in *Plasmodium yoelii nigeriensis:* A transmission electron microscope study. *Proc. R. Soc. London, Ser. B* **193**, 55–76.

Sodeman, T., Schnitzer, B., Durkee, T., and Contacos, P. (1970). Fine structure of the exoerythrocytic stages of *Plasmodium cynomolgi*. *Science* **170**, 340–341.

Sterling, C. R., Aikawa, M., and Nussenzweig, R. S. (1972). Morphological divergence in a mammalian malarial parasite: The fine structure of *Plasmodium brasilianum*. *Proc. Helminthol. Soc. Wash.* **39**, 109–129.

Terzakis, J. A. (1972). Virus-like particles and sporozoite budding. *Proc. Helminthol. Soc. Wash.* **39**, 129–136.

Terzakis, J. A., Sprinz, H., and Ward, R. A. (1967). The transformation of the *Plasmodium gallinaceum* oocyst in *Aedes aegypti* mosquitoes. *J. Cell Biol.* **34**, 311–326.

Vanderberg, J., Rhodin, J., and Yoeli, M. (1967). Electron microscopic and histochemical studies of sporozoite formation on *Plasmodium berghei*. *J. Protozool*. **14**, 82–103.

Wessells, N. K., Spoones, B. S., Ash, J. F., Bradley, M. O., Luduena, M. A., Taylor, E. L., Wrenn, J. T., and Yamada, K. M. (1971). Microfilaments in cellular and developmental processes. *Science* **171**, 135.

Young, M. D., Clyles, D. E., Burgess, R. W., and Jeffery, G. M. (1955). Experimental testing of the immunity of negroes to *Plasmodium vivax*. *J. Parasitol*. **41**, 315–318.

Biochemistry of Malarial Parasites

C. A. Homewood and K. D. Neame

I. INTRODUCTION

> The feeling on me grows and grows
> That hardly anybody knows
> If those are these or these are those.
>   (Milne, 1927)

The biochemistry of malarial parasites is still poorly understood in spite of many years of research. This is not for lack of effort, but because many of the published data are invalid for one reason or another.

The difficulty of investigating the biochemistry of these parasites makes it tempting to perform fewer experiments than should be considered acceptable in any field of biochemistry. Indeed, many published papers are of little value because they report the results of an inadequate number of observations from only single experiments, and controls were also inadequate or else nonexistent.

More frequently, papers are invalidated because the results described were quite possibly due more to host cells than to parasites. The importance of distinguishing between parasites and host cells has been stressed by other reviewers (Danforth, 1967; Fletcher and Maegraith, 1972; Oelshlegel and Brewer, 1975).

In this introduction we set out the various causes of error peculiar to this type of research.

A. Contamination of Intraerythrocytic Parasites by Host Material

The apparent simplicity of working with the intraerythrocytic stages of malarial parasites has led many investigators to consider that parasitized blood is equivalent merely to normal blood with parasites added. This inevitably leads to attempts to determine the metabolism or composition of the parasite simply by comparing infected blood with normal blood, but this is likely to give misleading results because of the many changes which take place in the blood of the host as a result of infection. Thus it is possible to attribute to the parasite itself changes in the overall metabolism of blood following infection, when these changes are in fact the result of alterations in the plasma, white cells, red cells, or platelets.

1. Blood Plasma

There are many changes in the enzymes and other constituents of the plasma of infected animals (Sadun *et al.*, 1966). The consequences of this can be (but are not always) avoided by working with washed cells rather than with whole blood.

2. White Cells

The number of white cells in the bloodstream of an infected animal may be greatly increased; the increase appears to be particularly marked in rodents

(Broun, 1961; Kretschmar, 1961) but may be less significant in primates (e.g., Ball *et al.,* 1948; Hickman, 1969).

The error caused by white cells depends to a large extent on the type of investigation. Determination of the biochemical composition of parasites, for example, may be little affected by the presence of white cells. Investigations of metabolic activity, however, may be completely invalidated by the contribution from relatively few white cells, because they have a greater range of metabolic activities than red cells, and the activity of a given enzyme or process may be many times higher (compare Cline, 1965, with Brewer, 1974). In addition, the interfering effects of white cells can be more serious in some species of animals than in others (Richards and Williams, 1973).

Many early workers ignored the presence of white cells (experiments have been reported in which the number of white cells was as much as 1% of the number of parasitized cells), and even now white cells are often not removed, or else the methods used for their removal are inadequate. Frequently, a method shown to be effective in removing leukocytes from the blood of healthy animals of one species is applied without further test to the blood of a malaria-infected animal of a different species. No method can be accepted as satisfactory until it has been thoroughly tested on the blood of the appropriate animal infected with the chosen parasite, and the results of the test reported. This has been done for the cellulose powder method of Fulton and Grant (1956), which effectively removes white cells from the blood of *Plasmodium berghei*-infected mice (Homewood and Neame, 1976) and *P. berghei*-infected rats and *P. knowlesi*-infected monkeys (Williams and Richards, 1973). Without such supporting evidence, the use of an unproved method, accompanied by a statement that ''leukocytes were removed,'' cannot be accepted as proof of an uncontaminated parasite preparation.

The method of removal of white cells must be checked by a standard method of counting using a counting chamber, and not, for example, by comparing a film of infected whole blood with a film made from washed cells suspended in a medium other than plasma, since the distribution of white cells can be quite different in the two types of films.

In some cases, leukocytes are deliberately not removed because their numbers are similar in infected and uninfected blood, or corrections are made by applying to infected blood calculations based on the activities of leukocytes of normal blood. It is possible, however, that the metabolic activities of white cells in infected blood may differ from those of the white cells in the blood of uninfected animals, and this must be checked before such calculations are considered valid. For example, activated or phagocytosing macrophages show marked changes in several of their biochemical functions (Iyer *et al.,* 1961; Karnovsky *et al.,* 1975).

3. Immature Red Cells

This source of interference is less obvious and less easily corrected for. During the course of an infection, there are marked changes in various properties of the erythrocytes (see Kreier *et al.*, 1972; Seed and Kreier, 1972), and it is apparent that there must be considerable change in their metabolism. The lysis of red cells caused by the progress of the infection inevitably leads to a population of cells younger than that of uninfected animals, especially when high parasitemias (commonly used in biochemical experiments) are reached. These younger cells are in many respects more metabolically active than mature erythrocytes (Lowenstein, 1959; Augustin, 1961; Rapoport, 1961; Bunn, 1972). It has often been stated that the blood of an animal used in an experiment had only a low percentage of reticulocytes as determined by standard histological methods. However, the histological staining of reticulocytes does not necessarily correlate well with the levels of enzyme activity of immature red cells. It is possible to have increases in the enzymes or metabolic activities of red cells without corresponding increases in the percentage of detectable reticulocytes or polychromatophils (Silverman *et al.*, 1944; Goetze and Rapoport, 1954; Schröter *et al.*, 1967; Momen *et al.*, 1975). In addition, Howells and Maxwell (1973b) have shown that *P. berghei*, which does not itself possess isocitrate dehydrogenase, can cause an increase in the activity of this enzyme in reticulocytes of mice. It is therefore necessary, before attributing a metabolic activity to a parasite, to make certain that the activity did not originate in immature red cells.

4. Platelets

The high rate of metabolism of platelets, and their possession of metabolic pathways not found in erythrocytes (Marcus and Zucker, 1965), can in some cases cause misleading results. The number of platelets falls during infection with *P. berghei* in the mouse (Fabiani *et al.*, 1958), but there is evidence that the opposite is true of *P. knowlesi* infections in the monkey (Reid and Sucharit, 1972).

B. Contamination of Free Parasites by Host Material

Experiments using free parasites can be particularly misleading if it is always assumed that the parasites are free of erythrocytic contamination. Most methods of preparing free parasites leave at least part of the red cell membrane around the parasite (Cook *et al.*, 1969; Killby and Silverman, 1969; Aikawa and Cook, 1972; Trager *et al.*, 1972; Seed *et al.*, 1973; Kreier, 1977). Many enzymes are firmly attached to this membrane (Schrier, 1963; Green *et al.*, 1970), including some, such as the enzymes of glycolysis, which are normally considered soluble although a change in pH or salt concentration may release them (Green *et al.*, 1970). The residual membrane may also trap organelles of the host red cells so that these contaminate the free parasite preparation. In addition, organelles freed from other lysed host cells will be collected with the free parasites during centrifugation unless special care is taken. This will be particularly true for avian parasites, whose host cells contain more organelles than are found in the erythrocytes of mammals. Most free parasites of the avian species are contaminated with nuclei, and preparations of nuclei can themselves contain a considerable number of enzymes (Allfrey and Mirsky, 1959; Roodyn, 1959, 1963).

C. Viability of Parasites *in Vitro*

Even with a completely uncontaminated preparation of parasites or parasitized cells, misleading results can still be obtained. Malarial parasites are organisms with a high rate of metabolism, and an incubation medium whose composition remains virtually constant when it contains only normal red cells may change considerably when it contains parasitized cells. Two types of change are particularly important, one being the reduction in the concentration of a nutrient such as glucose, and the other being a change in pH. A common practice is to incubate a concentrated suspension of parasites or parasitized cells for up to several hours at 37°C, either in plasma or in a simplified medium. It is almost certain that in such circumstances the parasites will be dead long before the end of the incubation period, because of the disappearance of glucose due to metabolism to lactic acid and because of the consequent fall in pH. It is possible that, in a medium whose pH is poorly controlled, the metabolism of any white cells present could become predominant, since they appear to be more tolerant of acid conditions; for example, a fall in pH reduces the rate of glucose metabolism by white cells less than that by red cells (Graubarth *et al.*, 1953) and possibly less than that by parasites. If the pH becomes low enough, the white cells will break down and release degradative enzymes. An alteration in pH can be reduced by increasing the concentration of the buffer in the medium, but the rapid disappearance of glucose cannot be prevented if the density of the parasites is high.

It will be seen in this chapter that many of the errors discussed above are surprisingly common. In many papers, a lack of experimental detail makes it impossible to decide whether or not such errors have been avoided. The conclusions drawn from the experiments described may be correct but, unfortunately, where there is any doubt they cannot be accepted. Mistakes will inevitably be made at some time by most experimenters, but until more work on the biochemistry of malarial parasites is carried out with the caution and thoroughness characteristic at present of only a few investigations, the metabolism of the parasite will never be fully understood.

Because an attempt has been made to assess the reliability of experiments, only those papers which give full experimental details have been reviewed. Abstracts, communications at conferences, and laboratory demonstrations have therefore been omitted. In addition the biochemistry of only the intraerythrocytic stages of rodent, primate, and avian parasites has been discussed. So little is known of the metabolism of any stage of saurian parasites that it has been impossible to include them, and the small amount of information on the non-erythrocytic stages of mammalian and avian parasites has also been omitted.

II. CARBOHYDRATE UTILIZATION AND GLYCOLYSIS

A. Carbohydrate Reserves

The intraerythrocytic stages of malarial parasites have few, if any, reserves of glycogen or other polysaccharide (rodent: Sen Gupta et al., 1955; Ciucă et al., 1963; primate: Christophers and Fulton, 1938; Dasgupta, 1960; avian: Lillie, 1947; Dasgupta, 1960).

B. Substrates Used

Glucose is the main substrate of carbohydrate metabolism by malarial parasites (see Section II,C for references), but it has been reported that they can also use a variety of other substances, particularly lactate, glycerol and intermediates of the citric acid cycle (primate: Fulton, 1939; Maier and Coggeshall, 1941; Wendel and Kimball, 1942; Wendel, 1943; McKee et al., 1946; avian: Bovarnick et al., 1946a,b; Speck et al., 1946; Marshall, 1948; Moulder, 1948, 1949).

Often the only test for the utilization of a substrate has been the measurement of an increase in oxygen uptake on addition of the substrate to washed blood cells from infected animals. This may not be a valid test because, as will be discussed in Section V,A, there is insufficient evidence that all or even some of the measured respiration was from the parasite itself and not from contaminating host blood cells.

A better test is the ability of a given substrate to support growth of the parasite in vitro in the absence of glucose. By this criterion, glycerol, which is at least as effective as glucose in stimulating respiration of P. knowlesi (Fulton, 1939; Maier and Coggeshall, 1941; McKee et al., 1946), cannot be used by the parasite (Anfinsen et al., 1946). Of other substances tested, only maltose was effective in supporting growth of P. falciparum and P. vivax (Bass and Johns, 1912).

C. Glucose Utilization

Normal red cells use very little glucose, whereas cells infected with malarial parasites consume glucose at a high rate (rodent: Fulton and Spooner, 1956; Bowman et al., 1960; Cenedella and Jarrell, 1970; Cenedella et al., 1970;

Coombs and Gutteridge, 1975; Oelshlegel *et al.*, 1975; primate: Christophers and Fulton, 1938; Maier and Coggeshall, 1941; Wendel, 1943; McKee *et al.*, 1946; Ball *et al.*, 1948; Scheibel and Miller, 1969b; Scheibel and Pflaum, 1970; Shakespeare and Trigg, 1973; Oelshlegel *et al.*, 1975; avian: Silverman *et al.*, 1944; Ceithaml and Evans, 1946; Manwell and Feigelson, 1949; Moulder, 1949; Warren and Manwell, 1954; Khabir and Manwell, 1955).

The erythrocytes of both ducks and mice have a low permeability to glucose, and Herman *et al.*, (1966) suggested that a high rate of glucose utilization could only be maintained if the permeability of the host cell were altered. Sherman and Tanigoshi (1974b) showed that the rate of entry of glucose into the duck red cell increased on parasitization and that this was due to an increase in the rate of diffusion. In *P. berghei*-infected mice, a similar change in the permeability of red cells (Neame and Homewood, 1975) was shown to be limited to cells which contained parasites (Homewood and Neame, 1974). It is not known whether such changes in permeability also occur in primate erythrocytes, which normally have a high permeability to glucose (Christensen, 1975).

It is difficult to determine precisely the rate at which glucose is used by the parasite itself, for several reasons (1) the rate of utilization may depend on the initial concentration of glucose in the medium (primate: Scheibel and Miller, 1969b), although this may appear not to be the case if the initial concentration is high (primate: Christophers and Fulton, 1938); (2) conditions of incubation are sometimes far from ideal (e.g., a progressive decrease in the concentration of glucose in the medium and a decrease in pH due to the production of lactic acid can affect the rate of utilization); (3) white cells, with their high rate of glucose utilization, may be present in the parasite preparation; for example, rabbit white cells metabolize glucose at up to 500 times the rate of normal red cells (Guest *et al.*, 1953); (4) the presence of immature red cells, which in mammals (Jones *et al.*, 1953; Rubinstein *et al.*, 1956; Bernstein, 1959; Rapoport, 1961; Momen, 1979b) and birds (Manwell and Feigelson, 1949; Khabir and Manwell, 1955) have increased glycolytic activity, can contribute significantly to measured values; (5) the amount of glucose used by a preparation of free parasites is nearly always less than that used by the same number of parasitized cells (rodent: Bryant *et al.*, 1964; Bowman *et al.*, 1960, 1961; Cenedella, 1968; Cenedella and Jarrell, 1970; Cenedella *et al.*, 1970; avian: Speck *et al.*, 1946), either because the parasites have been damaged during their release from the red cell or because the contribution to glucose metabolism by host cells has been reduced.

D. End Products of Glucose Metabolism

1. Lactate

Part of the glucose used by malarial parasites is converted to lactate. The proportion so converted varies greatly and appears to depend partly on the species studied and partly on the conditions of incubation. The percentage of utilized glucose metabolized to lactate has been reported to be between about 40 and 100% for rodent malarial parasites (Fulton and Spooner, 1956; Bowman *et al.*, 1960, 1961; Cenedella and Jarrell, 1970; Cenedella *et al.*, 1970; Coombs and Gutteridge, 1975; Momen, 1979b), between about 6 and 106% for primate parasites (Wendel, 1943; Ball *et al.*, 1948; Scheibel and Miller, 1969b; Shakespeare and Trigg, 1973; Trigg and Shakespeare, 1976), and between 0 and about 200% for avian parasites (Silverman *et al.*, 1944; Ceithaml and Evans, 1946; Speck *et al.*, 1946; Marshall, 1948).

2. *Other End Products*

An early attempt to detect end products of glucose metabolism other than lactate was that of Wendel and Kimball (1942) who claimed that *P. knowlesi*-parasitized monkey erythrocytes excreted pyruvate. This could not be confirmed by Scheibel and Pflaum (1970) who, however, reported the conversion to acetate of a considerable fraction of the glucose used. Polet *et al.* (1969) reported that label from radioactive glucose was found in aspartate, glutamate, and alanine from the protein of *P. knowlesi;* they felt, however, that complete removal of white cells would be necessary before these metabolic conversions could be attributed with certainty to the parasite, since white cell protein also contained label in these amino acids.

For *P. berghei,* significant quantities of end products other than lactate have not been detected. The small amounts of succinate and acetate produced by *P. berghei*-infected rat reticulocytes were considered by Fulton and Spooner (1956) to be produced by host cells. Bryant *et al.* (1964) could not account for about 70% of the glucose used by *P. berghei*-infected mouse cells; they attributed this to a loss of volatile end products but did not investigate further. The metabolized glucose unaccounted for was not stored as 2,3-diphosphoglycerate, since Ali and Fletcher (1974) showed that the level of this compound fell in heavily infected mouse blood.

With avian malarial parasites, the interpretation of results is even more difficult because of the more complex metabolism of the host red cell. *Plasmodium lophurae*-infected duck erythrocytes and free parasites metabolized glucose not only to lactate but also to succinate and amino acids (mainly glutamate, with some alanine and aspartate) (Sherman *et al.*, 1969b); this pattern of glucose metabolism was the same as that of the host erythrocyte, but the amount of glucose used was very much greater in parasitized cells.

E. Enzymes of Glycolysis

The conversion of glucose at least partly to lactate indicates that the malarial parasite must contain the enzymes of the glycolytic pathway. The first enzyme of the pathway, hexokinase, was shown by Speck and Evans (1945) to be present in extracts of free parasites of *P. gallinaceum* (stated by the authors, however, to be contaminated with white cells and red cell nuclei, for which no allowance was made). This enzyme also showed increased activity in *P. berghei*-infected blood (Fraser and Kermack, 1957). It is difficult to know in both these cases the extent to which the measured activities were due to the host cells. The activity of hexokinase is higher in immature than in mature red cells of humans (Hutton, 1972), although Fraser and Kermack (1957) found the activity to be the same in both mature and immature red cells of mice.

Using electrophoretic methods, Carter (1973) showed the presence of hexokinase in rodent parasites. Although no controls for white cells or immature red cells were used, different strains of parasite gave bands of different electrophoretic mobility. By similar means, glucosephosphate isomerase was also found in rodent parasites (Carter, 1970, 1973, 1978; Momen, 1979a) and in *P. falciparum* (Carter and McGregor, 1973; Carter and Voller, 1973, 1975; see also Carter and Walliker, 1977).

Aldolase was detected by direct measurement in extracts of free parasites of *P. gallinaceum* (Speck and Evans, 1945), but these extracts were again contaminated with host material.

An increase in phosphoglycerate kinase activity in the red cells of ducks on infection with *P. lophurae* was found to be present even after the removal of white cells (Trager, 1967).

Pyruvate kinase of *P. berghei* and *P. knowlesi* was investigated by Oelshlegel *et al.* (1975) who found isoenzymes in infected cells that did not occur in normal blood. However, the method used for the removal of leukocytes has been shown to be inefficient for *P. berghei*-infected mouse blood (Homewood and Neame, 1976), and it is known that human leukocytes contain a pyruvate kinase whose electrophoretic mobility differs from that of the enzyme of erythrocytes (Koler *et al.*, 1964).

Trager (1967) found a rise in the activity of pyruvate kinase in duck cells infected with *P. lophurae* and showed that the extra activity was destroyed by freezing and thawing, suggesting a different isoenzyme; the activity which could have been due to contaminating white cells was calculated.

Lactate dehydrogenase activity was shown to be present in extracts of *P. gallinaceum,* but the extracts were contaminated with host material (Speck and Evans, 1945). Sherman (1961, 1962) showed that lactate dehydrogenase activity increased in the red cells of ducks infected with *P. lophurae* and of mice infected with *P. berghei;* in each case activity was also present in free parasites. An additional isoenzyme of lactate dehydrogenase was detected after electrophoresis of extracts both of *P. lophurae* and of *P. berghei,* but a comparison with immature red cells was not made. More convincingly, Carter (1973) showed that lactate dehydrogenases from different strains of *P. vinckei* had different electrophoretic mobilities, and Carter and Voller (1973) in a similar way detected lactate dehydrogenases in two strains of *P. falciparum* maintained in monkeys (see also Carter and Walliker, 1977). Lactate dehydrogenase was also shown to be present in *P. falciparum* by the detection of separate isoenzymes in different strains of the parasite in Africa (Carter and McGregor, 1973; Carter and Voller, 1975). Tsukamoto (1974) separated by electrophoresis all possible isoenzymes of mouse lactate dehydrogenase and then showed an additional band of enzyme activity after electrophoresis of extracts of *P. berghei*. The enzyme was also found in rodent parasites by Carter (1978) and Momen (1979a).

Phisphumvidhi and Langer (1969) claimed to have detected the lactate dehydrogenase of *P. berghei* and to have shown that the enzyme of the parasite had a higher affinity for pyruvate than that shown by the enzyme of mouse red cells. However, the enzyme preparation was probably not pure, since white cells (with their high lactate dehydrogenase activity) were removed by a method which was ineffective in other laboratories (Homewood and Neame, 1976) and immature red cells were not taken into account. In addition, examination of the published figures for the affinity of the enzyme for pyruvate do not reveal the large differences in K_m which were claimed.

In summary, it seems that, although all the enzymes of the glycolytic pathway must be present in malarial parasites, only hexokinase, glucosephosphate isomerase and lactate dehydrogenase have been definitely detected. Nothing is known of the properties of any of the enzymes, in spite of the importance of this pathway to the parasites.

III. PENTOSE PHOSPHATE PATHWAY

The activity of the pentose phosphate pathway appears to be low in all species of malaria studied. Bowman *et al.* (1961) found, by measuring carbon dioxide production, that less than 2% of the glucose metabolized by *P. berghei* (either free or within the host cell) was metabolized by this pathway, and Bryant *et al.* (1964) could not detect conversion of glucose to 6-phosphogluconate by free parasites. In avian (Herman *et al.*, 1966) and primate species (Scheibel and Miller, 1969b; Shakespeare and Trigg, 1973) the activity of the pathway is also relatively low, although Sherman *et al.* (1970) found relatively greater activity of the pathway in *P. lophurae*.

A. Enzymes of the Pathway

1. Glucose-6-Phosphate Dehydrogenase

The activity of this enzyme is much higher in immature than in mature red cells of mammals (Hutton, 1972; Rozenszajn *et al.*, 1972), and the enzymes of the two types of cell behave differently when examined by electrophoresis (Walter *et al.*, 1965); white cells, also, have a pentose phosphate pathway (Beck, 1958). Avian erythrocytes also contain glucose-6-phosphate dehydrogenase (Bell, 1971).

The glucose-6-phosphate dehydrogenase attributed by Carter (1973) to *P. berghei* may, as later suggested by Carter himself (quoted by Killick-Kendrick, 1974), have originated from host cells, since immature red cells and white cells were not taken into account. Similarly, the enzyme which Langer *et al.* (1967) detected in free parasites of *P. berghei,* although electrophoretically distinct from the enzyme of normal red cells, may also have been derived from host material.

Several authors have reported the absence of glucose-6-phosphate dehydrogenase from malarial parasites. Although the activity of the enzyme increased in the red cells of infected animals, no activity could be detected in free parasites of *P. knowlesi* by Fletcher and Maegraith (1962), nor could Tsukamoto (1974), Fletcher *et al.* (1977) or Momen (1979a) detect it by electrophoresis in extracts of *P. berghei*. In addition, activity of the enzyme could not be detected in malarial parasites by electron microscope histochemistry, although it was clearly present in the red cells (rodent: Theakston and Fletcher, 1971, 1973a; primate: Theakston and Fletcher, 1971, 1973a; Theakston *et al.*, 1976; avian: Theakston and Fletcher, 1971).

Further evidence that the glucose-6-phosphate dehydrogenase of infected cells was solely in the erythrocyte was the finding that, while the parasite was increasing in size and the red cell cytoplasm was being destroyed, the activity of the enzyme in infected cells was falling (rodent: Jung *et al.*, 1975; Picard-Maureau *et al.*, 1975). Sherman (1965) reported, on the other hand, that there was no decrease in the activity of glucose-6-phosphate dehydrogenase in red cells from animals infected with *P. berghei* or *P. lophurae* until the parasitemia had reached high levels, but it is possible that the simple dye test used may not apply without correction to the complicated mixture of cells obtained from infected animals.

A comparison of the actions of oxidative agents on *P. berghei* and on erythrocytes deficient in glucose-6-phosphate dehydrogenase led Pollack *et al.* (1966) to the conclusion that the similarity of the effects which they found might indicate a similar enzyme deficiency in both types of cell, although it was also possible that the oxidative agents had other, unrelated, effects on the parasite.

2. 6-Phosphogluconate Dehydrogenase

This enzyme has been detected in malarial parasites by electrophoresis (rodent: Carter, 1970, 1973, 1978; Carter and Walliker, 1977; Fletcher *et al.*, 1977; Momen, 1979a; primate: Carter and McGregor, 1973; Carter and Voller, 1973, 1975; Carter and Walliker, 1977) and by electron microscopy (rodent: Theakston and Fletcher, 1973b; primate: Theakston and Fletcher, 1973b; Theakston *et al.*, 1976; avian: Theakston and Fletcher, 1973b). Langer *et al.* (1967) measured the activity of this and other enzymes of the pentose phosphate pathway in free parasites of *P. berghei*, but it is possible that some of the activity found was due to host material. The only doubt as to the presence of the enzyme was expressed by Fletcher and Maegraith (1962) who could not detect its activity in free parasites of *P. knowlesi*, although this group later detected it in the parasite by electron microscopy (see above).

B. Reduced Glutathione

Decreased activity of the pentose phosphate pathway of the red cells affects their ability to keep glutathione in the reduced state. It was reported that monkey erythrocytes containing *P. knowlesi* in the later stages of the intraerythrocytic cycle showed some decrease in the amount of reduced glutathione present (Fletcher and Maegraith, 1970), but with *P. vinckei,* in contrast, the level of reduced glutathione rose during growth of the parasite (Picard-Maureau *et al.,* 1975). Towards the end of an infection with *P. berghei,* when the parasitemia was high, reduced glutathione of the blood cells increased (Fletcher and Maegraith, 1970), but the high level of glutathione in immature red cells (Wagenknecht, 1961; Hopkins and Tudhope, 1973) and in white cells (Hardin *et al.,* 1954) may have contributed to the increase.

It thus appears that malarial parasites do not themselves have a complete pentose phosphate pathway, since at least one enzyme, glucose-6-phosphate dehydrogenase, is absent. It has been suggested by Motulsky (1964) that the parasite is able to make use of the pentose phosphate pathway of the host. It may be, however, that the intraerythrocytic parasite is able to survive without a complete pathway, obtaining preformed from the host the substances whose synthesis *de novo* would require a functioning cycle. It is also perhaps possible that part of the cycle is present in malarial parasites, as it is in *Tetrahymena,* in which it can be used in the metabolism of pentose sugars (Eldan and Blum, 1975).

IV. CITRIC ACID CYCLE

It is widely believed that avian malarial parasites possess a functioning citric acid cycle and that mammalian ones do not (Danforth, 1967; Peters, 1969, 1970; von Brand, 1973; Oelshlegel and Brewer, 1975), but this has been questioned (Homewood, 1977).

The belief that avian parasites alone have a citric acid cycle is based on (1) structure of the mitochondria, (2) stimulation of oxygen uptake by intermediates of the cycle, (3) utilization of intermediates of the cycle, (4) end products of glucose metabolism, and (5) detection of enzymes of the cycle.

A. Structure of Mitochondria

The mitochondria of intraerythrocytic avian malarial parasites are cristate, whereas those of most mammalian parasites are not. However, in most mitochondria the enzymes of the citric acid cycle are not part of the structure of the cristae, and the presence of cristae therefore does not prove the presence of a functioning cycle. (For references, see Section V,B.)

B. Stimulation of Oxygen Uptake

Although several reports claim that oxygen uptake of avian malarial parasites is increased by pyruvate, lactate and intermediates of the citric acid cycle (Bovarnick et al., 1946a,b; Silverman et al., 1944; Speck et al., 1946; Marshall, 1948; Moulder, 1948, 1949), there is little clear evidence that all, or indeed any, of the increase can be attributed to the parasite (see Section V,A). In addition, stimulation of oxygen uptake by lactate has been reported for *P. knowlesi* (Wendel, 1943; McKee et al., 1946), although it is believed that this parasite does not have a functioning cycle.

C. Utilization of Intermediates

It has been reported that avian parasites can metabolize pyruvate, lactate and various intermediates of the cycle *in vitro* (Silverman et al., 1944; Speck et al., 1946), but it is difficult to know the extent to which host cells, which have a citric acid cycle (Rubinstein and Denstedt, 1953; Dajani and Orten, 1958), participated in the observed metabolism. In addition, these observations cannot be taken as proof that only avian parasites have a citric acid cycle, because *P. knowlesi*, believed to lack a cycle, has also been reported to utilize lactate (Wendel and Kimball, 1942; Wendel, 1943; McKee et al., 1946). The results obtained could have been due either to utilization by the parasite (thus suggesting a citric acid cycle in the parasite) or to utilization by host cells.

Clarke (1952b) and Trager (1952) observed that malate prolonged the life of extracellular *P. lophurae:* this could, however, have been due, not to the use of malate itself by the parasite, but to substances derived from malate by enzymes of the red cell extract which was a component of the culture medium.

D. End Products of Glucose Metabolism

These have been discussed in Section II,D. In most experiments, both avian and mammalian parasites metabolized to lactate a large part of the glucose utilized. Usually, little of the glucose used by rodent, primate or avian parasites was metabolized to carbon dioxide (rodent: Bowman *et al.*, 1961; primate: Scheibel and Miller, 1969b; Scheibel and Pflaum, 1970; Shakespeare and Trigg, 1973; avian: Silverman *et al.*, 1944; Herman *et al.*, 1966), indicating little activity of the citric acid cycle. The most convincing evidence in favor of the operation of the cycle in avian parasites was provided by Sherman *et al.* (1970) who found that free parasites of *P. lophurae* metabolized a considerable proportion of glucose to carbon dioxide (over 20% of the glucose used).

Lack of carbon dioxide production from glucose does not necessarily indicate the absence of a citric acid cycle. It is possible that, even if the cycle were present, it would be little used either by the parasite or by the host cell in many experiments, because of the low availability of oxygen together with the relatively high initial concentration of glucose. [A Pasteur effect has been demonstrated for mammalian reticulocytes (Ghosh and Sloviter, 1973) and for white cells (Cline, 1965).]

E. Enzymes of the Citric Acid Cycle

1. Malate Dehydrogenase

Nagarajan (1968a) detected malate dehydrogenase activity in free parasites of *P. berghei,* although reticulocyte stroma, used as a control in these experiments, also contained the enzyme.

Carter (1970, 1973), Momen *et al.* (1975), and Momen (1979a) detected, in addition to the malate dehydrogenase of the erythrocyte, other isoenzymes in cells of mice infected with *P. berghei.* One of these isoenzymes was considered by Momen *et al.* (1975) to originate in immature red cells, but both groups agreed that one of the isoenzymes in *P. berghei*-parasitized cells was of parasite origin. Momen *et al.* (1975) and Momen (1979a) failed to find the enzyme in one strain of *P. berghei* and suggested that it was therefore not essential to the normal metabolism of the parasite; failure to find the enzyme may, however, have been due to technical difficulties rather than to its absence from the parasite.

The presence of malate dehydrogenase in *P. berghei* has also been reported as a result of the electrophoretic investigations of Sherman (1966) and Tsukamoto (1974), but in the former case white cells were not removed, and in both cases there was no examination of immature red cells, which have been shown to contain an isoenzyme electrophoretically distinct from that in mature red cells (Momen *et al.*, 1975).

Malate dehydrogenase has not been detected in primate parasites, or with certainty in avian ones; although Sherman (1966) reported its presence in *P. lophurae,* no comparisons were made with immature red cells.

2. Succinate Dehydrogenase

Howells (1970) was unable to detect succinate dehydrogenase by electron microscope histochemistry in *P. berghei,* nor could Nagarajan (1968a) measure activity of either this enzyme or several others of the cycle in free parasites in spite of the observation that respiration was stimulated by succinate. Seaman (1953) claimed to have found succinate dehydrogenase in *P. lophurae,* although in this case contaminating host cell material could well have been the source of the enzyme. No attempt has been made to detect the enzyme in avian parasites by histochemical methods.

3. Isocitrate Dehydrogenase

Isocitrate dehydrogenase specific to the intraerythrocytic parasite was not detected after electrophoresis of extracts of *P. berghei* (Howells and Maxwell, 1973a).

Experiments on oxygen uptake, substrate utilization, and end product formation thus fail to provide evidence for a functioning citric acid cycle in malarial parasites. It is fairly certain that rodent and primate parasites contain malate dehydrogenase, but this enzyme is also found in mature red cells of mammals, which lack the cycle (Brewer, 1974).

The only general conclusion that can be drawn is that rodent malarial parasites do not contain a functioning citric acid cycle and that there is little convincing proof for either its presence or its absence in primate and avian parasites.

F. Carbon Dioxide Fixation

It has been reported that avian and mammalian parasites can fix carbon dioxide, and some of the enzymes involved have been investigated.

Preparations of *P. berghei* (free or within the rat reticulocyte) were able to incorporate carbon dioxide into organic acids (chiefly malate) and amino acids (aspartate and glutamate) (Nagarajan, 1968c). Although this incorporation may have been carried out by the parasite, the detection of radioactivity from labeled carbon dioxide in glutamate and aspartate (possible only by operation of the citric acid cycle, which is absent from this parasite) suggests contamination with host material. A large increase in the amount of radioactive carbon dioxide fixed by cells of duck blood on infection with *P. lophurae* was reported by Sherman and Ting (1966) and Ting and Sherman (1966); here, too, label was found in glutamate and aspartate, and also in acids of the citric acid cycle. Incorporation of carbon dioxide by *P. knowlesi* was also claimed by Sherman and Ting (1968), but in these experiments white cells, which are known to fix carbon dioxide (Cline, 1965), were not removed.

The enzymes involved in carbon dioxide fixation have been studied in *P.*

berghei in some detail. Phosphenolpyruvate carboxylase (Siu, 1967; Forrester and Siu, 1971; McDaniel and Siu, 1972) and phosphenolpyruvate carboxykinase (Siu, 1967) have been found, but malic enzyme could not be detected in free parasites (Nagarajan, 1968a; Tsukamoto, 1974). Phosphoenolpyruvate carboxylase has never been found in mammalian cells (Lane *et al.*, 1969), so that at least one enzyme able to fix carbon dioxide must be present in *P. berghei*.

V. OXYGEN UTILIZATION AND ELECTRON TRANSPORT

A. Oxygen Utilization

The utilization of oxygen by malarial parasites suggests the presence of an electron transport chain but, although a belief that the parasites respire is widely held, there is little convincing evidence for it.

To prove that parasites use oxygen it would be essential to have a preparation completely free of host material, or for which it could be incontrovertibly shown that contaminating material does not introduce significant error. The importance of distinguishing between the metabolism of parasite and of host was demonstrated by Jones *et al.* (1951) who showed that, although the respiratory rate of *P. berghei*-infected rat reticulocytes increased as the percentage of parasitized cells increased, oxygen uptake continued to rise even after the parasitemia had begun to fall.

White cells, because of their high rate of oxygen consumption (see Cline, 1965), must be completely removed in all experiments on parasite respiration. A number of experiments (rodent: Jones *et al.*, 1951; Cho and Aviado, 1968; primate: Christophers and Fulton, 1938, 1939; Fulton, 1939; Coggeshall, 1940; Coggeshall and Maier, 1941; Maier and Coggeshall, 1941; Wendel, 1943; McKee *et al.*, 1946; avian: Maier and Coggeshall, 1941; Velick, 1942; Silverman *et al.*, 1944; Bovarnick *et al.*, 1946a,b; Speck *et al.*, 1946; Marshall, 1948; Moulder, 1948, 1949) have been invalidated by the use of whole blood or the failure to remove white cells efficiently.

The rate of oxygen utilization by immature red cells of mammals is much higher than that of mature cells (Jones *et al.*, 1953; Lowenstein, 1959); for example, the respiratory rate of rabbit reticulocytes is over 30 times that of mature red cells (Ramsey and Warren, 1933). In experiments which demonstrate the utilization of oxygen by reticulocytes infected with rodent parasites it is therefore particularly difficult to be certain of the origin of the respiration (Jones *et al.*, 1951; Fulton and Spooner, 1956; Bowman *et al.*, 1960). A puzzling observation is that of Nagarajan (1968a) who found that *P. berghei* freed from rat reticulocytes used oxygen only with succinate as substrate, even after removal of white cells and after it was shown that reticulocyte stroma did not use oxygen.

Succinate dehydrogenase could not be detected in the free parasites, and it is therefore difficult to explain the mechanism of oxygen utilization in this case.

Experiments with avian parasites are complicated by the fact that in birds even mature red cells use oxygen and immature ones use it at an even higher rate (Silverman *et al.*, 1944; Khabir and Manwell, 1955; Augustin, 1961; Doktorandenkollektiv des Physiologisch-Chemischen Institutes, Berlin, 1962; Bell, 1971); furthermore, an increase in the rate of oxygen consumption by avian red cells can occur without a detectable increase in the percentage of reticulocytes (Silverman *et al.*, 1944). In addition, avian parasites freed from the red cell are often contaminated by host cell organelles such as nuclei; preparations of nuclei, made by a method similar to that used in preparing free parasites, have been shown to respire (Laskowski, 1942), presumably because of contamination with mitochondria.

The belief that malarial parasites use oxygen was apparently supported by the observation that the rate of utilization increased as the parasites grew in size (primate: Maier and Coggeshall, 1941; Ball *et al.*, 1948; avian: Maier and Coggeshall, 1941; Velick, 1942). However, this was only seen with parasites removed from the host at intervals throughout the cycle; with parasites cultured *in vitro* the increase in respiration did not occur, even though the same amount of growth took place (primate: Ball *et al.*, 1948), suggesting that variations in contaminating host cells were at least partly responsible for the observed changes.

B. Electron Transport

Mitochondria have been detected in *P. berghei* by staining with janus green which also apparently gave some evidence for oxidative reactions (Sen Gupta *et al.*, 1955). By electron microscopy it can be seen that the mitochondria of rodent and primate parasites, with the exception of *P. malariae* (Smith and Theakston, 1970), *P. traguli* (Cadigan *et al.*, 1972) and *P. brasilianum* (Sterling *et al.*, 1972), are acristate (rodent: Ladda, 1969; Blackburn and Vinijchaikul, 1970; Howells, 1970; primate: Rudzinska and Trager, 1968; Rudzinska and Vickerman, 1968; Collins and Aikawa, 1977); those of avian parasites, on the other hand, have well-defined cristae (Aikawa, 1966; Aikawa *et al.*, 1966a,b, 1967; Rudzinska and Vickerman, 1968), although Ristic and Kreier (1964) did not detect cristate mitochondria in *P. gallinaceum*. [The structure of malarial parasites, including the mitochondria of intraerythrocytic stages, has been reviewed by Aikawa (1971, 1977) and Collins and Aikawa (1977).] The absence of cristae is usually taken to indicate that cytochromes (and therefore electron transport) are absent, but mitochondria-like organelles can lack cristae and yet possess a complete set of cytochromes (Ritter and André, 1975).

Attempts have been made to demonstrate various components of the mitochondrial electron transport chain in malarial parasites.

NADH dehydrogenase was detected cytochemically in *P. berghei* by Theakston *et al.* (1970b), but it could not be detected biochemically in the free parasite by Nagarajan (1968a).

The ubiquinones of mammalian blood infected with malarial parasites have only been shown to differ quantitatively from those of normal blood (rodent: Skelton *et al.*, 1970; primate: Skelton *et al.*, 1969, 1970). Increased synthesis of ubiquinones took place in blood infected with *P. knowlesi* (Skelton *et al.*, 1969) and also with *P. falciparum*, although the rate of synthesis was not proportional to the parasitemia (Schnell *et al.*, 1971). Blood infected with *P. lophurae* contained ubiquinones 8 and 9, which are absent from normal duck blood as reported by Rietz *et al.* (1967). These authors believed that these ubiquinones were synthesized by the parasite, since they thought it unlikely that white cells could be the source. However, ubiquinones different from those of normal blood are found in the blood of mice infected with Friend leukemia virus (Casey and Bliznakov, 1973), and it must therefore be shown that similar changes cannot take place in the ubiquinones of blood cells after malarial infection if the synthesis of ubiquinones by the parasite is to be firmly established.

The only other component of the electron transport chain which has been investigated is cytochrome oxidase. This enzyme has been shown cytochemically in *P. berghei* (Howells *et al.*, 1969; Theakston *et al.*, 1969) and *P. gallinaceum* (Theakston *et al.*, 1969), but examination of the method used (Seligman *et al.*, 1967) makes it doubtful whether the specificity was high enough to establish the presence of the enzyme. The effect of cyanide was used as evidence for the presence of the enzyme in parasites, but the concentration used (10^{-2} M) was not specific for cytochrome oxidase (Dixon and Webb, 1964).

Cytochrome oxidase activity was detected biochemically in free parasites of *P. berghei* and *P. knowlesi* by Scheibel and Miller (1969a,b) after careful removal of white cells and platelets, but it has been suggested that mitochondria (which can contaminate free parasites) may be present in red cells of mice infected with *P. berghei* (Momen *et al.*, 1975). Nagarajan (1968a), who removed white cells but not platelets from *P. berghei*-infected rat blood, showed that free parasite preparations could transfer electrons from ascorbic acid to oxygen, but this is not considered completely specific for cytochrome oxidase and, as Scheibel and Miller (1969a) pointed out, the presence of platelets could give misleading results.

The functioning of a possible electron transport chain has also been investigated by indirect means. It has been shown that inhibitors of electron transport affect the chloroquine-induced clumping of pigment in *P. berghei* (Homewood *et al.*, 1972a); although clumping is a synthetic and therefore energy-requiring process (Warhurst *et al.*, 1971), its inhibition by high concentrations of inhibitors, as well as the complications introduced by the use of chloroquine (whose mode of action is not understood), makes it impossible to draw firm conclusions about electron transport mechanisms from such experiments. It may, however, be significant that clumping can take place in the absence of oxygen (Homewood *et al.*, 1972a).

Nagarajan (1968b) showed that incorporation of inorganic phosphate into high-energy phosphates by free parasites of *P. berghei* was inhibited by cyanide and azide, but ATP could not be detected. ATP and other nucleotides were, however, measured by Van Dyke *et al.* (1977b). The synthesis of ATP by parasites was demonstrated by Carter *et al.* (1972), but inhibitors were not tested.

The malarial parasite may depend to some extent on the ATP of the red cell, since higher levels of ATP apparently favored its development (primate: Brewer and Powell, 1965; Eaton and Brewer, 1969), and growth of free parasites of *P. lophurae in vitro* was improved by ATP (Trager, 1950). The ATP levels of red cells of rats fell during the course of infection with *P. berghei* (Brewer and Coan, 1969), although in monkeys infected with *P. knowlesi* an increase in the ATP level of the red cells was seen up to the onset of nuclear division of the parasite (Fletcher *et al.*, 1970). The levels of ATP in the red cells of ducks infected with *P. lophurae* were lower than in uninfected cells (Trager, 1967), and bongkrekic acid, an inhibitor of adenine nucleotide translocase of mitochondria, prevented development of the extracellular parasites *in vitro* and also reduced the incorporation of proline but had less effect on the incorporation of methionine. The concentration of bongkrekic acid which was effective against *P. lophurae* was similar to that needed for inhibition of the translocase of mitochondria, but atractyloside, which acts at the same site although by a different mechanism, had no effect on the development of free parasites of *P. lophurae*. Development of *P. falciparum* within the red cell was also inhibited *in vitro* by bongkrekic acid. It was suggested from the foregoing evidence that the malarial parasite may have a transport system in its outside membrane which uses the ATP of the red cell (Trager, 1972, 1973).

It is impossible to draw firm conclusions about the presence of electron transport in malarial parasites; it has almost certainly not been proved that they need, in the short term at least, to use oxygen.

VI. BREAKDOWN OF HEMOGLOBIN AND METABOLISM OF AMINO ACIDS

A. Malarial Pigment (Hemozoin)

Early workers considered that the malarial pigment which accumulates in the digestive vacuoles of the parasite was melanin or a melanin derivative, but in 1891 Carbone suggested that it might consist of hematin, and in 1911 Brown proposed that the pigment was formed from hemoglobin by digestion of the protein part of the molecule by a proteolytic enzyme. In support of this, several workers showed that, although hemoglobin itself was destroyed during growth of the parasite, the total amount of iron porphyrin in a parasitized cell was the same as in a normal cell (primate: Ball *et al.*, 1948; Morrison and Jeskey, 1948; avian: Groman, 1951). Groman (1951) further showed that part of the iron porphyrin of infected cells was in an insoluble form, in contrast to the ''soluble'' heme in the hemoglobin of normal cells. Later Theakston *et al.* (1970a) and Eckman *et al.* (1977) provided evidence for the derivation of pigment from heme.

Much of the work of the first half of this century appeared to show fairly conclusively that malarial pigment was identical to hematin or was a closely related derivative (rodent: Fulton and Rimington, 1953; primate: Glasunow, 1925; Ghosh and Nath, 1934; Sinton and Ghosh, 1934a,b; Devine and Fulton, 1941; Morrison and Anderson, 1942; Rimington *et al.*, 1947; avian: Devine and Fulton, 1942; Rimington *et al.*, 1947), although Wats and White (1932) could not detect the absorption bands of hematin in pigment extracted from infected blood or spleen. In addition, iron was detected in the pigment (primate: Ghosh and Nath, 1934; Ghosh and Sinton, 1934), and hematin crystals were prepared from it (primate: Sinton and Ghosh, 1934b; Rimington *et al.*, 1947). During this period there were one or two dissenting voices, such as that of Warasi (1927) who believed that the pigment might be closer to an iron-containing melanin than to hematin and that the final amount of pigment in each parasite was greater than the total amount of hematin that could have been derived from the hemoglobin of the red cell (primate: Warasi, 1928).

More recently it has been proposed that the pigment may be hematin combined with some other component. Deegan and Maegraith (1956a,b) suggested that the methods previously used for extraction (for example, the use of sodium hydroxide, sodium carbonate, acids, or phenol) were too harsh and that the hematin was released by breakdown of the pigment. They found that, when extracted with borate buffer at pH 9.2, the pigment of primate parasites could be shown to consist of hematin in combination with some other, probably nitrogenous, material which might be denatured protein or polypeptide.

Subsequent work by another group (Sherman and Hull, 1960; Sherman *et al.*, 1965, 1968) showed that preparations of the pigment from *P. lophurae* contained protein, suggesting that it might consist simply of partially digested and denatured hemoglobin. However, these pigment preparations were later found by electron microscopy to be contaminated by cell membranes (Sherman, 1977b). Nevertheless, the pigment may contain remnants of globin. Theakston *et al.* (1970a) showed autoradiographically that leucine, but not methionine, from hemoglobin was associated with the pigment in the digestive vacuole of the parasite, and Homewood *et al.* (1975) found that only about 10% of the purified pigment appeared to consist of hematin (measured either as extracted hematin or as iron).

The molecular weight of the pigment was reported by Sherman *et al.* (1968) to be about 40,000, but the impurity of the preparations makes this value doubtful. Homewood *et al.* (1972b) claimed that its molecular weight was higher than that of hemoglobin, but this also cannot be relied upon, since, as pointed out by Sherman (1977b), the method used could have given an anomalously high molecular weight. The regular structure of the purified pigment was demonstrated by Moore and Boothroyd (1974) who showed by electron microscopy that the iron atoms were arranged in the form of a regular lattice.

As discussed by Sherman (1977b), it is difficult to be certain that pigment extracted from the malarial parasite is identical to the pigment as it occurs in the parasite. During extraction, attempts must be made to remove cell debris and membranes, and it is likely that any protein or polypeptide forming part of the native pigment but not tightly bound will be removed at the same time. In addition, extraction procedures may be selective in removing only part of the pigment, or may cause alteration of its structure. Alternatively, it is possible that a combination of the pigment with protein or with other material might occur during extraction and that, as Sherman (1977b) believes, the pigment in the parasite consists simply of hematin.

Another view is that the pigment consists not of one well-defined molecule but of a series of transition molecules between hemoglobin and a final degradation product. In support of this, Morselt *et al.* (1973) showed that individual grains of pigment in a parasite had different absorption spectra, possibly representing different stages of breakdown to a final product of unknown composition.

B. Digestion of Protein

The hemoglobin content of infected cells falls during growth of the malarial parasite, the amount destroyed during each intraerythrocytic cycle apparently depending on the species of parasite (primate: Christophers and Fulton, 1938; Ball *et al.*, 1948; Morrison and Jeskey, 1948; avian: Groman, 1951). The parasite incorporates amino acids from the hemoglobin into its own protein (rodent: Theakston *et al.*, 1970a; primate: Fulton and Grant, 1956; avian: Sherman and Tanigoshi, 1970) and must therefore possess enzymes capable of digesting globin. However, investigation of these enzymes is complicated by the fact that proteases are also present in white cells (Cline, 1965) and immature red cells of mammals (Goetze and Rapoport, 1954; Ellis *et al.*, 1956); even mature erythrocytes of mammals contain several proteases bound to the membrane (Pennell, 1974).

Moulder and Evans (1946) reported the detection in *P. gallinaceum* of a protease which hydrolyzed acid-denatured hemoglobin faster than native hemoglobin, but white cells present may have contributed to the activity. Ball *et al.* (1948) could not detect proteolytic activity (pH unspecified) in *P. knowlesi-*infected monkey erythrocytes, but Cook *et al.* (1961), on the other hand, found two soluble proteases in *P. knowlesi* (pH optima about 5 and 8) and also in *P. berghei* (pH optima about 4 and 8); in both species the enzyme with an acid pH optimum was the less stable and the less active of the two. These proteases were attributed to the parasites, but doubts were later cast on the accuracy of the method used for their assay (Cook *et al.*, 1969; Sherman, 1977b). Cook *et al.* (1969) measured the protease activity (at pH 7.5) of extracts of free parasites of *P. knowlesi* and found that the activity was in the soluble fraction; the enzyme therefore differed from the membrane-bound proteases of normal erythrocytes.

The acid proteases of *P. berghei*, *P. knowlesi* and *P. falciparum* have been investigated by Levy and co-workers. White cells were removed, but by a method which has been found to be relatively inefficient for *P. berghei*-infected mouse erythrocytes (Homewood and Neame, 1976). The enzyme of *P. berghei* was similar to that of normal mouse erythrocytes in several respects, namely, K_m for hemoglobin, molecular weight, and sensitivity to several inhibitors, and there was only a slight difference in the pH optima of the enzymes of parasite and host cell (Levy and Chou, 1973, 1974). The enzyme of the parasite appeared to be similar to cathepsin D, which is present both in white cells (Mounter and Atiyeh, 1960) and in immature red cells (Goetze and Rapoport, 1954; Ellis *et al.*, 1956), but acid phosphatase, found together with cathepsin D in the lysosomes of host cells, was not present in free parasites of *P. berghei*, *P. knowlesi*, or *P. falciparum* (Levy and Chou, 1973; Levy *et al.*, 1974). [These results incidentally give support to the view of Scorza *et al.* (1972) that acid phosphatase is not present in malarial parasites, and contrast with the reports of Sen Gupta *et al.* (1955) and of Aikawa and Thompson (1971).] With *P. knowlesi* and *P. falciparum* there were greater differences between the pH optima of the proteases attributed to the parasite and host, the enzyme of the parasite having an optimum of 3.6 and that of the red cell 2–2.5. An unusual feature of the malarial enzymes was their inhibition by both pepstatin and chymostatin, and to a lesser extent by antipain and leupeptin, inhibitors which are usually specific for different types of proteases (Levy and Chou, 1974; Levy *et al.*, 1974). Furthermore, protein synthesis by intracellular *P. berghei* (as measured by incorporation of isoleucine) was inhibited by pepstatin, chymostatin, and phenylmethanesulfonyl fluoride (Levy and Chou, 1975), presumably because the parasite was prevented from obtaining amino acids from hemoglobin. All the inhibitors must have crossed the membranes not only of the parasite but also of the red cell, and this suggests a marked change in the permeability of the parasitized red cell, since pepstatin (a pentapeptide) is not known to cross the membrane of any other cell (Dean, 1975).

An alkaline protease from *P. berghei*-infected mouse red cells was separated by Chan and Lee (1974) into three fractions. One fraction was equally active against both mouse and human hemoglobin, but the other two acted only against the hemoglobin of mice. However, white cells were removed by a method only shown to be effective for normal human and chicken blood, and immature red cells were not investigated, so that it is not possible to be certain which, if any, of the proteases originated in the parasite.

The breakdown of hemoglobin may leave a surplus of some amino acids after the parasite has satisfied its requirements for protein synthesis. Christophers and Fulton (1938) found little or no increase in amino nitrogen in *P. knowlesi*-infected cells, but Moulder and Evans (1946) and Groman (1951), working with *P. gallinaceum* in chicken red cells (contaminated with white cells), showed the production of amino nitrogen *in vitro*. Cenedella *et al.* (1968) reported that *P. berghei*-infected cells produced amino acids. In most cases, however, the conditions of incubation of the parasitized cells (concentrated suspensions incubated for long periods) must have led to the early death of the parasites; this, and the presence of white cells, make it difficult to attribute the amino acid production solely to the normal metabolic activities of the parasites.

C. Amino Acid Metabolism

1. Incorporation into Protein

The intraerythrocytic malarial parasite can obtain the amino acids which it needs either from the digestion of red cell protein (probably the main source) or from the free amino acids in the plasma.

The incorporation of exogenous amino acids into the protein of the parasite has been shown many times and has frequently been used as an indicator of growth (rodent: Richards and Williams, 1973; Williams and Richards, 1973; primate: Cohen *et al.*, 1969; Butcher and Cohen, 1971; Gutteridge *et al.*, 1972; Phillips *et al.*, 1972; Siddiqui *et al.*, 1974; Diggs *et al.*, 1975; Richards and Williams, 1975; Mitchell *et al.*, 1976; avian: Sherman *et al.*, 1971a; Trager, 1971). The rate of incorporation of amino acids by *P. lophurae* in duck cells or by free parasites was little affected by changing from a medium high in sodium to one high in potassium (Sherman *et al.*, 1969a). In synchronous infections, the rate of incorporation of amino acids into protein was constant throughout most of the cycle but diminished during schizogony (primate: Polet and Barr, 1968a,b; McColm *et al.*, 1976).

Primate parasites must obtain part of their requirement of isoleucine and methionine from outside the red cell (Polet and Conrad, 1968, 1969a,b; Siddiqui *et al.*, 1969; Trigg and Gutteridge, 1971; Siddiqui and Schnell, 1972). Nevertheless, it has been calculated that about 80% of the methionine in the protein of *P. knowlesi* is derived from the red cell (Fulton and Grant, 1956). Part of the methionine taken up into the parasitized cell appears to be used by the parasite as a source of cysteine (Fulton and Grant, 1956).

Not all the amino acids taken up by the parasite are incorporated directly into protein. Free parasites of *P. lophurae* incorporated methionine and the basic amino acids arginine and lysine, and probably also proline, mainly into protein, but they metabolized glutamate mainly to carbon dioxide (Sherman and Tanigoshi, 1971).

2. Enzymes of Amino Acid Metabolism

Glutamate dehydrogenase is apparently present in *P. lophurae*. Sherman *et al.* (1971b) showed that infected cells and free parasites contained a form of the enzyme not present in uninfected duck cells; this enzyme could use either NAD or NADP as cofactor. The same enzyme purified from *P. chabaudi* was specific for NADP, and no glutamate dehydrogenase specific for NAD was found (Walter *et al.*, 1974). Tsukamoto (1974) found that the enzyme from *P. berghei* was also NADP-specific, but Langer *et al.* (1970) and Picard-Maureau *et al.* (1975) found in contrast that the glutamate dehydrogenase of *P. berghei* and *P. vinckei*, although having greater activity with NADP, also had appreciable activity with NAD. The activity of the *P. berghei* enzyme with NADP as cofactor was not affected by ADP or ATP, suggesting that the NADP-specific enzyme was not of mammalian origin (Langer *et al.*, 1970). Carter (1978) proved that this enzyme was present in the parasite by showing electrophoretic differences among the enzymes of different species of rodent malarial parasites. Picard-Maureau *et al.* (1975) used a different approach: The activity of glutamate dehydrogenase in *P. vinckei*-infected mouse erythrocytes increased during the intraerythrocytic cycle, suggesting that it originated in the growing parasite and not in the red cell undergoing destruction.

Plasmodium berghei may contain aspartate aminotransferase (Tsukamoto, 1974), but it is possible that the enzyme detected was that of immature red cells since human reticulocytes are known to contain an isoenzyme of aspartate aminotransferase not present in mature erythrocytes (Fiorelli *et al.*, 1969).

3. Transport of Amino Acids

The amino acid content of infected red cells differs from that of normal red cells, presumably as a result both of hemoglobin breakdown by the parasite and of changes in transport across the erythrocyte membrane. The concentrations of most amino acids in duck erythrocytes rose on infection with *P. lophurae*, but the level of cysteine fell to about two-thirds of the normal red cell value (Siddiqui and Trager, 1967). Sherman and Mudd (1966) found that increases in the concentrations of amino acids in infected cells could be accounted for almost entirely by the amino acids within the parasites themselves.

As discussed by Sherman (1977a), data on the entry of exogenous amino acids into parasites are particularly difficult to interpret, since the amino acids must cross not only the membrane of the red cell but also the membranes surrounding the parasite. In any case, reliable kinetic analysis is impossible without sufficient accurate data obtained over a suitable range of concentrations of substrate (Neame and Richards, 1972), and such information is seldom available.

On infection of duck erythrocytes with *P. lophurae,* changes take place in the method of entry of amino acids. Many amino acids (alanine, arginine, cysteine, glycine, histidine, leucine, lysine, methionine, serine, and threonine) entered the normal erythrocyte by carrier-mediated transport, but after infection some of these (alanine, cysteine, histidine, leucine and methionine) entered by diffusion, and those that were still transported had a raised K_m. With free parasites, however, most amino acids entered by diffusion, the exceptions being arginine, aspartate, cysteine, glutamate and lysine; aspartate and glutamate shared the same carrier (Sherman and Tanigoshi, 1972, 1974a).

It was claimed by Sherman and Tanigoshi (1974a) that these changes in the transport properties of the erythrocyte could to some extent be produced in normal cells by incubating them in an extract of parasitized cells. The results of this experiment could, however, be interpreted as showing that the kinetic constants of cells incubated with extract were changed less from the normal than were those of cells incubated without it.

The equilibrium distribution ratios of most amino acids changed only slightly on infection with *P. lophurae;* those most affected were alanine, serine, and threonine, which entered the infected cell less readily, and proline and methionine, which reached a higher distribution ratio in infected than in normal cells (Sherman *et al.,* 1967, 1971a). It has, on the other hand, been reported (McCormick, 1970) that monkey erythrocytes infected with *P. knowlesi* accumulated not only methionine but also isoleucine against a concentration gradient, in contrast to cystine, histidine and leucine which developed a distribution ratio of about unity, as in normal cells. Free parasites of *P. lophurae,* however, appeared to be able to accumulate several amino acids against a concentration gradient (Sherman *et al.,* 1967), although this was later shown to be transient in most cases (Sherman *et al.,* 1971a).

The malarial parasite therefore digests the protein (mainly hemoglobin) of the red cell, incorporating the amino acids into its own protein and leaving an insoluble residue of pigment, which contains hematin but whose structure is otherwise uncertain. The parasite can also use amino acids from the plasma and, in particular, part of its requirement for methionine and isoleucine must be satisfied by amino acids from outside the red cell. On infection, the transport properties of the erythrocyte are changed, so that more amino acids enter by diffusion.

VII. NUCLEIC ACIDS

A. Properties of Nucleic Acids

DNA and RNA have been demonstrated in malarial parasites (rodent: Sen Gupta *et al.*, 1955; Ciucă *et al.*, 1963; Bahr, 1966; primates: Deane, 1945; Lewert, 1952a; avian: Lewert, 1952a; Bahr, 1966), and nuclear structure has been further studied by a number of workers (rodent: Aikawa *et al.*, 1972; Bahr and Mikel, 1972; avian: Chen, 1944; Aikawa *et al.*, 1972).

The amount of DNA in a malarial parasite (*P. berghei, P. knowlesi* and *P. lophurae*) is about 10^{-13} g (Whitfeld, 1952, 1953; Bahr, 1966; Gutteridge and Trigg, 1972); it should be noted that a higher value earlier attributed to Whitfeld by Homewood (1978) is incorrect.

The DNA of primate malarial parasites has been shown to consist of a major and a minor component with buoyant densities of 1.697 and 1.679 g/ml, respectively. Initially, the DNA of both rodent and avian parasites appeared to consist of only one component, that of rodent parasites having a buoyant density of 1.683–1.685 g/ml and that of avian parasites 1.680 g/ml (rodent: Chance *et al.*, 1978; rodent, primate, avian: Gutteridge *et al.*, 1969, 1971; Gutteridge and Trigg, 1972; avian: Walsh and Sherman, 1968a; DNA of parasites has been reviewed by Borst and Fairlamb, 1976). However, closer examination of the DNA of *P. lophurae* revealed a second component consisting of circular mitochondrial DNA which had the same density as the nuclear DNA (Kilejian, 1975). The major component of the DNA of all the parasites was shown to be double-stranded and linear and contained no unusual bases.

Each parasite contained about two (rodent: Whitfeld, 1953) to five (rodent: Bahr, 1966; primate: Gutteridge and Trigg, 1972) times more RNA than DNA.

A ribosomal fraction which could be used for protein synthesis *in vitro* was isolated from *P. knowlesi* by Cook *et al.* (1969). The monosomes of *P. knowlesi* and *P. lophurae* were shown to have sedimentation coefficients of about 80 S, that of the larger subparticle being about 60 S and of the smaller subparticle about 40 S; the sedimentation coefficient of the rRNA derived from the larger subparticle was about 25 S and from the smaller one about 17 S (primate: Warhurst and Williamson, 1970; Cook *et al.*, 1971; Sherman *et al.*, 1975; Trigg *et al.*, 1975; Sherman, 1976; avian: Sherman and Jones, 1977). The corresponding values of the rRNA of mammals are 28 and 18 S, respectively (Davidson, 1976). The value of 25 S for the rRNA of the larger ribosomal subparticle of plasmodia is thus intermediate between that of mammals and bacteria. However, protein synthesis *in vitro* with ribosomes isolated from *P. knowlesi* was sensitive to puromycin and cycloheximide, as was protein synthesis by the intact parasite, but synthesis was not inhibited by chloramphenicol (Cook *et al.*, 1971; Schnell and Siddiqui, 1972; Sherman, 1976; Sherman and Jones, 1976). Although protein synthesis of *P. lophurae* was inhibited not only by cycloheximide but also by chloramphenicol (Sherman *et al.*, 1971a), the concentration of the latter was too high to be specific (Schnell and Siddiqui, 1972). In appearance the ribosomes of *P. knowlesi* resembled those of eukaryotes more than those of prokaryotes (Aikawa and Cook, 1971). It thus seems that the ribosomes of malarial parasites are more like those of mammals than those of bacteria. An interesting difference between the malarial and the mammalian cell is shown by the effect of the antiviral agent arabinosyladenine which, although ineffective against mammalian cells, inhibits protein synthesis by *P. berghei in vivo* and *in vitro* and also changes the pattern of proteins produced (Ilan *et al.*, 1977).

Tokuyasu *et al.* (1969) found it impossible to label the rRNA of the larger subparticle of the *P. berghei* ribosome with ^{32}P or radioactive orotic acid, although the smaller subparticle was easily labeled; these authors therefore suggested that the parasite may be able to use the 60 S ribosomal subparticle of the host. However, as pointed out above, the 60 S subparticle has been detected in primate and avian parasites and, in addition, that of *P. knowlesi* could be labeled with radioactive adenosine, showing that this subparticle was synthesized by the parasite itself (Sherman and Jones, 1977). Cook *et al.* (1971) pointed out that the 60 S subparticle of *P. knowlesi* was unstable outside a narrow range of concentrations of Mg^{2+} and that if the same were true for *P. berghei,* the larger subparticle could have been synthesized by the parasite but might have been broken down during the extraction procedure used by Tokuyasu *et al.* (1969). Finally, Sherman *et al.* (1975) found that the base composition of the rRNA of *P. knowlesi* and of the reticulocytes of monkeys was different (G + C contents 37 and 67%, respectively), proving that *P. knowlesi* at least does not obtain rRNA from host ribosomes.

Ilan *et al.* (1969) suggested that *P. berghei* could use the tRNA of the host as well as synthesize its own (Tokuyasu *et al.*, 1969), since they found that the parasite aminoacyl-tRNA synthetases, unlike those of mammals, were relatively nonspecific.

B. Nucleic Acid Precursors

There are three possible sources of bases or nucleosides for nucleic acid synthesis by the intraerythrocytic parasite: material derived from the degradation of macromolecules of the host, synthesis from simpler precursors, and material from outside the cell.

Degradation of the nucleus of the host red cell during the growth of *P. gallinaceum* has been suggested by Lewert (1952b), but there is no evidence for the transfer of material from the host nucleus to the parasite. An RNase was found in extracts of *P. gallinaceum* (Miller and Kozloff, 1947), but this could well have been derived from host material.

1. Purines

Plasmodium lophurae cannot synthesize purines *de novo* to any great extent (Walsh and Sherman, 1968b; Booden and Hull, 1973), nor can *P. knowlesi* in culture (Trigg and Gutteridge, 1971).

If parasites cannot synthesize purines, they must be able to obtain them from the host. In support of this, Gutteridge and Trigg (1971) reported that the growth of intraerythrocytic *P. knowlesi in vitro* was improved if purines were present, but Siddiqui *et al.* (1969) and Trigg (1969) found that the parasite could grow in the absence of exogenous purines.

Measurements of the incorporation of purines and pyrimidines into parasite nucleic acids are simplified by a relatively small amount of interference from the host cells. Mature red cells of mammals do not contain either DNA or RNA, and reticulocytes, although containing RNA (Lowenstein, 1959), cannot incorporate exogenous uridine (Borsook, 1964) or adenosine (Van Dyke *et al.*, 1969).

Mature red cells of birds are also unable to synthesize RNA and DNA (Allfrey and Mirsky, 1952; Cameron and Prescott, 1963; Walsh and Sherman, 1968a). Immature avian red cells can, however, incorporate uridine to a limited extent (Cameron and Prescott, 1963).

White cells of mammals and birds can synthesize RNA and DNA using exogenous purines and pyrimidines (Cameron and Prescott, 1963; Cline, 1965; Büngener and Nielsen, 1967), but ^{32}P from exogenous phosphate was not incorporated into the DNA of duck leukocytes (Walsh and Sherman, 1968a). It has been shown also that the rate of incorporation of adenosine into a white cell is less than into a malarial parasite (Büngener and Nielsen, 1967), and the error contributed by white cells may therefore be no more than proportionate to their numbers. Nevertheless, there are situations in which failure to remove white cells can give misleading results, and their presence should never be ignored unless it is first shown that they do not interfere.

Intraerythrocytic malarial parasites use exogenous purines for nucleic acid synthesis, and the rate of incorporation is often used simply as a measure of growth (rodent: Büngener and Nielsen, 1967, 1968, 1969; Van Dyke and Szustkiewicz, 1969; Van Dyke *et al.*, 1969, 1970a,b; Lantz *et al.*, 1971; Carter and Van Dyke, 1972; Theakston *et al.*, 1972; Lukow *et al.*, 1973; Neame *et al.*, 1974; Van Dyke, 1975; primate: Polet and Barr, 1968a,b; Gutteridge and Trigg, 1970; Gutteridge *et al.*, 1971, 1972; Trigg *et al.*, 1971; Gutteridge and Trigg, 1972; Booden and Hull, 1973; McCormick *et al.*, 1974; avian: Gutteridge *et al.*, 1971; Tracy and Sherman, 1972; Sherman and Jones, 1977).

Plasmodium berghei can also use the purines of the red cell pool (Büngener and Nielsen, 1969), as shown by preloading mouse red cells with radioactive adenosine and subsequently finding incorporation of label by the parasite. However, as mouse cells can carry out several interconversions of purines (Miyazaki and Minaki, 1972), it is not certain from which of the possible purines or derivatives the label was actually derived.

Although it is unlikely that the parasite membrane is permeable to nucleotides, Lantz et al. (1971) reported that free parasites of P. berghei incorporated more radioactivity into nucleic acids from added AMP than from added adenosine. However, these authors considered that adenosine was released from the AMP by phosphorylase of the serum in the incubation medium and that it was adenosine that was actually taken up by the parasites. They felt that the adenosine slowly released from the AMP was more readily available to the parasites than the adenosine present in the medium, owing to rapid deamination of the latter.

Manandhar and Van Dyke (1975) and Van Dyke et al. (1977a) suggested that, of the purines, the parasite preferentially took up hypoxanthine. They believed that exogenous adenosine was metabolized to hypoxanthine on the outside of the parasite before being taken up and converted to AMP via IMP. Part of the evidence for this was the finding that, after incubation of free parasites of P. berghei with labeled adenosine, radioactivity appeared inside the parasite mainly in phosphorylated derivatives, while outside the cell radioactivity was found in adenosine, inosine and hypoxanthine. Before attributing these extracellular reactions with certainty to the parasite, however, it would be necessary to demonstrate that enzymes of contaminating host material are not involved, since enzymes able to convert adenosine to inosine and hypoxanthine are present in mouse erythrocytes (Miyazaki and Minaki, 1972) and in human erythrocytes and lymphocytes (Parks et al., 1975).

Plasmodium berghei incorporates exogenous hypoxanthine readily, as well as adenosine and inosine, but adenine is less well utilized (Van Dyke, 1975). On the other hand, P. lophurae freed from or within the host cell, incorporates hypoxanthine, adenosine, and inosine at similar rates (Tracy and Sherman (1972).

Büngener also suggested that hypoxanthine was the purine nucleoside most readily used by P. vinckei. He observed that treatment of P. vinckei-infected rats with allopurinol caused a faster rise in the parasitemia (Büngener, 1974a) by shortening the length of the cycle (Büngener, 1974b). This may have been due to increased levels in the red cell of hypoxanthine, whose breakdown is inhibited by allopurinol, but it is probable that levels of other purines were also affected.

It may be that adenosine is the purine most readily available to the parasite, as this is probably the form in which purines are carried by the red cell from the liver to other parts of the body (Pritchard et al., 1975).

The utilization of exogenous purines indicates that the parasite must possess at least some of the enzymes of the salvage pathway for purines (Fig. 1).

Free parasites of P. chabaudi (white cells removed) contain all the enzymes listed in Fig. 1 (Lukow et al., 1973). Adenosine kinase (Schmidt et al., 1974), hypoxanthine-guanine phosphoribosyltransferase and adenine phosphoribosyltransferase (Walter and Königk, 1974b) have been isolated from P. chabaudi.

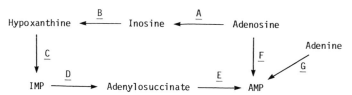

FIG. 1. The salvage pathway for purines. *A*, Adenosine deaminase; *B*, inosine phosphorylase; *C*, hypoxanthine-guanine phosphoribosyltransferase; *D*, adenylosuccinate synthetase; *E*, adenylosuccinase; *F*, adenosine kinase; *G*, adenine phosphoribosyltransferase.

Adenosine deaminase and purine nucleoside phosphorylase of *P. berghei* were shown by Büngener (1967) to have electrophoretic mobilities which differed from those of the same enzyme of *P. vinckei* (in the same host), confirming their presence in the parasite. (The salvage pathway of rodent malarial parasites has been reviewed by Königk, 1977.)

Many of the enzymes of the salvage pathway are present in mature red cells of mammals, and some of them have been demonstrated in the red cells of birds (Bishop, 1960; Miyazaki and Minaki, 1972; Brewer, 1974), but different species of animal show variations in the number of reactions they can carry out.

2. *Pyrimidines*

Most authors have found that exogenous pyrimidines, in contrast to purines, are not used by the intraerythrocytic stages of malarial parasites. When parasites were incubated with radioactive pyrimidine bases or nucleosides, label was in most cases not incorporated into nucleic acids (rodent: Büngener and Nielsen, 1967; Van Dyke *et al.*, 1970b; Walter *et al.*, 1970; Theakston *et al.*, 1972; Neame *et al.*, 1974; primate: Gutteridge and Trigg, 1970; Trigg and Gutteridge, 1971; avian: Booden and Hull, 1973), but Conklin *et al.* (1973) measured the incorporation of thymidine and uridine into nucleic acids of blood cells from monkeys infected with *P. knowlesi,* and Theakston *et al.* (1972) detected by autoradiography the incorporation of uridine by *P. berghei.*

It is not certain whether exogenous pyrimidines are necessary for growth *in vitro;* Siddiqui *et al.* (1969) found that they improved the growth of *P. knowlesi,* whereas Trigg and Gutteridge (1971) found that they did not.

The reason for the failure of the parasites to use exogenous pyrimidines could be either that pyrimidine bases and nucleosides do not cross the cell membrane of the red cell and/or the parasite, or that the parasites lack the enzymes of a salvage pathway for pyrimidines.

Pyrimidines can pass through the red cell membrane (Lieu *et al.*, 1971; Oliver and Paterson, 1971; Neame *et al.*, 1974) but, as pointed out by Sherman (1977a), the rate of entry may be slow. Nevertheless, even free parasites are unable to incorporate pyrimidines (rodent: Walter *et al.*, 1970), so that impermeability of the membrane of the host cell does not entirely explain the lack of utilization.

Pyrimidines may, however, be unable to penetrate the membrane of the parasite itself, as shown by experiments with free parasites of *P. berghei* in which adenosine entered the parasite but thymidine appeared not to (Van Dyke *et al.,* 1970b). This result could be explained, however, if both nucleosides entered the parasite but only adenosine were phosphorylated. During subsequent washing, the phosphorylated adenosine would remain within the parasite, but unphosphorylated thymidine would diffuse out.

It is likely that malarial parasites are unable to use thymidine because they cannot phosphorylate it. This is probably the case with *P. chabaudi,* since it has been shown that this parasite lacks thymidine kinase (Walter *et al.,* 1970), although it does possess deoxycytidine kinase (Königk, 1976).

If malarial parasites are unable to utilize exogenous pyrimidines, they must be able to synthesize them. There is some evidence that this is so, although the enzymes involved have been little investigated (see Fig. 2).

Plasmodium lophurae presumably has all the enzymes of the pathway shown in Fig. 2, since it was able to incorporate carbon dioxide into nucleic acids (Ting and Sherman, 1966) and, specifically, into pyrimidines (Walsh and Sherman, 1968b).

The level of aspartate transcarbamylase in the whole blood of rats infected with *P. berghei* increased as the parasitemia rose and was present in free parasites (Van Dyke *et al.,* 1970b). Increased activity of dihydroorotate dehydrogenase in mouse red cells on infection with *P. berghei* or *P. vinckei,* and high levels of activity in free parasites, have also been reported (Krooth *et al.,* 1969). However, both these enzymes are present in reticulocytes (Lotz and Smith, 1962; Van Dyke *et al.,* 1970b) and in the particulate fraction of human white cells (Smith and Baker, 1959). Both *P. knowlesi* (Polet and Barr, 1968b; Gutteridge and Trigg, 1970; Trigg and Gutteridge, 1971) and *P. lophurae* can form pyrimidines from orotic acid.

Walsh and Sherman (1968b) showed that free parasites of *P. lophurae* contained orotidine-5'-monophosphate pyrophosphorylase activity, and deoxycytidylate aminohydrolase was found in *P. chabaudi* (Königk, 1976).

The only other enzyme of pyrimidine biosynthesis which has been investigated is thymidylate synthetase. The activity of this enzyme is higher in cells infected with *P. lophurae* than in normal duck erythrocytes, and it is present in free parasites (Walsh and Sherman, 1968b). The enzyme has also been detected in preparations of *P. chabaudi* by Walter *et al.* (1970); although it is not stated that white cells were removed, human lymphocytes do not contain the enzyme (Silber *et al.,* 1963), but mouse reticulocytes do (Reid and Friedkin, 1973b). The activity of thymidylate synthetase of *P. chabaudi* was highest during the later part of the intraerythrocytic cycle, rising rapidly just before the first nuclear division

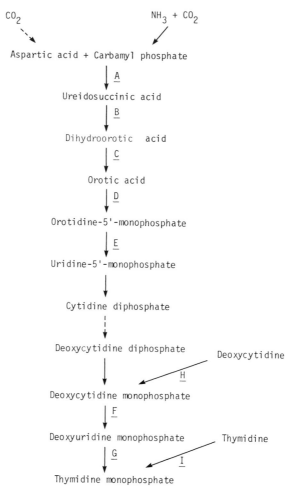

FIG. 2. Biosynthesis of pyrimidines. *A*, Aspartate transcarbamylase; *B*, dihydroorotase; *C*, dihydroorotate dehydrogenase; *D*, orotidine-5'-monophosphate pyrophosphorylase; *E*, orotidine decarboxylase; *F*, deoxycytidylate aminohydrolase; *G*, thymidylate synthetase; *H*, deoxycytidine kinase; *I*, thymidine kinase.

(Walter and Königk, 1971a). Thymidylate synthetase of *P. berghei* has been distinguished from the host enzyme, the parasite enzyme having an apparent molecular weight of over 100,000, in contrast to the 68,000 of the enzyme of mouse reticulocytes (Reid and Friedkin, 1973b).

3. Nucleic Acid Synthesis and the Intraerythrocytic Cycle

Attempts have been made to determine if the rate of synthesis of nucleic acids by the malarial parasite varies in the different stages of the cycle, but results are equivocal. This may be partly because of the different methods used, some workers removing parasites from the host at different stages of the cycle and others cultivating them *in vitro* for the whole cycle.

Several authors have shown that DNA synthesis, as measured by the incorporation of labeled precursors, is fastest in schizonts (primate: Polet and Barr, 1968b; Conklin *et al.*, 1973; avian: Tracy and Sherman, 1972). Gutteridge and Trigg (1970), however, found no clear evidence of periodicity in the synthesis of DNA by *P. knowlesi*. Walsh and Sherman (1968a) found that incorporation of ^{32}P into the DNA of *P. lophurae* appeared to continue at the same rate throughout the cycle but suggested that this was because division was not completely synchronous. In an investigation of asynchronous parasites, Jung *et al.* (1975) separated the different stages of *P. vinckei* by means of a Ficoll gradient. They found that DNA synthesis was fastest in old ring forms and young trophozoites but was much slower in schizonts and young ring forms.

The synthesis of RNA (total or ribosomal) by *P. knowlesi*-infected erythrocytes occurred throughout the cycle (Polet and Barr, 1968a,b; Gutteridge and Trigg, 1970; Conklin *et al.*, 1973; Trigg *et al.*, 1975). Synthesis of RNA by parasites *in vitro* may, however, differ from that *in vivo*, since Trigg and Gutteridge (1972) have found that one of the indications of deterioration of *P. knowlesi* during cultivation *in vitro* is a progressive reduction in the rate of RNA synthesis; later, DNA and protein synthesis are also affected. The pattern of RNA synthesis by *P. vinckei* is similar to that of DNA synthesis by this parasite (see above: Jung *et al.*, 1975).

Clarke (1952a) measured the incorporation of ^{32}P into nucleic acids of *P. gallinaceum* but did not attempt to relate it to different stages.

Malarial parasites, then, are probably unable to synthesize purines but possess a salvage pathway and are therefore able to use preformed bases and nucleosides from the host. Pyrimidines, in contrast, can be synthesized by the parasite, although little is known about the enzymes involved. The parasites probably cannot use most pyrimidines supplied by the host owing to a lack of the appropriate kinases. The evidence relating the rate of synthesis of DNA to the stage of the parasite in the red cell is conflicting, but most reports suggest, as might be expected, a more rapid rate of synthesis during nuclear division than during other parts of the cycle.

VIII. LIPIDS

The content of total lipid and of various lipid fractions is higher in infected erythrocytes than in normal ones (rodent: Lawrence and Cenedella, 1969; Rao *et al.*, 1970; primate: Ball *et al.*, 1948; Morrison and Jeskey, 1948; Rock *et al.*, 1971a; Angus *et al.*, 1972; avian: Lewert, 1952a; Seed and Kreier, 1972; Beach *et al.*, 1977).

Analysis of the lipid composition of the parasite is complicated by the problem of obtaining parasites completely free of contaminating host cell membranes, and even of deciding whether the membrane of the parasitophorous vacuole should be included as part of the parasite. Attempts to avoid the problem by determining the lipid composition of the parasite from a comparison of parasitized red cells with normal ones may not be valid because of changes in the lipid composition of the host cell on infection. One way to minimize errors is to prepare free parasites which are as pure as possible, followed by a comparison of their lipid composition with that of the membranes of the host cells from which they have been released. This method can often indicate the extent of contamination with host cell material and has been used with success, notably by Rock and co-workers.

A. Lipid Composition

The lipids of *P. knowlesi* contain a greater proportion of phospholipid than the monkey red cell. Rock (1971b) found that the lipids of the parasite contained 65% phospholipid and 25% neutral lipid, and the lipids of the red cell 60% phospholipid and 33% neutral lipid, while Angus *et al.* (1972) found that phospholipid was 65% of the total lipid of parasitized red cells and only 50% in normal cells or in uninfected red cells of infected monkeys.

The two major phospholipids of both the erythrocyte membrane (of the infected cell) and *P. knowlesi* were phosphatidylethanolamine and phosphatidylcholine, although the proportion of phosphatidylethanolamine was rather higher in *P. knowlesi,* but the erythrocyte and the parasite showed more differences in the proportions of other phospholipids. There was much less sphingomyelin and phosphatidylserine in the parasite (2–4% of the total lipid, and almost nil, respectively) than in the host cell (both roughly 12% of the total lipid). In fact, it was considered that phosphatidylserine was probably absent from the parasite and that the small amount present was an indication of host cell contamination (Rock *et al.,* 1971a; De Zeeuw *et al.,* 1972). Beckwith *et al.* (1975) also found that phosphatidylserine was absent not only from *P. knowlesi* but also from *P. berghei*. Phosphatidylinositol, which was low in the erythrocyte, was a higher proportion of the lipids of *P. knowlesi* (Rock *et al.,* 1971a; De Zeeuw *et al.,* 1972). Similar results were found for *P. knowlesi* by McClean *et al.* (1976) who showed in addition that there were quite marked variations in the phospholipid composition not only of the erythrocytes but also of the parasites obtained from different monkeys.

The neutral lipids of *P. knowlesi* differed somewhat from those of the red cell membrane. There were a smaller proportion of the total lipid of *P. knowlesi* (25%) than of the red cell (33%), mainly because of a reduction in cholesterol (Rock, 1971a). The neutral lipids of *P. knowlesi* were cholesterol, 40.9% of the total neutral lipid fraction; free fatty acids, 25%; triglycerides, 15.9%; cholesterol esters, 12.4%; and diglycerides, 5.8% (Rock, 1971a). Angus *et al.* (1972)

also found a smaller proportion of cholesterol (free and combined) in parasitized cells (15–25% of total lipids) than in normal erythrocytes (30%).

The commonest fatty acids of the total lipids of free parasites, parasitized cells and red cell membranes were palmitic (16:0), stearic (18:0), oleic (18:1), and linoleic (18:2) (Rock, 1971b; Angus *et al.,* 1972). Palmitic acid was about the same percentage of the total in both parasites and red cell membranes (about 29 and 26%, respectively), whereas the unsaturated oleic and linoleic acids were higher in parasites than in red cells (oleic about 28 and 17%, respectively, and linoleic about 24 and 17%, respectively). Stearic acid was somewhat lower in parasites than in red cells (about 8 and 14%), whereas arachidonic (20:4) was much lower (about 4 compared with 13%) (Rock, 1971b).

The lipids of *P. knowlesi* thus differ from those of the red cell in having (1) a smaller proportion of neutral lipids, the decrease being mainly in cholesterol, (2) considerably less sphingomyelin, (3) probably no phosphatidylserine, (4) a greater proportion of phosphatidylinositol, and (5) a higher proportion of octadecenoic acids.

Beckwith *et al.* (1975) found that the lipids of *P. berghei* were qualitatively similar to those of *P. knowlesi,* notably in lacking phosphatidylserine.

Wallace *et al.* (1965) found that *P. berghei* (and *P. lophurae*) contained phospholipids, sterols, free fatty acids, and small amounts of triglycerides and sterol esters but did not attempt further analysis.

The lipid content of *P. berghei*-infected rat cells was found to be higher than that of uninfected reticulocytes, the increase in phospholipids being relatively greater than the increase in cholesterol (Lawrence and Cenedella, 1969; Rao *et al.,* 1970). A comparison of *P. berghei*-infected rat reticulocytes with uninfected reticulocytes showed that phosphatidylethanolamine as a proportion of the phospholipids was higher in the infected cell, sphingomyelin and lysophosphatidylcholine were lower, and phosphatidylserine was about the same in spite of being absent from the parasites themselves (see above). In addition, choline lipids were found to be the commonest phospholipids of free parasites of *P. berghei,* but in infected reticulocytes their proportion was less than in uninfected cells (Rao *et al.,* 1970). It thus appears that calculation of the lipid composition of parasites from a comparison of infected with uninfected cells may not be reliable, presumably because of changes in the host erythrocyte. Indeed, Rao *et al.* (1970) calculated that the lipids of *P. berghei* contributed only about 6% to the total lipids of the infected rat reticulocyte. The data of Lawrence and Cenedella (1969), on the other hand, showed that the parasites from a given number of infected reticulocytes contained about five times as much lipid as the same number of uninfected reticulocytes.

During infection with *P. gallinaceum* the phospholipid content of the red cells rose and, at least before the parasitemia became very high, the increase could be accounted for by the phospholipids of the parasite (Seed and Kreier, 1972).

Wallace *et al.* (1965), referred to above, found that *P. lophurae* contained various lipid classes, and of these Hardy *et al.* (1975) showed that phospholipids accounted for about 70% of the total lipids.

Further analysis (Beach *et al.*, 1977) showed that *P. lophurae* resembled *P. knowlesi* in that the proportion of phospholipid was higher in the free parasites than in the host cells (86% compared with 74%) and that of neutral lipid lower (12% compared with 21%), the decrease being mainly due to the low proportion of cholesterol in the parasite (only 8% as compared with 20% in the duck erythrocyte). Of the phospholipids, phosphatidylcholine was the commonest, being the same percentage of the total lipid of both parasite and host cell (40%). Phosphatidylethanolamine, the second most common, was higher in the free parasite than in the duck erythrocyte (36% compared with 20%). As with *P. knowlesi*, sphingomyelin was much lower in the parasite than in the host cell (2% compared with 11%), and phosphatidylserine was virtually absent from the parasite (less than 1% of the total lipid) but, in contrast to monkey cells, this phospholipid was almost absent from duck red cells also.

The fatty acids of lipids in *P. lophurae* were examined by Beach *et al.* (1977). The most common fatty acids in all classes of lipid examined were palmitic (16:0), stearic (18:0), oleic (18:1), and linoleic (18:2); pentadecanoic acid (15:0) was higher in the free fatty acids than in any other lipid class of the parasite. Wallace *et al.* (1965) and Wallace (1966) also found that the same fatty acids were present in the highest proportions in the lipids of free parasites of *P. lophurae* (and *P. berghei*).

The proportion of octadecenoic acids in the lipids of *P. lophurae*-infected duck erythrocytes was much higher than in uninfected cells and was also high in free parasites (Holz *et al.*, 1977). Of these fatty acids, oleic [18:1 $(n - 9)$] and *cis*-vaccenic [18:1 $(n - 7)$] acids have been shown to lyze erythrocytes *in vitro*, and it has been suggested that these two fatty acids are implicated in producing the changes in fragility and related properties observed in the red cells of malaria-infected animals; this topic has recently been discussed by Holz (1977) and Holz *et al.* (1977).

Beach *et al.* (1977) showed that the content of glycosphingolipids was less in *P. lophurae*-infected erythrocytes than in normal cells; of this fraction, McLaughlin and McGhee (1972) found that the same neutral glycosylceramides were present in infected and uninfected duck erythrocytes but that quantities differed in the two types of cell. Changes in the glycosphingolipids of erythrocytes upon infection could lead to changes in the immunological properties of these cells, but this has not been investigated further.

B. Biosynthesis of Lipids

Phospholipids can be synthesized by *P. knowlesi*. The glyceryl backbone can be obtained from glucose or glycerol (Rock, 1971a), and inorganic phosphate can also be incorporated, all three precursors entering mainly into phosphatidyl-choline, phosphatidylethanolamine and phosphatidylinositol (Rock, 1971a; Rock *et al.*, 1971b). The acyl portion of the phospholipid molecule is probably made up almost entirely of fatty acids obtained from the host, although the parasite can incorporate acetate into this portion of the molecule, mostly into phos-phatidylethanolamine (Rock, 1971a). This incorporation of acetate is stimulated by various cofactors involved in chain elongation, which suggests that the para-site is able to carry out the necessary reactions, but the activity of this pathway is low (Rock, 1971a). *Plasmodium knowlesi* can rapidly incorporate fatty acids into phospholipids, the rate of incorporation of the fatty acids tested being in the order: palmitic > stearic > oleic (Rock, 1971b). About 88% of the palmitic acid incorporated by the parasite was found in phospholipid, mainly in phosphatidyl-choline and phosphatidylethanolamine (each roughly 40% of the incorporation) and also in phosphatidylinositol (about 8%); the remainder was incorporated into neutral lipids. The dependence of the parasite on exogenous fatty acids is suggested by the fact that at least one fatty acid (stearic) improves the growth of *P. knowlesi* in culture (Siddiqui *et al.*, 1967; Trigg, 1969). It is possible that other parts of the phospholipid molecule are also derived ready-formed from the host; this is suggested by the rapid incorporation of ethanolamine and choline into their respective phospholipids (Rock, 1971a).

Part of the glucose and glycerol incorporated by *P. knowlesi* into lipid was found in neutral lipids, almost entirely in the glyceryl moiety of di- and tri-glycerides (Rock, 1971a). Part of the palmitate incorporated was also found in neutral lipids (about 12% of the total incorporation into lipid), again mostly in di- and triglycerides (6.7% and 4.5%, respectively.)

Cholesterol is probably obtained preformed from the host. *Plasmodium knowlesi*-parasitized cells were unable to synthesize cholesterol to any extent from acetate or mevalonic acid, but they could readily incorporate the exogenous sterol into lipid (Trigg, 1968), and cholesterol added to the medium improved growth *in vitro* (Trigg, 1969).

Less reliable information is available on the synthesis of lipids by rodent and avian parasites, partly because interference from the host cannot always be eliminated. For example, white cells are 100 to 1000 times more active than red cells in incorporating acetate into lipid, and glucose and phosphate are also incorporated (see Cline, 1965).

Cenedella (1968) reported the synthesis of lipids from glucose by *P. berghei*-infected cells and free parasites *in vitro*. Most of the incorporation was into phospholipids, with only a small proportion into neutral lipids. Almost all the incorporation into the phospholipids was into the glyceryl backbone, only about 4% being found in the acyl portion. The highest incorporation by free parasites was into sphingomyelin and lysophosphatides (grouped together in the analysis), followed by phosphatidylethanolamine (cephalins) and then phosphatidylcholine and phosphatidic acid. The extent of the incorporation of glucose into the sphingomyelin and lysophosphatide fraction (about 39% of the total) is in contrast to the results obtained with *P. knowlesi* (see above).

Cenedella *et al.* (1969b) attempted to avoid long incubations *in vitro* by infusing precursors, in this case glucose and oleic acid, into *P. berghei*-infected rats for up to 18 hours. They reported that the parasite incorporated both these compounds into phospholipids (mainly phosphatidylcholine and phosphatidylethanolamine) but that the fatty acids of the parasite lipid were not derived from the glucose. However, incorporation into contaminating leukocytes and platelets cannot be disregarded and, as pointed out by Holz (1977), the possibility of metabolism by the host during such infusions makes it difficult to be certain of the immediate precursors of the parasite lipids. Similar considerations apply to the experiments of Gutierrez (1966) who injected radioactive acetate into *P. fallax*-infected turkeys and removed parasitized cells 7 hours later for analysis of lipids. Experiments *in vitro* (Gutierrez, 1966) showed incorporation of acetate not only into phospholipids and free fatty acids but also into cholesterol. Fatty acids (palmitic, oleic and stearic) were incorporated into the same lipid fractions. Again, white cells and platelets may have contributed to the results.

Hardy *et al.* (1975) found that, in *P. lophurae*-infected cells *in vitro*, acetate was incorporated mainly into phospholipids, with varying amounts being taken up into free fatty acids, diglycerides and lipid alcohols. Little or no acetate was incorporated into sterols or sterol esters. Brundage *et al.* (1969), in similar experiments, found that *P. lophurae*-infected cells incorporated about 16 times more acetate into total lipids than normal cells; a large part of the acetate was incorporated into phospholipids, and it was also incorporated into monoglycerides, sterols, free fatty acids, triglycerides and sterol esters.

The above results might suggest that cholesterol can be synthesized by *P. lophurae* (Brundage *et al.*, 1969) and *P. fallax* (Gutierrez, 1966), but not by *P. knowlesi* (Trigg, 1968). However, the experimental uncertainties already mentioned make it difficult to be certain that there is a species difference.

Cenedella *et al.* (1969a) reported that *P. berghei in vitro* released free fatty acids, presumably by digestion of the host's lipids. However, the parasitized cells were incubated as a concentrated suspension for 4 hours, and it is possible that some breakdown of the parasites occurred, thereby contributing to the total free fatty acids. Phospholipase A was also demonstrated in the parasitized cells, but white cells, which contain phospholipases (Elsbach and Rizack, 1963), were also present.

In summary, *P. knowlesi* can synthesize part of its lipid, being able to make the glyceryl backbone of phospholipids and glycerides and to incorporate phosphate into phospholipids; however, it obtains cholesterol, most of its fatty acids, and probably ethanolamine and choline, from the host. It is, however, difficult to draw equally firm conclusions as to the biosynthesis of lipids by rodent and avian parasites.

IX. FOLATES

The susceptibility of malarial parasites to sulfonamides suggests that they contain the pathway for synthesis *de novo* of folate cofactors, and this is supported by the finding that growth of the parasites requires *p*-aminobenzoate (pABA) (rodent: Jacobs, 1964; primate: Anfinsen *et al.*, 1946). In addition, suppression of the growth of *P. berghei* by feeding only milk to the host (Maegraith *et al.*, 1952) was shown (rodent: Hawking, 1954; primate: Hawking, 1954; Kretschmar and Voller, 1973) to be due to the absence of pABA from milk.

The enzymes required for the synthesis of tetrahydrofolate are shown in Fig. 3. Mammals and birds are unable to synthesize dihydrofolate from the pteridine precursors but obtain dihydrofolate from folates in the diet (Woods and Tucker, 1958). 2-Amino-4-hydroxymethyldihydropteridine pyrophosphokinase activity has been shown in rodent parasites (Ferone, 1973; Walter and König, 1974a). Dihydropteroate synthetase activity has been found in rodent (Walter and König, 1971b, 1974a; Ferone, 1973; McCullough and Maren, 1974), primate and avian parasites (Ferone, 1973). Although Ferone (1973) was able partially to separate the proteins which had these two enzyme activities, Walter and König (1974a) were unable to do so. The dihydropteroate synthetase and 2-amino-4-hydroxy-6-hydroxymethyldihydropteridine pyrophosphokinase combined had a molecular weight of about 200,000–250,000, but it is not known if this is the molecular weight of each separate enzyme or of a complex of the two (Walter and König, 1974a).

Dihydropteroate synthetase from *P. berghei* can also use *p*-aminobenzoyl-glutamate (pAGA) to form dihydrofolate (Ferone, 1973), but the K_m is about 100 times higher than for pABA. It therefore seems that the pathway involving pABA is the one predominantly used by the parasite, although R. Ferone and S. Roland (unpublished observations, quoted by Ferone, 1977) were unable to detect dihydrofolate synthetase.

Dihydrofolate reductase is present in rodent (Ferone *et al.*, 1969, 1970; Gerzeli and Polver, 1969; Diggens *et al.*, 1970; Ferone, 1970; Walter and König, 1971a; Schoenfeld *et al.*, 1974), primate (Gutteridge and Trigg, 1971) and avian (Platzer, 1974) malarial parasites. (Dihydrofolate reductases of parasites have been reviewed by Jaffe, 1972.) Dihydrofolate reductase is also present in the host, but the enzyme of the parasites differs from that of mammals and birds in having a much higher molecular weight, about 200,000 in *P. knowlesi* and in rodent parasites and about 100,000 in *P. lophurae,* compared with the approximately 20,000 of mammalian and avian enzymes (rodent: Ferone *et al.*, 1969;

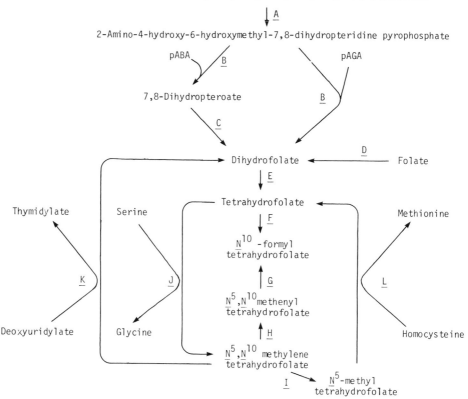

FIG. 3. Folate metabolic pathways. *A*, 2-Amino-4-hydroxy-6- hydroxymethyldihydropteridine pyrophosphokinase; *B*, dihydropteroate synthetase; *C*, dihydrofolate synthetase; *D*, folate reductase; *E*, dihydrofolate reductase; *F*, formyltetrahydrofolate synthetase; *G*, methenyltetrahydrofolate cyclohydrolase; *H*, methylenetetrahydrofolate dehydrogenase; *I*, methylenetetrahydrofolate reductase; *J*, serine hydroxymethyltransferase; *K*, thymidylate synthetase; *L*, tetrahydropteroylglumate methyltransferase.

primate: Gutteridge and Trigg, 1971; avian: Platzer, 1974). Another striking difference between the enzymes of parasite and host is that the K_m for pyrimethamine of the parasite enzyme is very much lower than in the case of the host (Ferone *et al.*, 1969), thus accounting for the selective action of the drug.

The activity of dihydrofolate reductase, like that of thymidylate synthetase (see Section VII,B,2), increases during the intraerythrocytic cycle, beginning to rise just before the first nuclear division (rodent: Walter and Königk, 1971a).

Free parasites of *P. berghei* are almost unable to produce dihydrofolate from folate, indicating that they lack folate reductase and that the dihydrofolate reductase of the parasite, unlike that of some other organisms (Brown, 1970), cannot reduce folate (Ferone and Hitchings, 1966). It is therefore not surprising that folate is less effective than pABA in reversing the effects of sulfonamides on the parasites (rodent: Thurston, 1954; primate; McCormick et al., 1971; avian: Rollo, 1955). However, cultivation in vitro is enhanced by folate and folinate (N^5-formyltetrahydrofolate) (primate: Trager, 1958; avian: Glenn and Manwell, 1956; Trager, 1958), as is the synthesis of nucleic acids (primate: McCormick et al., 1971), but, as pointed out by Ferone (1977), this may be due to utilization by the parasites not of the intact molecules but of breakdown products or contaminating pteridines, etc.

Trager (1959) showed that the level of folate and folinate was much higher in P. lophurae-infected duck erythrocytes than in normal cells, but that the levels in free parasites were low, suggesting that the increase was therefore due to changes in the host cell. Siddiqui and Trager (1966) found that most of the increase was due to a raised concentration of folinate during division of the parasites in vivo, but that during the same amount of development in vitro there was a much smaller increase. The types of folate compounds in infected and uninfected cells were the same (Siddiqui and Trager, 1964).

Plasmodium berghei can synthesize some folate cofactors from dihydrofolate, as shown by the production by free parasites of substances promoting the growth of Pediococcus cerevisiae (presumably cofactor forms of tetrahydrofolate such as folinate) from dihydrofolate (Ferone and Hitchings, 1966). Reid and Friedkin (1973a) showed that, although there was a slight increase in the total folate of P. berghei-infected mouse blood, the most marked change was in the types of folates present.

Further synthesis of folate cofactors has not been investigated in rodent malarial parasites. Extracts of P. lophurae contain serine hydroxymethyltransferase, whose molecular weight of about 68,000 is less than that of the duck enzyme (>100,000) (Platzer, 1972; Platzer and Campuzano, 1976) and which produces N^5,N^{10}-methylenetetrahydrofolate, used in the methylation of deoxyuridylate to form thymidylate by thymidylate synthetase. The functioning of both these enzymes in P. knowlesi (in whole monkey blood) was shown by Smith et al. (1976) who found that radioactivity from L-[3-^{14}C]serine was found in thymidylate. In the same experiments, almost the same amount of label from serine was found in methionine, suggesting the action of methylenetetrahydrofolate reductase and tetrahydropteroylglutamate methyltransferase. However, attempts to confirm this by forming labeled methionine from N^5-methyl-[^{14}C]tetrahydrofolate gave inconclusive results and, although label from [^{35}S]homocysteine was found in methionine, about 10 times as much homocysteine as serine was needed for an equivalent amount of labeling, suggesting that homocysteine had difficulty in reaching the enzyme. Synthesis of methionine from homocysteine has also been shown in P. berghei (Langer, et al., 1969), although this reaction is probably of limited importance in malarial parasites since they need an exogenous supply of methionine (see Section VI,C,1).

Platzer (1972) showed that the activities of formyltetrahydrofolate synthetase and methylenetetrahydrofolate dehydrogenase were lower in *P. lophurae*-infected duck erythrocytes than in normal cells and that the activity of neither enzyme could be detected in free parasites. *Plasmodium lophurae,* therefore, would be unable to form N^{10}-formyltetrahydrofolate, which is required for purine synthesis. The absence of these enzymes is therefore consonant with the apparent inability of malarial parasites to synthesize purines.

Investigation of the enzymes of folate production by malarial parasites is simplified by the inability of the host to synthesize dihydrofolate from pteridine precursors, so that any enzymes of this pathway which are detected can safely be attributed to the parasite. Several of these enzymes have been detected, confirming the synthesis of dihydrofolate by the parasite, probably by the pathway incorporating pABA rather than pAGA.

Both host and parasite produce tetrahydrofolate from dihydrofolate, but the enzymes which carry out the reaction have markedly different properties. Further synthesis of folate cofactors by the parasite appears to be somewhat limited. It is able to produce N^5, N^{10}-methylenetetrahydrofolate, used in the thymidylate synthetase cycle, but is unable to produce N^{10}-formyltetrahydrofolate which is required for the synthesis of purines. The parasite is apparently able to synthesize methionine from serine and must therefore possess the relevant enzymes, but the activity of this pathway is probably low.

REFERENCES

Aikawa, M. (1966). The fine structure of the erythrocytic stages of three avian malarial parasites, *Plasmodium fallax, P. lophurae,* and *P. cathemerium. Am. J. Trop. Med. Hyg.* **15,** 449–471.

Aikawa, M. (1971). *Plasmodium:* The fine structure of malarial parasites. *Exp. Parasitol.* **30,** 284–320.

Aikawa, M. (1977). Variations in structure and function during the life cycle of malarial parasites. *Bull. W. H. O.* **55,** 139–156.

Aikawa, M., and Cook, R. T. (1971). Ribosomes of the malarial parasite, *Plasmodium knowlesi.* II. Ultrastructural features. *Comp. Biochem. Physiol. B* **39,** 913–917.

Aikawa, M., and Cook, R. T. (1972). *Plasmodium:* Electron microscopy of antigen preparations. *Exp. Parasitol.* **31,** 67–74.

Aikawa, M., and Thompson, P. E. (1971). Localization of acid phosphatase activity in *Plasmodium berghei* and *P. gallinaceum:* An electron microscopic observation. *J. Parasitol.* **57,** 603–610.

Aikawa, M., Hepler, P. K., Huff, C. G., and Sprinz, H. (1966a). The feeding mechanism of avian malarial parasites. *J. Cell Biol.* **28,** 355–373.

Aikawa, M., Huff, C. G., and Sprinz, H. (1966b). Comparative feeding mechanisms of avian and primate malarial parasites. *Mil. Med.* **131,** 969–983.

Aikawa, M., Huff, C. G., and Sprinz, H. (1967). Fine structure of the asexual stages of *Plasmodium elongatum. J. Cell Biol.* **34,** 229–249.

Aikawa, M., Sterling, C. R., and Rabbege, J. (1972). Cytochemistry of the nucleus of malarial parasites. *Proc. Helminthol. Soc. Wash.* **39**, 174–194.

Ali, S. N., and Fletcher, K. A. (1974). The concentration of 2,3-diphosphoglycerate in malarial blood (*P. berghei* malaria). *Int. J. Biochem.* **5**, 17–19.

Allfrey, V., and Mirsky, A. E. (1952). The incorporation of N^{15}-glycine by avian erythrocytes and reticulocytes in vitro. *J. Gen. Physiol.* **35**, 841–846.

Allfrey, V., and Mirsky, A. E. (1959). Biochemical properties of the isolated nucleus. *In* "Subcellular Particles" (T. Hayashi, ed.), pp. 186–204. Ronald Press, New York.

Anfinsen, C. B., Geiman, Q. M., McKee, R. W., Ormsbee, R. A., and Ball, E. G. (1946). Studies on malarial parasites. VIII. Factors affecting the growth of Plasmodium knowlesi in vitro. *J. Exp. Med.* **84**, 607–621.

Angus, M. G. N., Fletcher, K. A., and Maegraith, B. G. (1972). Studies on the lipids of *Plasmodium knowlesi*-infected rhesus monkeys (*Macaca mulatta*). IV. Changes in erythrocyte lipids. *Ann. Trop. Med. Parasitol.* **65**, 429–439.

Augustin, W. (1961). Reifungsvorgänge bei Hühnererythrozyten. *Folia Haematol. (Leipzig)* **78**, 436–440.

Bahr, G. F. (1966). Quantitative cytochemical study of erythrocytic stages of *Plasmodium lophurae* and *Plasmodium berghei*. *Mil. Med.* **131**, 1064–1070.

Bahr, G. F., and Mikel, U. (1972). The arrangement of DNA in the nucleus of rodent malaria parasites. *Proc. Helminthol. Soc. Wash.* **39**, 361–372.

Ball, E. G., McKee, R. W., Anfinsen, C. B., Cruz, W. O., and Geiman, Q. M. (1948). Studies on malarial parasites. IX. Chemical and metabolic changes during growth and multiplication in vivo and in vitro. *J. Biol. Chem.* **175**, 547–571.

Bass, C. C., and Johns, F. M. (1912). The cultivation of malarial plasmodia (Plasmodium vivax and Plasmodium falciparum) in vitro. *J. Exp. Med.* **16**, 567–579.

Beach, D. H., Sherman, I. W., and Holz, G. G., Jr. (1977). Lipids of *Plasmodium lophurae*, and of erythrocytes and plasmas of normal and *P. lophurae*-infected Pekin ducklings. *J. Parasitol.* **63**, 62–75.

Beck, W. S. (1958). Occurrence and control of phosphogluconate oxidation pathway in normal and leukemic leukocytes. *J. Biol. Chem.* **232**, 271–283.

Beckwith, R., Schenkel, R. H., and Silverman, P. H. (1975). Qualitative analysis of phospholipids isolated from nonviable plasmodium antigen. *Exp. Parasitol.* **37**, 164–172.

Bell, D. J. (1971). Metabolism of the erythrocyte. *In* "Physiology and Biochemistry of the Domestic Fowl" (D. J. Bell, ed.), Vol. 2, pp. 863–872. Academic Press, New York.

Bernstein, R. E. (1959). Alterations in metabolic energetics and cation transport during aging of red cells. *J. Clin. Invest.* **38**, 1572–1586.

Bishop, C. (1960). Purine metabolism in human and chicken blood, *in vitro*. *J. Biol. Chem.* **235**, 3228–3232.

Blackburn, W. R., and Vinijchaikul, K. (1970). Experimental mammalian malaria. I. The asexual development of *Plasmodium berghei* trophozoites in inbred mice. *Lab. Invest.* **22**, 417–431.

Booden, T., and Hull, R. W. (1973). Nucleic acid precursor synthesis by *Plasmodium lophurae* parasitizing chicken erythrocytes. *Exp. Parasitol.* **34**, 220–228.

Borsook, H. (1964). DNA, RNA and protein synthesis after acute, severe, blood loss: A picture of erythropoiesis at the combined morphological and molecular levels. *Ann. N.Y. Acad. Sci.* **119**, 523–539.

Borst, P., and Fairlamb, A. H. (1976). DNA of parasites, with special reference to kinetoplast DNA. *In* "Biochemistry of Parasites and Host-Parasite Relationships" (H. Van den Bossche, ed.), pp. 169–191. North-Holland Publ., Amsterdam.

Bovarnick, M. R., Lindsay, A., and Hellerman, L. (1946a). Metabolism of the malarial parasite, with reference particularly to the action of antimalarial agents. I. Preparation and properties of

Plasmodium lophurae separated from the red cells of duck blood by means of saponin. *J. Biol. Chem.* **163**, 523–533.

Bovarnick, M. R., Lindsay, A., and Hellerman, L. (1946b). Metabolism of the malarial parasite, with reference particularly to the action of antimalarial agents. II. Atabrine (quinacrine) inhibition of glucose oxidation in parasites initially depleted of substrate. Reversal by adenylic acid. *J. Biol. Chem.* **163**, 535–551.

Bowman, I. B. R., Grant, P. T., and Kermack, W. O. (1960). The metabolism of *Plasmodium berghei*, the malaria parasite of rodents. I. The preparation of the erythrocytic form of *P. berghei* separated from the host cell. *Exp. Parasitol.* **9**, 131–136.

Bowman, I. B. R., Grant, P. T., Kermack, W. O., and Ogston, D. (1961). The metabolism of *Plasmodium berghei*, the malaria parasite of rodents. 2.·An effect of mepacrine on the metabolism of glucose by the parasite separated from its host cell. *Biochem. J.* **78**, 472–478.

Brewer, G. J. (1974). Red cell metabolism and function. *In* "The Red Blood Cell" (D. MacN. Surgenor, ed.), 2nd ed., Vol. 1, pp. 473–508. Academic Press, New York.

Brewer, G. J., and Coan, C. C. (1969). Interaction of red cell ATP levels and malaria, and the treatment of malaria with hyperoxia. *Mil. Med.* **134**, 1056–1067.

Brewer, G. J., and Powell, R. D. (1965). A study of the relationship between the content of adenosine triphosphate in human red cells and the course of falciparum malaria: A new system that may confer protection against malaria. *Proc. Natl. Acad. Sci. U.S.A.* **54**, 741–745.

Broun, G. (1961). Enzymes érythrocytaires et infestation a *Plasmodium berghei* chez la souris. *Rev. Fr. Etud. Clin. Biol.* **6**, 695–699.

Brown, G. M. (1970). Biogenesis and metabolism of folic acid. *In* "Metabolic Pathways" (D. M. Greenberg, ed.), 3rd ed., Vol. 4, pp. 383–410. Academic Press, New York.

Brown, W. H. (1911). Malarial pigment (so-called melanin): Its nature and mode of production. *J. Exp. Med.* **13**, 290–299.

Brundage, W. G., Hyland, C. M., Sr., and Dimopoullos, G. T. (1969). *In vitro* biosynthesis of lipids in blood from ducks infected with *Plasmodium lophurae*. *Am. J. Trop. Med. Hyg.* **18**, 657–661.

Bryant, C., Voller, A., and Smith, M. J. H. (1964). The incorporation of radioactivity from [^{14}C] glucose into the soluble metabolic intermediates of malaria parasites. *Am. J. Trop. Med. Hyg.* **13**, 515–519.

Büngener, W. (1967). Adenosindeaminase und Nucleosidphosphorylase bei Malariaparasiten. *Z. Tropenmed. Parasitol.* **18**, 48–52.

Büngener, W. (1974a). Influence of allopurinol on the multiplication of rodent malaria parasites. *Tropenmed. Parasitol.* **25**, 309–312.

Büngener, W. (1974b). Einfluss von Allopurinol auf Zyklusdauer und Vermehrungsrate von Plasmodium vinckei in der Ratte. *Tropenmed. Parasitol.* **25**, 464–468.

Büngener, W., and Nielsen, G. (1967). Nukleinsäurenstoffwechsel bei experimenteller Malaria. 1. Untersuchungen über den Einbau von Thymidin, Uridin und Adenosin in Malariaparasiten (Plasmodium berghei und Plasmodium vinckei). *Z. Tropenmed. Parasitol.* **18**, 456–462.

Büngener, W., and Nielsen, G. (1968). Nukleinsäurenstoffwechsel bei experimenteller Malaria. 2. Einbau von Adenosin und Hypoxanthin in die Nukleinsäuren von Malariaparasiten (Plasmodium berghei und Plasmodium vinckei). *Z. Tropenmed. Parasitol.* **19**, 185–197.

Büngener, W., and Nielsen, G. (1969). Nukleinsäurenstoffwechsel bei experimenteller Malaria. 3. Einbau von Adenin aus dem Adeninnukleotidpool der Erythrozyten in die Nukleinsäuren von Malariaparasiten. *Z. Tropenmed. Parasitol.* **20**, 66–73.

Bunn, H. F. (1972). Erythrocyte destruction and hemoglobin catabolism. *Semin. Hematol.* **9**, 3–17.

Butcher, G. A., and Cohen, S. (1971). Short-term culture of *Plasmodium knowlesi. Parasitology* **62**, 309–320.

Cadigan, F. C., Jr., Colley, F. C., and Zaman, V. (1972). Observations on the fine structure of *Plasmodium traguli*. *Proc. Helminthol. Soc. Wash.* **39**, 137–148.

Cameron, I. L., and Prescott, D. M. (1963). RNA and protein metabolism in the maturation of the nucleated chicken erythrocyte. *Exp. Cell Res.* **30**, 609–612.

Carbone, T. (1891). *G. Accad. Med. Torino* **39**, 901 (quoted by Sinton and Ghosh, 1934a).

Carter, G., and Van Dyke, K. (1972). Drug effects on the phosphorylation of adenosine and its incorporation into nucleic acids of chloroquine sensitive and resistant erythrocyte-free malarial parasites. *Proc. Helminthol. Soc. Wash.* **39**, 244–249.

Carter, G., Van Dyke, K., and Mengoli, H. F. (1972). Energetics of the malarial parasite. *Proc. Helminthol. Soc. Wash.* **39**, 241–243.

Carter, R. (1970). Enzyme variation in *Plasmodium berghei*. *Trans. R. Soc. Trop. Med. Hyg.* **64**, 401–406.

Carter, R. (1973). Enzyme variation in *Plasmodium berghei* and *Plasmodium vinckei*. *Parasitology* **66**, 297–307.

Carter, R. (1978). Studies on enzyme variation in the murine malaria parasites *Plasmodium berghei*, *P. yoelii*, *P. vinckei* and *P. chabaudi* by starch gel electrophoresis. *Parasitology* **76**, 241–267.

Carter, R., and McGregor, I. A. (1973). Enzyme variation in *Plasmodium falciparum* in the Gambia. *Trans. R. Soc. Trop. Med. Hyg.* **67**, 830–837.

Carter, R., and Voller, A. (1973). Enzyme typing of malaria parasites. *Br. Med. J.* **1**, 149–150.

Carter, R., and Voller, A. (1975). The distribution of enzyme variation in populations of *Plasmodium falciparum* in Africa. *Trans. R. Soc. Trop. Med. Hyg.* **69**, 371–376.

Carter, R., and Walliker, D. (1977). Biochemical markers for strain differentiation in malarial parasites. *Bull. W. H. O.* **55**, 339–345.

Casey, A. C., and Bliznakov, E. G. (1973). Coenzymes Q levels in liver, spleen, and blood of mice with Friend leukemia virus infection. *Cancer Res.* **33**, 1183–1186.

Ceithaml, J., and Evans, E. A., Jr. (1946). The biochemistry of the malaria parasite. IV. The in vitro effects of X-rays upon *Plasmodium gallinaceum*. *J. Infect. Dis.* **78**, 190–197.

Cenedella, R. J. (1968). Lipid synthesis from glucose carbon by *Plasmodium berghei in vitro*. *Am. J. Trop. Med. Hyg.* **17**, 680–684.

Cenedella, R. J., and Jarrell, J. J. (1970). Suggested new mechanisms of antimalarial action for DDS involving inhibition of glucose utilization by the intraerythrocytic parasite. *Am. J. Trop. Med. Hyg.* **19**, 592–598.

Cenedella, R. J., Rosen, H., Angel, C. R., and Saxe, L. H. (1968). Free amino-acid production *in vitro* by *Plasmodium berghei*. *Am. J. Trop. Med. Hyg.* **17**, 800–803.

Cenedella, R. J., Jarrell, J. J., and Saxe, L. H. (1969a). *Plasmodium berghei*: Production *in vitro* of free fatty acids. *Exp. Parasitol.* **24**, 130–136.

Cenedella, R. J., Jarrell, J. J., and Saxe, L. H. (1969b). Lipid synthesis *in vivo* from 1-^{14}C-oleic acid and 6-^{3}H-glucose by intraerythrocytic *Plasmodium berghei*. *Mil. Med.* **134**, 1045–1055.

Cenedella, R. J., Saxe, L. H., and Van Dyke, K. (1970). An automated method of mass drug testing applied to screening for antimalarial activity. *Chemotherapy (Basel)* **15**, 158–176.

Chan, V. L., and Lee, P. Y. (1974). Host-cell specific proteolytic enzymes in *Plasmodium berghei* infected erythrocytes. *Southeast Asian J. Trop. Med. Public Health* **5**, 447–449.

Chance, M. L., Momen, H., Warhurst, D. C., and Peters, W. (1978). The chemotherapy of rodent malaria. XXIX. DNA relationships within the subgenus *Plasmodium* (Vinckeia). *Ann. Trop. Med. Parasitol.* **72**, 13–22.

Chen, T.-T. (1944). The nuclei in avian malaria parasites. I. The structure of nuclei in *Plasmodium elongatum* with some considerations on technique. *Am. J. Hyg.* **40**, 26–34.

Cho, Y. W., and Aviado, D. M. (1968). Pathologic physiology and chemotherapy of *Plasmodium berghei*. IV. Influence of chloroquine on oxygen uptake of red blood cells infected with sensitive or resistant strains. *Exp. Parasitol.* **23**, 143–150.

Christensen, H. N. (1975). "Biological Transport," 2nd ed., p. 203. Benjamin, Reading, Massachusetts.

Christophers, S. R., and Fulton, J. D. (1938). Observations on the respiratory metabolism of malaria parasites and trypanosomes. *Ann. Trop. Med. Parasitol.* **32,** 43–75.

Christophers, S. R., and Fulton, J. D. (1939). Experiments with isolated malaria parasites (*Plasmodium knowlesi*) free from red cells. *Ann. Trop. Med. Parasitol.* **33,** 161–170.

Ciucă, M., Ciplea, Al. Gh., Bona, C., Poszgi, N., Isfan, Tr., and Iuga, G. (1963). Études cytochimiques sanguines dans l'infection expérimentale avec *Plasmodium berghei* de la souris blanche. I. Structure cytochimique du parasite, des globules rouges et observations effectuées au microscope à contraste de phase. *Arch. Roum. Pathol. Exp. Microbiol.* **22,** 503–514.

Clarke, D. H. (1952a). The use of phosphorus 32 in studies on Plasmodium gallinaceum. I. The development of a method for the quantitative determination of parasite growth and development in vitro. *J. Exp. Med.* **96,** 439–450.

Clarke, D. H. (1952b). The use of phosphorus 32 in studies on Plasmodium gallinaceum. II. Studies on conditions affecting parasite growth in intact cells and in lysates. *J. Exp. Med.* **96,** 451–463.

Cline, M. J. (1965). Metabolism of the circulating leukocyte. *Physiol. Rev.* **45,** 674–720.

Coggeshall, L. T. (1940). The selective action of sulfanilamide on the parasites of experimental malaria in monkeys in vivo and in vitro. *J. Exp. Med.* **71,** 13–20.

Coggeshall, L. T., and Maier, J. (1941). Determination of the activity of various drugs against the malaria parasite. *J. Infect. Dis.* **69,** 108–113.

Cohen, S., Butcher, G. A., and Crandall, R. B. (1969). Action of malarial antibody *in vitro. Nature (London)* **223,** 368–371.

Collins, W. E., and Aikawa, M. (1977). Plasmodia of nonhuman primates. *In* "Parasitic Protozoa" (J. P. Kreier, ed.), Vol. 3, pp. 467–492. Academic Press, New York.

Conklin, K. A., Chou, S. C., Siddiqui, W. A., and Schnell, J. V. (1973). DNA and RNA syntheses by intraerythrocytic stages of *Plasmodium knowlesi. J. Protozool.* **20,** 683–688.

Cook, L., Grant, P. T., and Kermack, W. O. (1961). Proteolytic enzymes of the erythrocytic forms of rodent and simian species of malarial plasmodia. *Exp. Parasitol.* **11,** 372–379.

Cook, R. T., Aikawa, M., Rock, R. C., Little, W., and Sprinz, H. (1969). The isolation and fractionation of *Plasmodium knowlesi. Mil. Med.* **134,** 866–883.

Cook, R. T., Rock, R. C., Aikawa, M., and Fournier, M. J., Jr. (1971). Ribosomes of the malarial parasite, *Plasmodium knowlesi.* I. Isolation, activity and sedimentation velocity. *Comp. Biochem. Physiol. B* **39,** 897–911.

Coombs, G. H., and Gutteridge, W. E. (1975). Growth *in vitro* and metabolism of *Plasmodium vinckei chabaudi. J. Protozool.* **22,** 555–560.

Dajani, R. M., and Orten, J. M. (1958). A study of the citric acid cycle in erythrocytes. *J. Biol. Chem.* **231,** 913–924.

Danforth, W. F. (1967). Respiratory metabolism. *In* "Research in Protozoology" (T.-T. Chen, ed.), Vol. 1, pp. 201–306. Pergamon, Oxford.

Dasgupta, B. (1960). Polysaccharides in the different stages of the life-cycles of certain sporozoa. *Parasitology* **50,** 509–514.

Davidson, J. N. (1976). "The Biochemistry of the Nucleic Acids" (revised by R. L. P. Adams, R. H. Burdon, A. M. Campbell, and R. M. S. Smellie), 8th ed., pp. 22 and 231. Chapman & Hall, London.

Dean, R. T. (1975). Direct evidence of importance of lysosomes in degradation of intracellular proteins. *Nature (London)* **257,** 414–416.

Deane, H. W. (1945). Studies on malarial parasites. II. The staining of two primate parasites by the Feulgen technique. *J. Cell. Comp. Physiol.* **26,** 139–145.

Deegan, T., and Maegraith, B. G. (1956a). Studies on the nature of malarial pigment (haemozoin). I.

The pigment of the simian species, *Plasmodium knowlesi* and *P. cynomolgi. Ann. Trop. Med. Parasitol.* **50,** 194–211.

Deegan, T., and Maegraith, B. G. (1956b). Studies on the nature of malarial pigment (haemozoin). II. The pigment of the human species, *Plasmodium falciparum* and *P. malariae. Ann. Trop. Med. Parasitol.* **50,** 212–222.

Devine, J., and Fulton, J. D. (1941). Observations on the nature of the malarial pigment present in infections of monkeys (*Macacus rhesus*) with *Plasmodium knowlesi. Ann. Trop. Med. Parasitol.* **35,** 15–22.

Devine, J., and Fulton, J. D. (1942). The pigment formed by *Plasmodium gallinaceum* Brumpt, 1935, in the domestic fowl. *Ann. Trop. Med. Parasitol.* **36,** 167–170.

De Zeeuw, R. A., Wijsbeek, J., Rock, R. C., and McCormick, G. J. (1972). Composition of phospholipids in *Plasmodium knowlesi* membranes and in host Rhesus erythrocyte membranes. *Proc. Helminthol. Soc. Wash.* **39,** 412–418.

Diggens, S. M., Gutteridge, W. E., and Trigg, P. I. (1970). Altered dihydrofolate reductase associated with a pyrimethamine-resistant *Plasmodium berghei berghei* produced in a single step. *Nature (London)* **228,** 579–580.

Diggs, C., Joseph, K., Flemmings, B., Snodgrass, R., and Hines, F. (1975). Protein synthesis in vitro by cryopreserved *Plasmodium falciparum. Am. J. Trop. Med. Hyg.* **24,** 760–763.

Dixon, M., and Webb, E. C. (1964). "Enzymes," 2nd ed., pp. 337–341. Longmans, London.

Doktorandenkollektiv des Physiologisch-chemischen Institutes, Berlin 1959–1960 (1962). Vergleichende Enzymatik der roten Blutkörperchen. *Folia Haematol. (Leipzig)* **78,** 441–446.

Eaton, J. W., and Brewer, G. J. (1969). Red cell ATP and malaria infection. *Nature (London)* **222,** 389–390.

Eckman, J. R., Modler, S., Eaton, J. W., Berger, E., and Engel, R. R. (1977). Host heme catabolism in drug-sensitive and drug-resistant malaria. *J. Lab. Clin. Med.* **90,** 767–770.

Eldan, N., and Blum, J. J. (1975). Presence of nonoxidative enzymes of the pentose phosphate shunt in *Tetrahymena. J. Protozool.* **22,** 145–149.

Ellis, D., Sewell, C. E., and Skinner, L. G. (1956). Reticulocyte enzymes and protein synthesis. *Nature (London)* **177,** 190–191.

Elsbach, P., and Rizack, M. A. (1963). Acid lipase and phospholipase activity in homogenates of rabbit polymorphonuclear leukocytes. *Am. J. Physiol.* **205,** 1154–1158.

Fabiani, G., Orfila, J., and Prades, Cl. M. (1958). Les variations des plaquettes sanguines au cours du paludisme expérimental de la souris blanche. *C. R. Séances Soc. Biol. Ses. Fil.* **152,** 588–589.

Ferone, R. (1970). Dihydrofolate reductase from pyrimethamine-resistant *Plasmodium berghei. J. Biol. Chem.* **245,** 850–854.

Ferone, R. (1973). The enzymic synthesis of dihydropteroate and dihydrofolate by *Plasmodium berghei. J. Protozool.* **20,** 459–464.

Ferone, R. (1977). Folate metabolism in malaria. *Bull. W. H. O.* **55,** 291–298.

Ferone, R., and Hitchings, G. H. (1966). Folate cofactor biosynthesis by *Plasmodium berghei.* Comparison of folate and dihydrofolate as substrates. *J. Protozool.* **13,** 504–506.

Ferone, R., Burchall, J. J., and Hitchings, G. H. (1969). *Plasmodium berghei* dihydrofolate reductase. Isolation, properties, and inhibition by antifolates. *Mol. Pharmacol.* **5,** 49–59.

Ferone, R., O'Shea, M., and Yoeli, M. (1970). Altered dihydrofolate reductase associated with drug-resistance transfer between rodent plasmodia. *Science* **167,** 1263–1264.

Fiorelli, G., Alessio, L., Bragotti, R., Labina, G., and Dioguardi, N. (1969). Eletrophoretic pattern of some isoenzymes in reticulocyte preparations. *Folia Haematol. (Leipzig)* **91,** 46–49.

Fletcher, K. A., and Maegraith, B. G. (1962). Glucose-6-phosphate and 6-phosphogluconate dehydrogenase activities in erythrocytes of monkeys infected with *Plasmodium knowlesi. Nature (London)* **196,** 1316–1318.

Fletcher, K. A., and Maegraith, B. G. (1970). Erythrocyte reduced glutathione in malaria (*Plasmodium berghei* and *P. knowlesi*). Ann. Trop. Med. Parasitol. **64**, 481–486.

Fletcher, K. A., and Maegraith, B. G. (1972). The metabolism of the malaria parasite and its host. *Adv. Parasitol.* **10**, 31–48.

Fletcher, K. A., Fielding, C. M., and Maegraith, B. G. (1970). Studies on the role of adenosine phosphates in erythrocytes of *Plasmodium knowlesi*-infected monkeys. *Ann. Trop. Med. Parasitol.* **64**, 487–496.

Fletcher, K. A., Canning, M. V., and Theakston, R. D. G. (1977). Electrophoresis of glucose-6-phosphate and 6-phosphogluconate dehydrogenases in erythrocytes from malaria-infected animals. *Ann. Trop. Med. Parasitol.* **71**, 125–130.

Forrester, L. J., and Siu, P. M. L. (1971). P-enol pyruvate carboxylase from *Plasmodium berghei*. *Comp. Biochem. Physiol. B* **38**, 73–85.

Fraser, D. M., and Kermack, W. O. (1957). The inhibitory action of some antimalarial drugs and related compounds on the hexokinase of yeasts and *Plasmodium berghei*. *Br. J. Pharmacol. Chemother.* **12**, 16–23.

Fulton, J. D. (1939). Experiments on the utilization of sugars by malarial parasites (*Plasmodium knowlesi*). *Ann. Trop. Med. Parasitol.* **33**, 217–227.

Fulton, J. D., and Grant, P. T. (1956). The sulphur requirements of the erythrocytic form of *Plasmodium knowlesi*. *Biochem. J.* **63**, 274–282.

Fulton, J. D., and Rimington, C. (1953). The pigment of the malaria parasite *Plasmodium berghei*. *J. Gen. Microbiol.* **8**, 157–159.

Fulton, J. D., and Spooner, D. F. (1956). The *in vitro* respiratory metabolism of erythrocytic forms of *Plasmodium berghei*. *Exp. Parasitol.* **5**, 59–78.

Gerzeli, G., and Polver, P. De P. (1969). Un nuovo metodo citochimico per lo studio dell'attività tetraidrofolicoreduttasica in *Plasmodium berghei:* Analisi dell'effetto di inibitori specifici. *Riv. Parassitol.* **30**, 19–26.

Ghosh, A. K., and Sloviter, H. A. (1973). Glycolysis and the Pasteur effect in rat reticulocytes. *J. Biol. Chem.* **248**, 3035–3040.

Ghosh, B. N., and Nath, M. C. (1934). The chemical composition of malaria pigment (haemozoin). *Rec. Malar. Surv. India* **4**, 321–325.

Ghosh, B. N., and Sinton, J. A. (1934). Studies of malarial pigment (haemozoin). Part II. The reactions of haemozoin to tests for iron. *Rec. Malar. Surv. India* **4**, 43–59.

Glasunow, M. (1925). Chemisch-spektroskopische Eigenschaften des Malariapigmentes. *Virchow's Arch. Pathol. Anat. Physiol.* **255**, 295–302.

Glenn, S., and Manwell, R. D. (1956). Further studies on the cultivation of the avian malaria parasites. II. The effects of heterologous sera and added metabolites on growth and reproduction *in vitro*. *Exp. Parasitol.* **5**, 22–33.

Goetze, E., and Rapoport, S. (1954). Das Kathepsin der Kaninchenerythrozyten und seine Veränderungen bei der Zellreifung. *Biochem. Z.* **326**, 53–61.

Graubarth, H., Mackler, B., and Guest, G. M. (1953). Effects of acidosis on utilization of glucose in erythrocytes and leucocytes. *Am. J. Physiol.* **172**, 301–308.

Green, M. L., Boyle, J. A., and Seegmiller, J. E. (1970). Substrate stabilization: Genetically controlled reciprocal relationship of two human enzymes. *Science* **167**, 887–889.

Groman, N. B. (1951). Dynamic aspects of the nitrogen metabolism of *Plasmodium gallinaceum* in vivo and in vitro. *J. Infect. Dis.* **88**, 126–150.

Guest, G. M., Mackler, B., Graubarth, H., and Ammentorp, P. A. (1953). Rates of utilization of glucose in erythrocytes and leucocytes. *Am. J. Physiol.* **172**, 295–300.

Gutierrez, J. (1966). Effect of the antimalarial chloroquine on the phospholipid metabolism of avian malaria and heart tissue. *Am. J. Trop. Med. Hyg.* **15**, 818–822.

Gutteridge, W. E., and Trigg, P. I. (1970). Incorporation of radioactive precursors into DNA and RNA of *Plasmodium knowlesi* in vitro. *J. Protozool.* **17**, 89–96.

Gutteridge, W. E., and Trigg, P. I. (1971). Action of pyrimethamine and related drugs against *Plasmodium knowlesi in vitro*. *Parasitology* **62**, 431–444.

Gutteridge, W. E., and Trigg, P. I. (1972). Some studies on the DNA of *Plasmodium knowlesi*. *In* "Comparative Biochemistry of Parasites" (H. Van den Bossche, ed.), pp. 199–218. Academic Press, New York.

Gutteridge, W. E., Trigg, P. I., and Williamson, D. H. (1969). Base compositions of DNA from some malarial parasites. *Nature (London)* **224**, 1210–1211.

Gutteridge, W. E., Trigg, P. I., and Williamson, D. H. (1971). Properties of DNA from some malarial parasites. *Parasitology* **62**, 209–219.

Gutteridge, W. E., Trigg, P. I., and Bayley, P. M. (1972). Effects of chloroquine on *Plasmodium knowlesi in vitro*. *Parasitology* **64**, 37–45.

Hardin, B., Valentine, W. N., Follette, J. H., and Lawrence, J. S. (1954). Studies on the sulfhydryl content of human leukocytes and erythrocytes. *Am. J. Med. Sci.* **228**, 73–82.

Hardy, C. L. S., Hart, L. T., Dimopoullos, G. T., and Lambremont, E. N. (1975). *Plasmodium lophurae:* Quantitative *in vitro* incorporation of ^{14}C-1-acetate into lipids. *Exp. Parasitol.* **37**, 193–204.

Hawking, F. (1954). Milk, *p*-aminobenzoate, and malaria of rats and monkeys. *Br. Med. J.* **1**, 425–429.

Herman, Y. F., Ward, R. A., and Herman, R. H. (1966). Stimulation of the utilization of 1-^{14}C-glucose in chicken red blood cells infected with *Plasmodium gallinaceum. Am. J. Trop. Med. Hyg.* **15**, 276–280.

Hickman, R. L. (1969). The use of subhuman primates for experimental studies of human malaria. *Mil. Med.* **134**, 741–756.

Holz, G. G., Jr. (1977). Lipids and the malarial parasite. *Bull. W. H. O.* **55**, 237–248.

Holz, G. G., Jr., Beach, D. H., and Sherman, I. W. (1977). Octadecenoic fatty acids and their association with hemolysis in malaria. *J. Protozool.* **24**, 566–574.

Homewood, C. A. (1977). Carbohydrate metabolism of malarial parasites. *Bull. W. H. O.* **55**, 229–235.

Homewood, C. A. (1978). Biochemistry. *In* "Rodent Malaria" (R. Killick-Kendrick and W. Peters, eds.), pp. 169–211. Academic Press, New York.

Homewood, C. A., and Neame, K. D. (1974). Malaria and the permeability of the host erythrocyte. *Nature (London)* **252**, 718–719.

Homewood, C. A., and Neame, K. D. (1976). A comparison of methods used for the removal of white cells from malaria-infected blood. *Ann. Trop. Med. Parasitol.* **70**, 249–251.

Homewood, C. A., Warhurst, D. C., Peters, W., and Baggaley, V. C. (1972a). Electron transport in intraerythrocytic *Plasmodium berghei. Proc. Helminthol. Soc. Wash.* **39**, 382–386.

Homewood, C. A., Jewsbury, J. M., and Chance, M. L. (1972b). The pigment formed during haemoglobin digestion by malarial and schistosomal parasites. *Comp. Biochem. Physiol. B* **43**, 517–523.

Homewood, C. A., Moore, G. A., Warhurst, D. C., and Atkinson, E. M. (1975). Purification and some properties of malarial pigment. *Ann. Trop. Med. Parasitol.* **69**, 283–287.

Hopkins, J., and Tudhope, G. R. (1973). Red cell glutathione in anaemia. *Scott. Med. J.* **18**, 177–181.

Howells, R. E. (1970). Mitochondrial changes during the life cycle of *Plasmodium berghei. Ann. Trop. Med. Parasitol.* **64**, 181–187.

Howells, R. E., and Maxwell, L. (1973a). Further studies on the mitochondrial changes during the life cycle of *Plasmodium berghei:* Electrophoretic studies on isocitrate dehydrogenases. *Ann. Trop. Med. Parasitol.* **67**, 279–283.

Howells, R. E., and Maxwell, L. (1973b). Citric acid cycle activity and chloroquine resistance in rodent malaria parasites: The role of the reticulocyte. *Ann. Trop. Med. Parasitol.* **67**, 285–300.

Howells, R. E., Peters, W., and Fullard, J. (1969). Cytochrome oxidase activity in a normal and some drug-resistant strains of *Plasmodium berghei*—A cytochemical study. I. Asexual erythrocytic stages. *Mil. Med.* **134**, 893–915.

Hutton, J. J. (1972). Glucose-metabolizing enzymes of the mouse erythrocyte: Activity changes during stress erythropoiesis. *Blood* **39**, 542–553.

Ilan, J., Ilan, J., and Tokuyasu, K. (1969). Amino acid activation for protein synthesis in *Plasmodium berghei*. *Mil. Med.* **134**, 1026–1031.

Ilan, J., Pierce, D. R., and Miller, F. W. (1977). Influence of 9-β-D-arabinofuranosyladenine on total protein synthesis and on differential gene expression of unique proteins in the rodent malarial parasite *Plasmodium berghei*. *Proc. Natl. Acad. Sci. U.S.A.* **74**, 3386–3390.

Iyer, G. Y. N., Islam, D. M. F., and Quastel, J. H. (1961). Biochemical aspects of phagocytosis. *Nature (London)* **192**, 535–541.

Jacobs, R. L. (1964). Role of *p*-aminobenzoic acid in *Plasmodium berghei* infection in the mouse. *Exp. Parasitol.* **15**, 213–225.

Jaffe, J. J. (1972). Dihydrofolate reductases in parasitic protozoa and helminths. *In* "Comparative Biochemistry of Parasites" (H. Van den Bossche, ed.), pp. 219–233. Academic Press, New York.

Jones, E. S., Maegraith, B. G., and Sculthorpe, H. H. (1951). Pathological processes in disease. III. The oxygen uptake of blood from albino rats infected with *Plasmodium berghei*. *Ann. Trop. Med. Parasitol.* **45**, 244–252.

Jones, E. S., Maegraith, B. G., and Gibson, Q. H. (1953). Pathological processes in disease. IV. Oxidation in the rat reticulocyte, a host cell of *Plasmodium berghei*. *Ann. Trop. Med. Parasitol.* **47**, 431–437.

Jung, A., Jackisch, R., Picard-Maureau, A., and Heischkeil, R. (1975). DNA-, RNA- und Lipid-synthese sowie die spezifische Aktivität von Glucose-6-phosphatdehydrogenase und Glucose-6-phosphatase in den verschiedenen morphologischen Stadien von Plasmodium vinckei. *Tropenmed. Parasitol.* **26**, 27–34.

Karnovsky, M. L., Lazdins, J., and Simmons, S. R. (1975). Metabolism of activated mononuclear phagocytes at rest and during phagocytosis. *In* "Mononuclear Phagocytes in Immunity, Infection and Pathology" (R. Van Furth, ed.), pp. 423–438. Blackwell, Oxford.

Khabir, P. A., and Manwell, R. D. (1955). Glucose consumption of *Plasmodium hexamerium*. *J. Parasitol.* **41**, 595–603.

Kilejian, A. (1975). Circular mitochondrial DNA from the avian malarial parasite *Plasmodium lophurae*. *Biochim. Biophys. Acta* **390**, 276–284.

Killby, V. A. A., and Silverman, P. H. (1969). Isolated erythrocytic forms of *Plasmodium berghei*: An electron-microscopical study. *Am. J. Trop. Med. Hyg.* **18**, 836–859.

Killick-Kendrick, R. (1974). Parasitic protozoa of the blood of rodents: A revision of *Plasmodium berghei*. *Parasitology* **69**, 225–237.

Koler, R. D., Bigley, R. H., Jones, R. T., Rigas, D. A., Vanbellinghen, P., and Thompson, P. (1964). Pyruvate kinase: Molecular differences between human red cell and leukocyte enzyme. *Cold Spring Harbor Symp. Quant. Biol.* **29**, 213–221.

Königk, E. (1976). Comparative aspects of nucleotide biosynthesis in pathogenic protozoa. *In* "Biochemistry of Parasites and Host-Parasite Relationships" (H. Van den Bossche, ed.), pp. 51–58. North-Holland Publ., Amsterdam.

Königk, E. (1977). Salvage syntheses and their relationship to nucleic acid metabolism. *Bull. W. H. O.* **55**, 249–252.

Kreier, J. P. (1977). The isolation and fractionation of malaria-infected cells. *Bull. W. H. O.* **55**, 317–331.

Kreier, J. P., Seed, T., Mohan, R., and Pfister, R. (1972). *Plasmodium sp.*: The relationship between erythrocyte morphology and parasitization in chickens, rats, and mice. *Exp. Parasitol.* **31**, 19–28.

Kretschmar, W. (1961). Infektionsverlauf und Krankheitsbild bei mit Plasmodium berghei infizierten Mäusen des Stammen NMRI. *Z. Tropenmed. Parasitol.* **12**, 346–368.

Kretschmar, W., and Voller, A. (1973). Suppression of Plasmodium falciparum malaria in Aotus monkeys by milk diet. *Z. Tropenmed. Parasitol.* **24**, 51–59.

Krooth, R. S., Wuu, K.-D., and Ma, R. (1969). Dihydroorotic acid dehydrogenase: Introduction into erythrocyte by the malaria parasite. *Science* **164**, 1073–1075.

Ladda, R. L. (1969). New insights into the fine structure of rodent malarial parasites. *Mil. Med.* **134**, 825–865.

Lane, M. D., Maruyama, H., and Easterday, R. L. (1969). Phosphoenolpyruvate carboxylase from peanut cotyledons. *In* "Methods in Enzymology" (J. M. Lowenstein, ed.), Vol. 13, pp. 277–283. Academic Press, New York.

Langer, B. W., Jr., Phisphumvidhi, P., and Friedlander, Y. (1967). Malarial parasite metabolism: The pentose cycle in *Plasmodium berghei. Exp. Parasitol.* **20**, 68–76.

Langer, B. W., Jr., Phisphumvidhi, P., Jiampermpoon, D., and Weidhorn, R. P. (1969). Malarial parasite metabolism: The metabolism of methionine by *Plasmodium berghei. Mil. Med.* **134**, 1039–1044.

Langer, B. W., Jr., Phisphumvidhi, P., and Jiampermpoon, D. (1970). Malarial parasite metabolism: The glutamic acid dehydrogenase of *Plasmodium berghei. Exp. Parasitol.* **28**, 298–303.

Lantz, C. H., Van Dyke, K., and Carter, G. (1971). *Plasmodium berghei: In vitro* incorporation of purine derivatives into nucleic acids. *Exp. Parasitol.* **29**, 402–416.

Laskowski, M. (1942). Preparation of living nuclei from hen erythrocytes. *Proc. Soc. Exp. Biol. Med.* **49**, 354–356.

Lawrence, C. W., and Cenedella, R. J. (1969). Lipid content of *Plasmodium berghei*-infected rat red blood cells. *Exp. Parasitol.* **26**, 181–186.

Levy, M. R., and Chou, S.-C. (1973). Activity and some properties of an acid proteinase from normal and *Plasmodium berghei*-infected red cells. *J. Parasitol.* **59**, 1064–1070.

Levy, M. R., and Chou, S.-C. (1974). Some properties and susceptibility to inhibitors of partially purified acid proteases from *Plasmodium berghei* and from ghosts of mouse red cells. *Biochim. Biophys. Acta* **334**, 423–430.

Levy, M. R., and Chou, S.-C. (1975). Inhibition of macromolecular synthesis in the malarial parasites by inhibitors of proteolytic enzymes. *Experientia* **31**, 52–54.

Levy, M. R., Siddiqui, W. A., and Chou, S.-C. (1974). Acid protease activity in *Plasmodium falciparum* and *P. knowlesi* and ghosts of their respective host red cells. *Nature (London)* **247**, 546–549.

Lewert, R. M. (1952a). Nucleic acids in plasmodia and the phosphorus partition of cells infected with *Plasmodium gallinaceum. J. Infect. Dis.* **91**, 125–144.

Lewert, R. M. (1952b). Changes in nucleic acids and protein in nucleated erythrocytes infected with *Plasmodium gallinaceum* as shown by ultraviolet absorption measurements. *J. Infect. Dis.* **91**, 180–183.

Lieu, T. S., Hudson, R. A., Brown, R. K., and White, B. C. (1971). Transport of pyrimidine nucleosides across human erythrocyte membranes. *Biochim. Biophys. Acta* **241**, 884–893.

Lillie, R. D. (1947). Reactions of various parasitic organisms in tissues to the Bauer, Feulgen, Gram, and Gram-Weigert methods. *J. Lab. Clin. Med.* **32**, 76–88.

Lotz, M., and Smith, L. H., Jr. (1962). The effect of reticulocytosis in the rabbit on the activities of enzymes in pyrimidine biosynthesis. *Blood* **19**, 593–600.

Lowenstein, L. M. (1959). The mammalian reticulocyte. *Int. Rev. Cytol.* **8**, 135–174.

Lukow, I., Schmidt, G., Walter, R. D., and Königk, E. (1973). Adenosinmonophosphat-Salvage-Synthese bei Plasmodium chabaudi. *Z. Tropenmed. Parasitol.* **24**, 500–504.

McClean, S., Purdy, W. C., Kabat, A., Sampugna, J., and De Zeeuw, R. (1976). Analysis of the phospholipid composition of *Plasmodium knowlesi* and rhesus erythrocyte membranes. *Anal. Chim. Acta* **82**, 175–185.

McColm, A. A., Shakespeare, P. G., and Trigg, P. I. (1976). Protein synthesis in the erythrocytic stages of *Plasmodium knowlesi. In* "Biochemistry of Parasites and Host-Parasite Relationships" (H. Van den Bossche, ed.), pp. 59–65. North-Holland Publ., Amsterdam.

McCormick, G. J. (1970). Amino acid transport and incorporation in red blood cells of normal and *Plasmodium knowlesi*-infected rhesus monkeys. *Exp. Parasitol.* **27**, 143–149.

McCormick, G. J., Canfield, C. J., and Willet, G. P. (1971). *Plasmodium knowlesi: In vitro* evaluation of antimalarial activity of folic acid inhibitors. *Exp. Parasitol.* **30**, 88–93.

McCormick, G. J., Canfield, C. J., and Willet, G. P. (1974). *In vitro* antimalarial activity of nucleic acid precursor analogs in the simian malaria *Plasmodium knowlesi. Antimicrob. Agents & Chemother.* **6**, 16–21.

McCullough, J. L., and Maren, T. H. (1974). Dihydropteroate synthetase from *Plasmodium berghei:* Isolation, properties, and inhibition by dapsone and sulfadiazine. *Mol. Pharmacol.* **10**, 140–145.

McDaniel, H. G., and Siu, P. M. L. (1972). Purification and characterization of phosphoenolpyruvate carboxylase from *Plasmodium berghei. J. Bacteriol.* **109**, 385–390.

McKee, R. W., Ormsbee, R. A., Anfinsen, C. B., Geiman, Q. M., and Ball, E. G. (1946). Studies on malarial parasites. VI. The chemistry and metabolism of normal and parasitized (P. knowlesi) monkey blood. *J. Exp. Med.* **84**, 569–582.

McLaughlin, J., and McGhee, R. B. (1972). Changes in the neutral glycosyl ceramides of duck erythrocytes during infection with the avian malaria parasite, *Plasmodium lophurae. Life Sci.* **11** (Part 2), 397–404.

Maegraith, B. G., Deegan, T., and Jones, E. S. (1952). Suppression of malaria (P. berghei) by milk. *Br. Med. J.* **2**, 1382–1384.

Maier, J., and Coggeshall, L. T. (1941). Respiration of malaria plasmodia. J. Infect. Dis. **69**, 87–96.

Manandhar, M. S. P., and Van Dyke, K. (1975). Detailed purine salvage metabolism in and outside the free malarial parasite. *Exp. Parasitol.* **37**, 138–146.

Manwell, R. D., and Feigelson, P. (1949). Glycolysis in *Plasmodium gallinaceum. Proc. Soc. Exp. Biol. Med.* **70**, 578–582.

Marcus, A. J., and Zucker, M. B. (1965). "The Physiology of Blood Platelets," pp. 1–12. Grune & Stratton, New York.

Marshall, P. B. (1948). The glucose metabolism of *Plasmodium gallinaceum,* and the action of antimalarial agents. *Br. J. Pharmacol. Chemother.* **3**, 1–7.

Miller, Z. B., and Kozloff, L. M. (1947). The ribonuclease activity of normal and parasitized chick erythrocytes. *J. Biol. Chem.* **170**, 105–120.

Milne, A. A. (1927). "Winnie-the-Pooh," 3rd ed., p. 97. Methuen, London.

Mitchell, G. H., Butcher, G. A., Voller, A., and Cohen, S. (1976). The effect of immune IgG on the *in vitro* development of *Plasmodium falciparum. Parasitology* **72**, 149–162.

Miyazaki, H., and Minaki, Y. (1972). Metabolic significance of adenosine in the mouse erythrocytes. *J. Biochem. (Tokyo)* **71**, 173–183.

Momen, H. (1979a). Biochemistry of intraerythrocytic parasites. I. Identification of enzymes of parasite origin by starch-gel electrophoresis. *Ann. Trop. Med. Parasitol.* **73**, 109–115.

Momen, H. (1979b). Biochemistry of intraerythrocytic parasites. II. Comparative studies in carbohydrate metabolism. *Ann. Trop. Med. Parasitol.* **73**, 117–123.

Momen, H., Atkinson, E. M., and Homewood, C. A. (1975). An electrophoretic investigation of the malate dehydrogenase of mouse erythrocytes infected with *Plasmodium berghei. Int. J. Biochem.* **6**, 533–535.

Moore, G. A., and Boothroyd, B. (1974). Direct resolution of the lattice planes of malarial pigment. *Ann. Trop. Med. Parasitol.* **68**, 489.

Morrison, D. B., and Anderson, W. A. D. (1942). The pigment of the malaria parasite. *Public Health Rep.* **57**, 90–94.

Morrison, D. B., and Jeskey, H. A. (1948). Alterations in some constituents of the monkey erythrocyte infected with *Plasmodium knowlesi* as related to pigment formation. *J. Natl. Malar. Soc.* **7**, 259–264.

Morselt, A. F. W., Glastra, A., and James, J. (1973). Microspectrophotometric analysis of malarial pigment. *Exp. Parasitol.* **33**, 17–22.

Motulsky, A. G. (1964). Hereditary red cell traits and malaria. *Am. J. Trop. Med. Hyg.* **13**, 147–158.

Moulder, J. W. (1948). Effect of quinine treatment of the host upon the carbohydrate metabolism of the malarial parasite *Plasmodium gallinaceum*. *J. Infect. Dis.* **83**, 262–270.

Moulder, J. W. (1949). Inhibition of pyruvate oxidation in the malarial parasite *Plasmodium gallinaceum* by quinine treatment of the host. *J. Infect. Dis.* **85**, 195–204.

Moulder, J. W., and Evans, E. A., Jr. (1946). The biochemistry of the malaria parasite. VI. Studies on the nitrogen metabolism of the malaria parasite. *J. Biol. Chem.* **164**, 145–157.

Mounter, L. A., and Atiyeh, W. (1960). Proteases of human leukocytes. *Blood* **15**, 52–59.

Nagarajan, K. (1968a). Metabolism of *Plasmodium berghei*. I. Krebs cycle. *Exp. Parasitol.* **22**, 19–26.

Nagarajan, J. (1968b). Metabolism of *Plasmodium berghei*. II. $^{32}P_i$ incorporation into high-energy phosphates. *Exp. Parasitol.* **22**, 27–32.

Nagarajan, K. (1968c). Metabolism of *Plasmodium berghei*. III. Carbon dioxide fixation and role of pyruvate and dicarboxylic acids. *Exp. Parasitol.* **22**, 33–42.

Neame, K. D., and Homewood, C. A. (1975). Alterations in the permeability of mouse erythrocytes infected with the malaria parasite, *Plasmodium berghei*. *Int. J. Parasitol.* **5**, 537–540.

Neame, K. D., and Richards, T. G. (1972). "Elementary Kinetics of Membrane Carrier Transport," p. 50. Blackwell, Oxford.

Neame, K. D., Brownbill, P. A., and Homewood, C. A. (1974). The uptake and incorporation of nucleosides into normal erythrocytes and erythrocytes containing *Plasmodium berghei*. *Parasitology* **69**, 329–335.

Oelshlegel, F. J., Jr., and Brewer, G. J. (1975). Parasitism and the red cell. *In* "The Red Blood Cell" (D. MacN. Surgenor, ed.), 2nd ed., Vol. 2, pp. 1263–1302. Academic Press, New York.

Oelshlegel, F. J., Jr., Sander, B. J., and Brewer, G. J. (1975). Pyruvate kinase in malaria host-parasite interaction. *Nature (London)* **255**, 345–347.

Oliver, J. M., and Paterson, A. R. P. (1971). Nucleoside transport. I. A mediated process in human erythrocytes. *Can. J. Biochem.* **49**, 262–270.

Parks, R. E., Jr., Crabtree, G. W., Kong, C. M., Agarwal, R. P., Agarwal, K. C., and Scholar, E. M. (1975). Incorporation of analog purine nucleosides into the formed elements of human blood: Erythrocytes, platelets, and lymphocytes. *Ann. N.Y. Acad. Sci.* **255**, 412–433.

Pennel, R. B. (1974). Composition of normal human red cells. *In* "The Red Blood Cell" (D. MacN. Surgenor, ed.), 2nd ed., Vol. 1, pp. 93–146. Academic Press, New York.

Peters, W. (1969). Recent advances in the physiology and biochemistry of plasmodia. *Trop. Dis. Bull.* **66**, 1–29.

Peters, W. (1970). "Chemotherapy and Drug Resistance in Malaria," pp. 34–35. Academic Press, New York.

Phillips, R. S., Trigg, P. I., and Scott-Finnigan, T. J. (1972). Culture of *Plasmodium falciparum in vitro:* A subculture technique used for demonstrating antiplasmodial activity in serum from some Gambians, resident in an endemic malarious area. *Parasitology* **65**, 525–535.

Phisphumvidhi, P., and Langer, B. W., Jr. (1969). Malarial parasite metabolism: The lactic acid dehydrogenase of *Plasmodium berghei*. *Exp. Parasitol.* **24**, 37–41.

Picard-Maureau, A., Hempelmann, E., Krämmer, G., Jackisch, R., and Jung, A. (1975). Glutathionstatus in Plasmodium vinckei parasitierten Erythrozyten in Abhängigkeit vom intraerythrozytären Entwicklungsstadium des Parasiten. *Tropenmed. Parasitol.* **26**, 405–416.

Platzer, E. G. (1972). Metabolism of tetrahydrofolate in Plasmodium lophurae and duckling erythrocytes. *Trans. N.Y. Acad. Sci.* [2] **34**, 200–208.

Platzer, E. G. (1974). Dihydrofolate reductase in *Plasmodium lophurae* and duckling erythrocytes. *J. Protozool.* **21**, 400–405.

Platzer, E. G., and Campuzano, H. C. (1976). The serine hydroxymethyltransferase of *Plasmodium lophurae*. *J. Protozool.* **23**, 282–286.

Polet, H., and Barr, C. F. (1968a). DNA, RNA, and protein synthesis in erythrocytic forms of *Plasmodium knowlesi*. *Am. J. Trop. Med. Hyg.* **17**, 672–679.

Polet, H., and Barr, C. F. (1968b). Chloroquine and dihydroquinine: *In vitro* studies of their antimalarial effect upon *Plasmodium knowlesi*. *J. Pharmacol. Exp. Ther.* **164**, 380–386.

Polet, H., and Conrad, M. E. (1968). Malaria: Extracellular amino acid requirements for *in vitro* growth of erythrocytic forms of *Plasmodium knowlesi*. *Proc. Soc. Exp. Biol. Med.* **127**, 251–253.

Polet, H., and Conrad, M. E. (1969a). *In vitro* studies on the amino acid metabolism of *Plasmodium knowlesi* and the antiplasmodial effect of the isoleucine antagonists. *Mil. Med.* **134**, 939–944.

Polet, H., and Conrad, M. E. (1969b). The influence of three analogs of isoleucine on *in vitro* growth and protein synthesis of erythrocytic forms of *Plasmodium knowlesi*. *Proc. Soc. Exp. Biol. Med.* **130**, 581–586.

Polet, H., Brown, N. D., and Angel, C. R. (1969). Biosynthesis of amino acids from ^{14}C-U-glucose, pyruvate, and acetate by erythrocytic forms of *P. knowlesi, in vitro*. *Proc. Soc. Exp. Biol. Med.* **131**, 1215–1218.

Pollack, S., George, J. N., and Crosby, W. H. (1966). Effect of agents simulating the abnormalities of the glucose-6-phosphate dehydrogenase-deficient red cell on *Plasmodium berghei* malaria. *Nature (London)* **210**, 33–35.

Pritchard, J. B., O'Connor, N., Oliver, J. M., and Berlin, R. D. (1975). Uptake and supply of purine compounds by the liver. *Am. J. Physiol.* **229**, 967–972.

Ramsey, R., and Warren, C. O., Jr. (1933). The rate of respiration in erythrocytes. II. The rate in mature rabbit erythrocytes. *Q. J. Exp. Physiol.* **22**, 49–56.

Rao, K. N., Subrahmanyam, D., and Prakash, S. (1970). *Plasmodium berghei:* Lipids of rat red blood cells. *Exp. Parasitol.* **27**, 22–27.

Rapoport, S. (1961). Reifung und Alterungsvorgänge in Erythrozyten. *Folia Haematol. (Leipzig)* **78**, 364–381.

Reid, H. A., and Sucharit, P. (1972). Ancrod, heparin, and ε-aminocaproic acid in simian knowlesi malaria. *Lancet* **2**, 1110–1112.

Reid, V. E., and Friedkin, M. (1973a). *Plasmodium berghei:* Folic acid levels in mouse erythrocytes. *Exp. Parasitol.* **33**, 424–428.

Reid, V. E., and Friedkin, M. (1973b). Thymidylate synthetase in mouse erythrocytes infected with *Plasmodium berghei*. *Mol. Pharmacol.* **9**, 74–80.

Richards, W. H. G., and Williams, S. G. (1973). Malaria studies *in vitro*. II. The measurement of drug activities using leucocyte-free blood-dilution cultures of *Plasmodium berghei* and ^{3}H-leucine. *Ann. Trop. Med. Parasitol.* **67**, 179–190.

Richards, W. H. G., and Williams, S. G. (1975). Malaria studies *in vitro*. III. The protein synthesising activity of *Plasmodium falciparum in vitro* after drug treatment *in vivo*. *Ann. Trop. Med. Parasitol.* **69**, 135–140.

Rietz, P. J., Skelton, F. S., and Folkers, K. (1967). Occurrence of ubiquinones-8 and -9 in Plasmodium lophurae. *Int. J. Vitam. Res.* **37**, 405–411.

Rimington, C., Fulton, J. D., and Sheinman, H. (1947). The pigment of the malarial parasites *Plasmodium knowlesi* and *Plasmodium gallinaceum. Biochem. J.* **41**, 619–622.

Ristic, M., and Kreier, J. P. (1964). The fine structure of the erythrocytic forms of *Plasmodium gallinaceum* as revealed by electron microscopy. *Am. J. Trop. Med. Hyg.* **13**, 509–514.

Ritter, C., and André, J. (1975). Presence of a complete set of cytochromes despite the absence of cristae in the mitochondrial derivative of snail sperm. *Exp. Cell Res.* **92**, 95–101.

Rock, R. C. (1971a). Incorporation of ^{14}C-labelled non-lipid precursors into lipids of *Plasmodium knowlesi in vitro. Comp. Biochem. Physiol. B* **40**, 657–669.

Rock, R. C. (1971b). Incorporation of ^{14}C-labelled fatty acids into lipids of rhesus erythrocytes and *Plasmodium knowlesi in vitro. Comp. Biochem. Physiol. B* **40**, 893–906.

Rock, R. C., Standefer, J. C., Cook, R. T., Little, W., and Sprinz, H. (1971a). Lipid composition of *Plasmodium knowlesi* membranes: Comparison of parasites and microsomal subfractions with host Rhesus erythrocyte membranes. *Comp. Biochem. Physiol. B* **38**, 425–437.

Rock, R. C., Standefer, J., and Little, W. (1971b). Incorporation of ^{33}P-orthophosphate into membrane phospholipids of *Plasmodium knowlesi* and host erythrocytes of *Macaca mulatta. Comp. Biochem. Physiol. B* **40**, 543–561.

Rollo, I. M. (1955). The mode of action of sulphonamides, proguanil and pyrimethamine on *Plasmodium gallinaceum. Br. J. Pharmacol. Chemother.* **10**, 208–214.

Roodyn, D. B. (1959). A survey of metabolic studies on isolated mammalian nuclei. *Int. Rev. Cytol.* **8**, 279–344.

Roodyn, D. B. (1963). A comparative account of methods for the isolation of nuclei. *Biochem. Soc. Symp.* **23**, 20–36.

Rozenszajn, L. A., Shoham, D., and Menashi, T. (1972). Evaluation of glucose-6-phosphate dehydrogenase in single erythrocytes in human blood smears. *Acta Haematol.* **47**, 303–310.

Rubinstein, D., and Denstedt, O. F. (1953). The metabolism of the erythrocyte. III. The tricarboxylic acid cycle in the avian erythrocyte. *J. Biol. Chem.* **204**, 623–637.

Rubinstein, D., Ottolenghi, P., and Denstedt, O. F. (1956). The metabolism of the erythrocyte. XIII. Enzyme activity in the reticulocyte. *Can. J. Biochem. Physiol.* **34**, 222–235.

Rudzinska, M. A., and Trager, W. (1968). The fine structure of trophozoites and gametocytes in *Plasmodium coatneyi. J. Protozool.* **15**, 73–88.

Rudzinska, M. A., and Vickerman, K. (1968). The fine structure. *In* "Infectious Blood Diseases of Man and Animals" (D. Weinman and M. Ristic, eds.), Vol. 1, pp. 217–306. Academic Press, New York.

Sadun, E. H., Williams, J. S., and Martin, L. K. (1966). Serum biochemical changes in malarial infections in men, chimpanzees and mice. *Mil. Med.* **131**, 1094–1106.

Scheibel, L. W., and Miller, J. (1969a). Cytochrome oxidase activity in platelet-free preparations of *Plasmodium knowlesi. J. Parasitol.* **55**, 825–829.

Scheibel, L. W., and Miller, J. (1969b). Glycolytic and cytochrome oxidase activity in plasmodia. *Mil. Med.* **134**, 1074–1080.

Scheibel, L. W., and Pflaum, W. K. (1970). Carbohydrate metabolism in *Plasmodium knowlesi. Comp. Biochem. Physiol.* **37**, 543–553.

Schmidt, G., Walter, R. D., and Königk, E. (1974). Adenosine kinase from normal mouse erythrocytes and from Plasmodium chabaudi: Partial purification and characterization. *Tropenmed. Parasitol.* **25**, 301–308.

Schnell, J. V., and Siddiqui, W. A. (1972). The effects of antibiotics on ^{14}C-isoleucine incorporation by monkey erythrocytes infected with malarial parasites. *Proc. Helminthol. Soc. Wash.* **39**, 201–203.

Schnell, J. V., Siddiqui, W. A., and Geiman, Q. M. (1971). Biosynthesis of coenzymes Q by malarial parasites. 2. Coenzyme Q synthesis in blood cultures of monkeys infected with malarial parasites (*Plasmodium falciparum* and *P. knowlesi*). *J. Med. Chem.* **14**, 1026–1029.

Schoenfeld, C., Most, H., and Entner, N. (1974). Chemotherapy of rodent malaria: Transfer of resistance vs mutation. *Exp. Parasitol.* **36,** 265–277.

Schrier, S. L. (1963). Studies of the metabolism of human erythrocyte membranes. *J. Clin. Invest.* **42.** 756–766.

Schröter, W., Beckmann, H., Grundherr, G., and Neth, R. (1967). Biochemische und cytochemische Charakterisierung von Reticulocyten und Pseudoreticulocyten. *Klin. Wochenschr.* **45,** 312–313.

Scorza, J. V., De Scorza, C., and Monteiro, M. C. C. (1972). Cytochemical observations of three acid hydrolases in blood stages of malaria parasites. *Ann. Trop. Med. Parasitol.* **66,** 167–172.

Seaman, G. R. (1953). Inhibition of the succinic dehydrogenase of parasitic protozoans by an arsono and a phosphono analog of succinic acid. *Exp. Parasitol.* **2,** 366–373.

Seed, T. M., and Kreier, J. P. (1972). *Plasmodium gallinaceum:* Erythrocyte membrane alterations and associated plasma changes induced by experimental infections. *Proc. Helminthol. Soc. Wash.* **39,** 387–411.

Seed, T. M., Aikawa, M., and Sterling, C. R. (1973). An electron microscope-cytochemical method for differentiating membranes of host red cells and malaria parasites. *J. Protozool.* **20,** 603–605.

Seligman, A. M., Plapinger, R. E., Wasserkrug, H. L., Deb, C., and Hanker, J. S. (1967). Ultrastructural demonstration of cytochrome oxidase activity by the NADI reaction with osmiophilic reagents. *J. Cell Biol.* **34,** 787–800.

Sen Gupta, P. C., Ray, H. N., Dutta, B. N., and Chaudhuri, R. N. (1955). A cytochemical study of *Plasmodium berghei* Vincke and Lips, 1948. *Ann. Trop. Med. Parasitol.* **49,** 273–277.

Shakespeare, P. G., and Trigg, P. I. (1973). Glucose catabolism by the simian malaria parasite *Plasmodium knowlesi. Nature (London)* **241,** 538–540.

Sherman, I. W. (1961). Molecular heterogeneity of lactic dehydrogenase in avian malaria (Plasmodium lophurae). *J. Exp. Med.* **114,** 1049–1062.

Sherman, I. W. (1962). Heterogeneity of lactic dehydrogenase in intra-erythrocytic parasites. *Trans. N.Y. Acad. Sci.* [2] **24,** 944–953.

Sherman, I. W. (1965). Glucose-6-phosphate dehydrogenase and reduced glutathione in malaria-infected erythrocytes (*Plasmodium lophurae* and *P. berghei*). *J. Protozool.* **12,** 394–396.

Sherman, I. W. (1966). Malic dehydrogenase heterogeneity in malaria (*Plasmodium lophurae* and *P. berghei*). *J. Protozool.* **13,** 344–349.

Sherman, I. W. (1976). The ribosomes of the simian malaria *Plasmodium knowlesi.* II. A cell-free protein synthesizing system. *Comp. Biochem. Physiol. B* **53,** 447–450.

Sherman, I. W. (1977a). Transport of amino acids and nucleic acid precursors in malarial parasites. *Bull. W. H. O.* **55,** 211–225.

Sherman, I. W. (1977b). Amino acid metabolism and protein synthesis in malarial parasites. *Bull. W. H. O.* **55,** 265–276.

Sherman, I. W., and Hull, R. W. (1960). The pigment (hemozoin) and proteins of the avian malaria parasite *Plasmodium lophurae. J. Protozool.* **7,** 409–416.

Sherman, I. W., and Jones, L. A. (1976). Protein synthesis by a cell-free preparation from the bird malaria, *Plasmodium lophurae. J. Protozool.* **23,** 277–281.

Sherman, I. W., and Jones, L. A. (1977). The *Plasmodium lophurae* (avian malaria) ribosome. *J. Protozool.* **24,** 331–334.

Sherman, I. W., and Mudd, J. B. (1966). Malaria infection (*P. lophurae*): Changes in free amino acids. *Science* **154,** 287–289.

Sherman, I. W., and Tanigoshi, L. (1970). Incorporation of ^{14}C-amino-acids by malaria (*Plasmodium lophurae*). IV. *In vivo* utilization of host cell haemoglobin. *Int. J. Biochem.* **1,** 635–637.

Sherman, I. W., and Tanigoshi, L. (1971). Incorporation of ^{14}C-amino-acids by malaria (*Plasmodium lophurae*). III. Metabolic fate of selected amino-acids. *Int. J. Biochem.* **2,** 41–48.

Sherman, I. W., and Tanigoshi, L. (1972). Incorporation of ^{14}C-amino acids by malaria (*Plasmodium lophurae*). V. Influence of antimalarials on the transport and incorporation of amino acids. *Proc. Helminthol. Soc. Wash.* **39,** 250–260.

Sherman, I. W., and Tanigoshi, L. (1974a). Incorporation of ^{14}C-amino acids by malarial plasmodia (*Plasmodium lophurae*). VI. Changes in the kinetic constants of amino acid transport during infection. *Exp. Parasitol.* **35,** 369–373.

Sherman, I. W., and Tanigoshi, L. (1974b). Glucose transport in the malarial (*Plasmodium lophurae*) infected erythrocyte. *J. Protozool.* **21,** 603–607.

Sherman, I. W., and Ting, I. P. (1966). Carbon dioxide fixation in malaria (*Plasmodium lophurae*). *Nature (London)* **212,** 1387–1389.

Sherman, I. W., and Ting, I. P. (1968). Carbon dioxide fixation in malaria. II. *Plasmodium knowlesi* (monkey malaria). *Comp. Biochem. Physiol.* **24,** 639–642.

Sherman, I. W., Mudd, J. B., and Trager, W. (1965). Chloroquine resistance and the nature of malarial pigment. *Nature (London)* **208,** 691–693.

Sherman, I. W., Virkar, R. A., and Ruble, J. A. (1967). The accumulation of amino acids by *Plasmodium lophurae* (avian malaria). *Comp. Biochem. Physiol.* **23,** 43–57.

Sherman, I. W., Ting, I. P., and Ruble, J. A. (1968). Characterization of the malaria pigment (hemozoin) from the avian malaria parasite *Plasmodium lophurae*. *J. Protozool.* **15,** 158–164.

Sherman, I. W., Ruble, J. A., and Tanigoshi, L. (1969a). Incorporation of ^{14}C-amino acids by malaria (*Plasmodium lophurae*). 1. Role of ions and amino acids in the medium. *Mil. Med.* **134,** 954–961.

Sherman, I. W., Ruble, J. A., and Ting, I. P. (1969b). *Plasmodium lophurae*: [U-^{14}C]-glucose catabolism by free plasmodia and duckling host erythrocytes. *Exp. Parasitol.* **25,** 181–192.

Sherman, I. W., Ting, I. P., and Tanigoshi, L. (1970). *Plasmodium lophurae*: Glucose-1-^{14}C and glucose-6-^{14}C catabolism by free plasmodia and duckling host erythrocytes. *Comp Biochem. Physiol.* **34,** 625–639.

Sherman, I. W., Tanigoshi, L., and Mudd, J. B. (1971a). Incorporation of ^{14}C-amino-acids by malaria (*Plasmodium lophurae*). II. Migration and incorporation of amino acids. *Int. J. Biochem.* **2,** 27–40.

Sherman, I. W., Peterson, I., Tanigoshi, L., and Ting, I. P. (1971b). The glutamate dehydrogenase of *Plasmodium lophurae* (avian malaria). *Exp. Parasitol.* **29,** 433–439.

Sherman, I. W., Cox, R. A., Higginson, B., McLaren, D. J., and Williamson, J. (1975). The ribosomes of the simian malaria, *Plasmodium knowlesi*. I. Isolation and characterization. *J. Protozool.* **22,** 568–572.

Siddiqui, W. A., and Schnell, J. V. (1972). *In-vitro* and *in-vivo* studies with *Plasmodium falciparum* and *Plasmodium knowlesi*. *Proc. Helminthol. Soc. Wash.* **39,** 204–210.

Siddiqui, W. A., and Trager, W. (1964). Comparative bioautography of folic and folinic acids of erythrocytes and livers of normal ducks and ducks infected with malarial parasites. *J. Parasitol.* **50,** 753–756.

Siddiqui, W. A., and Trager, W. (1966). Folic and folinic acids in relation to the development of *Plasmodium lophurae*. *J. Parasitol.* **52,** 556–558.

Siddiqui, W. A., and Trager, W. (1967). Free amino-acids of blood plasma and erythrocytes of normal ducks and ducks infected with malarial parasite, *Plasmodium lophurae*. *Nature (London)* **214,** 1046–1047.

Siddiqui, W. A., Schnell, J. V., and Geiman, Q. M. (1967). Stearic acid as plasma replacement for intracellular in vitro culture of Plasmodium knowlesi. *Science* **156,** 1623–1625.

Siddiqui, W. A., Schnell, J. V., and Geiman, Q. M. (1969). Nutritional requirements for *in vitro* cultivation of a simian malarial parasite, *Plasmodium knowlesi*. *Mil. Med.* **134,** 929–938.

Siddiqui, W. A., Schnell, J. V., and Richmond-Crum, S. (1974). In vitro cultivation of *Plasmodium falciparum* at high parasitemia. *Am. J. Trop. Med. Hyg.* **23,** 1015–1018.

Silber, R., Gabrio, B. W., and Huennekens, F. M. (1963). Studies on normal and leukemic leukocytes. VI. Thymidylate synthetase and deoxycytidylate deaminase. *J. Clin. Invest.* **42,** 1913–1921.

Silverman, M., Ceithaml, J., Taliaferro, L. G., and Evans, E. A., Jr. (1944). The in vitro metabolism of *Plasmodium gallinaceum. J. Infect. Dis.* **75,** 212–230.

Sinton, J. A., and Ghosh, B. N. (1934a). Studies of malarial pigment (haemozoin). Part I. Investigation of the action of solvents on haemozoin and the spectroscopical appearances observed in the solutions. *Rec. Malar. Surv. India* **4,** 15–42.

Sinton, J. A., and Ghosh, B. N. (1934b). Studies of malarial pigment (haemozoin). Part III. Further researches into the action of solvents, and the results of observations on the action of oxidising and reducing agents, on optical properties, and on crystallisation. *Rec. Malar. Surv. India* **4,** 205–221.

Siu, P. M. L. (1967). Carbon dioxide fixation in plasmodia and the effect of some antimalarial drugs on the enzyme. *Comp. Biochem. Physiol.* **23,** 785–795.

Skelton, F. S., Lunan, K. D., Folkers, K., Schnell, J. V., Siddiqui, W. A., and Geiman, Q. M. (1969). Biosynthesis of ubiquinones by malarial parasites. I. Isolation of [^{14}C]ubiquinones from cultures of rhesus monkey blood infected with *Plasmodium knowlesi. Biochemistry* **8,** 1284–1287.

Skelton, F. S., Rietz, P. J., and Folkers, K. (1970). Coenzyme Q. CXXII. Identification of ubiquinone-8 biosynthesized by *Plasmodium knowlesi, P. cynomolgi* and *P. berghei. J. Med. Chem.* **13,** 602–606.

Smith, C. C., McCormick, G. J., and Canfield, C. J. (1976). *Plasmodium knowlesi: In vitro* biosynthesis of methionine. *Exp. Parasitol.* **40,** 432–437.

Smith, D. H., and Theakston, R. D. G. (1970). Comments on the ultrastructure of human erythrocytes infected with *Plasmodium malariae. Ann. Trop. Med. Parasitol.* **64,** 329.

Smith, L. H., Jr., and Baker, F. A. (1959). Pyrimidine metabolism in man. I. The biosynthesis of orotic acid. *J. Clin. Invest.* **38,** 798–809.

Speck, J. F., and Evans, E. A., Jr. (1945). The biochemistry of the malaria parasite. II. Glycolysis in cell-free preparations of the malaria parasite. *J. Biol. Chem.* **159,** 71–81.

Speck, J. F., Moulder, J. W., and Evans, E. A., Jr. (1946). The biochemistry of the malaria parasite. V. Mechanism of pyruvate oxidation in the malaria parasite. *J. Biol. Chem.* **164,** 119–144.

Sterling, C. R., Aikawa, M., and Nussenzweig, R. S. (1972). Morphological divergence in a mammalian malarial parasite: The fine structure of *Plasmodium brasilianum. Proc. Helminthol. Soc. Wash.* **39,** 109–129.

Theakston, R. D. G., and Fletcher, K. A. (1971). An electron cytochemical study of glucose-6-phosphate dehydrogenase activity in erythrocytes of malaria-infected mice, monkeys and chickens. *Life Sci.* **10** (Part 2), 701–711.

Theakston, R. D. G., and Fletcher, K. A. (1973a). A technique for the cytochemical demonstration in the electron microscope of glucose-6-phosphate dehydrogenase activity in erythrocytes of malaria-infected animals. *J. Microsc. (Oxford)* **97,** 315–320.

Theakston, R. D. G., and Fletcher, K. A. (1973b). An electron cytochemical study of 6-phosphogluconate dehydrogenase activity in infected erythrocytes during malaria. *Life Sci.* **13** (Part 1), 405–410.

Theakston, R. D. G., Howells, R. E., Fletcher, K. A., Peters, W., Fullard, J., and Moore, G. A. (1969). The ultrastructural distribution of cytochrome oxidase activity in *Plasmodium berghei* and *P. gallinaceum. Life Sci.* **8** (Part 2), 521–529.

Theakston, R. D. G., Fletcher, K. A., and Maegraith, B. G. (1970a). The use of electron microscope autoradiography for examining the uptake and degradation of haemoglobin by *Plasmodium berghei. Ann. Trop. Med. Parasitol.* **64,** 63–71.

Theakston, R. D. G., Fletcher, K. A., and Maegraith, B. G. (1970b). Ultrastructural localisation of

NADH- and NADPH-dehydrogenases in the erythrocytic stages of the rodent malaria parasite, *Plasmodium berghei*. *Life Sci.* **9** (Part 2), 421–429.

Theakston, R. D. G., Ali, S. N., and Moore, G. A. (1972). Electron microscope autographic studies on the effect of chloroquine on the uptake of tritiated nucleosides and methionine by *Plasmodium berghei*. *Ann. Trop. Med. Parasitol.* **66**, 295–302.

Theakston, R. D. G., Fletcher, K. A., and Moore, G. A. (1976). Glucose-6-phosphate and 6-phosphogluconate dehydrogenase activities in human erythrocytes infected with *Plasmodium falciparum*. *Ann. Trop. Med. Parasitol.* **70**, 125–127.

Thurston, J. P. (1954). The chemotherapy of *Plasmodium berghei*. II. Antagonism of the action of drugs. *Parasitology* **44**, 99–110.

Ting, I. P., and Sherman, I. W. (1966). Carbon dioxide fixation in malaria. I. Kinetic studies in *Plasmodium lophurae*. *Comp. Biochem. Physiol.* **19**, 855–869.

Tokuyasu, K., Ilan, J., and Ilan, J. (1969). Biogenesis of ribosomes in *Plasmodium berghei*. *Mil. Med.* **134**, 1032–1038.

Tracy, S. M., and Sherman, I. W. (1972). Purine uptake and utilization by the avian malaria parasite *Plasmodium lophurae*. *J. Protozool.* **19**, 541–549.

Trager, W. (1950). Studies on the extracellular cultivation of an intracellular parasite (avian malaria). I. Development of the organisms in erythrocyte extracts, and the favoring effect of adenosinetriphosphate. *J. Exp. Med.* **92**, 349–366.

Trager, W. (1952). Studies on the extracellular cultivation of an intracellular parasite (avian malaria). II. The effects of malate and of coenzyme A concentrates. *J. Exp. Med.* **96**, 465–476.

Trager, W. (1958). Folinic acid and non-dialyzable materials in the nutrition of malaria parasites. *J. Exp. Med.* **108**, 753–772.

Trager, W. (1959). The enhanced folic and folinic acid contents of erythrocytes infected with malaria parasites. *Exp. Parasitol.* **8**, 265–273.

Trager, W. (1967). Adenosine triphosphate and the pyruvic and phosphoglyceric kinases of the malaria parasite *Plasmodium lophurae*. *J. Protozool.* **14**, 110–114.

Trager, W. (1971). Malaria parasites (*Plasmodium lophurae*) developing extracellularly *in vitro:* Incorporation of labeled precursors. *J. Protozool.* **18**, 392–399.

Trager, W. (1972). Effects of bongkrekic acid on malaria parasites (*Plasmodium lophurae*) developing extracellularly in vitro. *In* "Comparative Biochemistry of Parasites" (H. Van den Bossche, ed.), pp. 343–350. Academic Press, New York.

Trager, W. (1973). Bongkrekic acid and the adenosinetriphosphate requirement of malaria parasites. *Exp. Parasitol.* **34**, 412–416.

Trager, W., Langreth, S. G., and Platzer, E. G. (1972). Viability and fine structure of extracellular *Plasmodium lophurae* prepared by different methods. *Proc. Helminthol. Soc. Wash.* **39**, 220–230.

Trigg, P. I. (1968). Sterol metabolism of *Plasmodium knowlesi in vitro*. *Ann. Trop. Med. Parasitol.* **62**, 481–487.

Trigg, P. I. (1969). Some factors affecting the cultivation *in vitro* of the erythrocytic stages of *Plasmodium knowlesi*. *Parasitology* **59**, 915–924.

Trigg, P. I., and Gutteridge, W. E. (1971). A minimal medium for the growth of *Plasmodium knowlesi* in dilution cultures. *Parasitology* **62**, 113–123.

Trigg, P. I., and Gutteridge, W. E. (1972). A rational approach to the serial culture of malaria parasites. Evidence for a deficiency in RNA synthesis during the first cycle *in vitro*. *Parasitology* **65**, 265–271.

Trigg, P. I., and Shakespeare, P. G. (1976). The effects of incubation *in vitro* on the susceptibility of monkey erythrocytes to invasion by *Plasmodium knowlesi*. *Parasitology* **73**, 149–160.

Trigg, P. I., Gutteridge, W. E., and Williamson, J. (1971). The effects of cordycepin on malaria parasites. *Trans. R. Soc. Trop. Med. Hyg.* **65**, 514–520.

Trigg, P. I., Shakespeare, P. G., Burt, S. J., and Kyd, S. I. (1975). Ribonucleic acid synthesis in *Plasmodium knowlesi* maintained both *in vivo* and *in vitro*. *Parasitology* **71**, 199–209.

Tsukamoto, M. (1974). Differential detection of soluble enzymes specific to a rodent malaria parasite, *Plasmodium berghei,* by electrophoresis on polyacrylamide gels. *Trop. Med.* **16**, 55–69.

Van Dyke, K. (1975). Comparison of tritiated hypoxanthine, adenine and adenosine for purine-salvage incorporation into nucleic acids of the malarial parasite, Plasmodium berghei. *Tropenmed. Parasitol.* **26**, 232–238.

Van Dyke, K., and Szustkiewicz, C. (1969). Apparent new modes of antimalarial action detected by inhibited incorporation of adenosine-8-³H into nucleic acids of *Plasmodium berghei. Mil. Med.* **134**, 1000–1006.

Van Dyke, K., Szustkiewicz, C., Lantz, C, H., and Saxe, L. H. (1969). Studies concerning the mechanism of action of antimalarial drugs—Inhibition of the incorporation of adenosine-8-³H into nucleic acids of *Plasmodium berghei. Biochem. Pharmacol.* **18**, 1417–1425.

Van Dyke, K., Szustkiewicz, C., Cenedella, R., and Saxe, L. H. (1970a). A unique antinucleic acid approach to the mass screening of antimalarial drugs. *Chemotherapy* **15**, 177–188.

Van Dyke, K., Tremblay, G. C., Lantz, C. H., and Szustkiewicz, C. (1970b). The source of purines and pyrimidines in *Plasmodium berghei. Am. J. Trop. Med. Hyg.* **19**, 202–208.

Van Dyke, K., Trush, M. A., Wilson, M. E., and Stealey, P. K. (1977a). Isolation and analysis of nucleotides from erythrocyte-free malarial parasites (*Plasmodium berghei*) and potential relevance to malaria chemotherapy. *Bull. W. H. O.* **55**, 253–264.

Van Dyke, K., Wilson, M., Trush, M., Taylor, M., and Stealey, P. (1977b). *Plasmodium berghei:* High pressure liquid chromatographic analysis of nucleotides from erythrocyte-free malarial parasites. *Exp. Parasitol.* **42**, 274–281.

Velick, S. F. (1942). The respiratory metabolism of the malaria parasite, *P. cathemerium,* during its developmental cycle. *Am. J. Hyg.* **35**, 152–161.

Von Brand, T. (1973). "Biochemistry of Parasites," 2nd ed., p. 144. Academic Press, New York.

Wagenknecht, C. (1961). Gehalt und intrazelluläre Verteilung des Glutathions in Kaninchen-Erythrozyten und Retikulozyten. *Folia Haematol. (Leipzig)* **78**, 345–348.

Wallace, W. R. (1966). Fatty acid composition of lipid classes in *Plasmodium lophurae* and *Plasmodium berghei. Am. J. Trop. Med. Hyg.* **15**, 811–813.

Wallace, W. R., Finerty, J. F., and Dimopoullos, G. T. (1965). Studies on the lipids of *Plasmodium lophurae* and *Plasmodium berghei. Am. J. Trop. Med. Hyg.* **14**, 715–718.

Walsh, C. J., and Sherman, I. W. (1968a). Isolation, characterization and synthesis of DNA from a malaria parasite. *J. Protozool.* **15**, 503–508.

Walsh, C. J., and Sherman, I. W. (1968b). Purine and pyrimidine synthesis by the avian malaria parasite, *Plasmodium lophurae. J. Protozool.* **15**, 763–770.

Walter, H., Selby, F. W., and Francisco, J. R. (1965). Altered electrophoretic mobilities of some erythrocytic enzymes as a function of their age. *Nature (London)* **208**, 76–77.

Walter, R. D., and Königk, E. (1971a). Synthese der Desoxythymidylat-Synthetase und der Dihydrofolat-Reduktase bei synchroner Schizogonie von Plasmodium chabaudi. *Z. Tropenmed. Parasitol.* **22**, 250–255.

Walter, R. D., and Königk, E. (1971b). Plasmodium chabaudi: Die enzymatische Synthese von Dihydropteroat und ihre Hemmung durch Sulfonamide. *Z. Tropenmed. Parasitol.* **22**, 256–259.

Walter, R. D., and Königk, E. (1947a). Biosynthesis of folic acid compounds in plasmodia: Purification and properties of the 7,8-dihydropteroate-synthesizing enzyme from *Plasmodium chabaudi. Hoppe-Seyler's Z. Physiol. Chem.* **355**, 431–437.

Walter, R. D., and Königk, E. (1974b). Hypoxanthine-guanine phosphoribosyltransferase and adenine phosphoribosyltransferase from Plasmodium chabaudi: Purification and properties. *Tropenmed. Parasitol.* **25**, 227–235.

Walter, R. D., Mühlpfordt, H., and Königk, E. (1970). Vergleichende Untersuchungen der Desoxythymidylatsynthese bei Plasmodium chabaudi, Trypanosoma gambiense und Trypanosoma lewisi. Z. Tropenmed. Parasitol. 21, 347–357.

Walter, R. D., Nordmeyer, J.-P., and Königk, E. (1974). NADP-specific glutamate dehydrogenase from Plasmodium chabaudi. Hoppe-Seyler's Z. Physiol. Chem. 355, 495–500.

Warasi, W. (1927). Das Malariapigment und seine chemische Natur. Arch. Schiffs- Trop.-Hyg. 31, 428–431.

Warasi, W. (1928). Über die Entstehung des Malariapigments. Arch. Schiffs- Trop.-Hyg. 32, 513–517.

Warhurst, D. C., and Williamson, J. (1970). Ribonucleic acid from Plasmodium knowlesi before and after chloroquine treatment. Chem.-Biol. Interact. 2, 89–106.

Warhurst, D. C., Robinson, B. L., Howells, R. E., and Peters, W. (1971). The effect of cytotoxic agents on autophagic vacuole formation in chloroquine-treated malaria parasites (Plasmodium berghei). Life Sci. 10 (Part 2), 761–771.

Warren, L., and Manwell, R. D. (1954). Rate of glucose consumption by malarial blood. Exp. Parasitol. 3, 16–24.

Wats, R. C., and White, W. I. (1932). The malarial pigment (haemozoin) in the spleen. Indian J. Med. Res. 19, 945–950.

Wendel, W. B. (1943). Respiratory and carbohydrate metabolism of malaria parasites (Plasmodium knowlesi). J. Biol. Chem. 148, 21–34.

Wendel, W. B., and Kimball, S. (1942). Formation of lactic acid and pyruvic acid in blood containing Plasmodium knowlesi. J. Biol. Chem. 145, 343–344.

Whitfeld, P. R. (1952). Nucleic acids in erythrocytic stages of a malaria parasite. Nature (London) 169, 751–752.

Whitfeld, P. R. (1953). Studies on the nucleic acids of the malaria parasite, Plasmodium berghei (Vincke & Lips). Aust. J. Biol. Sci. 6, 234–243.

Williams, S. G., and Richards, W. H. G. (1973). Malaria studies in vitro. I. Techniques for the preparation and culture of leucocyte-free blood-dilution cultures of Plasmodia. Ann. Trop. Med. Parasitol. 67, 169–178.

Woods, D. D., and Tucker, R. G. (1958). The relation of strategy to tactics: Some general biochemical principles. Symp. Soc. Gen. Microbiol. 8, 1–28.

Index